Burnout in Women Physicians

Cynthia M. Stonnington
Julia A Files
Editors

Burnout in Women Physicians

Prevention, Treatment,
and Management

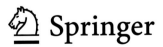 Springer

Editors
Cynthia M. Stonnington
Department of Psychiatry
and Psychology
Mayo Clinic
Scottsdale, AZ
USA

Julia A Files
Division of Women's Health
Internal Medicine
Mayo Clinic
Scottsdale, AZ
USA

ISBN 978-3-030-44458-7   ISBN 978-3-030-44459-4   (eBook)
https://doi.org/10.1007/978-3-030-44459-4

This Springer imprint is published by the registered company Springer Nature Switzerland AG
The registered company address is: Gewerbestrasse 11, 6330 Cham, Switzerland

Foreword

Sex as a Biological Variable

Medicine is experiencing a remarkable, truly historical change. For most of the last 500 years or so, western medicine operated on the assumption that, outside the body parts directly related to reproduction (i.e., outside "the bikini zone"), women and men possessed fundamentally identical biology. We assumed that when it comes to hearts, livers, bones, immune systems, brains, you name it, one need not worry about potential sex differences because, frankly, they did not exist. Any differences that were detected (such as in sex hormone function) were relegated to non-fundamental status, something we can figure out after we understand the supposedly fundamental (meaning "shared") features of human biology.

It is truly hard to overstate how deeply imbedded was this view, thus how large is the change now occurring. Driven by an ever-growing body of research findings, medicine is discovering that its 500-year-old assumption about sex differences is just plain wrong. Recognizing this fact, on January 25, 2016, the United States National Institute of Health (NIH) for the first time ever established a policy (called Sex as a Biological Variable, or SABV) requiring all research funded by them to carefully incorporate the study of potential male/female differences. And while this policy naturally generated resistance from many who do not want their research disturbed by having to consider females, it is truly a landmark moment. The NIH, we promise you, will not abandon this policy, and in effect tell all scientists/ medical doctors that it's ok to simply go back to ignoring potential differences in females compared to males.

It is now incumbent on all of us to explore sex influences on biology assiduously, and responsibly. Fear that sex differences research might be misused is no more a valid reason to avoid studying the topic than the fact that genetics has been misused historically is reason to stop studying genetics. Here we explore a portion of the burgeoning neuroscience literature especially relevant to the experience of women in the medical field, namely, sex differences in the neurobiology of stress responses, in particular social stress.

Fortunately, "social neuroscience" as a field is growing along with interest in sex influences. More and more studies, both involving animal and human subjects, examine stress responses not in subjects in isolation but in response to real social settings. These studies are of course particularly helpful in understanding sex differences in response to social situations encountered by those in the medical field. Both clinical and subclinical (animal) studies inform the discussion.

Animal research, sometimes dismissed by some as irrelevant to understanding sex differences in humans, in fact is a powerful tool for exploring biologically based sex differences in mammals that, while likely influenced to some degree by human culture, cannot be simply explained by human culture. And stated simply, these studies are beginning to identify sex-specific vulnerability as well as resilience in the brain mechanisms responding to stress.

Debra Bangasser and her colleagues at Temple University are among the leaders in this area. They have found that the center of the brain's arousal system, a small but powerful brainstem nucleus called the "locus coeruleus" (literally "blue place"), is far more sensitive to endogenous stress hormones, and less adaptable to their chronic hyper-secretion, in females than in males, effects that becomes apparent during puberty, and are strongly influenced by sex hormones. Other evidence suggests that females may be less sensitive than males to the disruptive effects of stress on attention. Evidence indicates that ovarian hormones can reduce or block the impairing effects of stress hormones on the functioning of attention-related brain systems seen in males. Many of these findings are relatively recent, since the original research was almost exclusively done in males.

Several lines of research reveal parallel findings in animal and human subject work, which of course are especially interesting. H. Elliot Albers and colleagues at Georgia State University examine similarities and differences between females and males in the effects of social interaction with either the same sex or the opposite sex. The existing data suggest that in both rodents and humans, females find same-sex interactions more rewarding than do males, a difference some evidence suggests is related to a differential action of the hormone oxytocin on brainstem circuits.

Also interesting and relevant are recent studies comparing the consequences of social defeat stress in females and males. Brian Trainor and colleagues at the University of California, Davis, were among the first to examine the effects of a social-defeat in female mice (almost all previous work having been done in male mice), and found clear differences. Social defeat induced social withdrawal in female, but not male, mice, an effect which was not related to circulating sex hormones. They next found that social defeat elevated levels of a key brain protein (called "BDNF") only in female mice. Social withdrawal is a key component of anxiety/depression disorders which predominate in women, thus these findings are likely relevant to understanding heightened susceptibility to depression in females.

Trainor and colleagues also report that stress reduces cognitive flexibility, but mainly in males. They first discovered that, in mice, social defeat stress reduced "cognitive flexibility" (i.e., the ability to adapt to novel learning situations), but only in male mice. Females were not impaired. They then showed the same effect in humans: An acute social stressor (called the TSST) elevated cortisol levels equally in healthy women and men, yet only impaired cognitive flexibility in the men.

In an interesting summary of their work, Trainor and colleagues observe that in females, the effects of social defeat are generally more consistent with *reactive* coping strategies (such as social withdrawal and reduced aggression), whereas behaviors in stressed males are generally more consistent with *proactive* coping strategies (such as social approach and aggression.)

These studies and many others prove the point: Sex matters, and it matters in ways we are only beginning to truly grasp, having avoided the issue for so long. Having advocated for the sex difference issue for almost 20 years now, I feel that what is truly needed now is a clear expression of the experiences of women, their individual successes and struggles moving into previously male-dominated fields like medicine. We need acknowledgement and acceptance and even celebration of sex differences, not their continued ideological denial. Consider this: If the entire structure of doctoral medicine was indeed created by and for its almost entirely male constituency (as it was), and if sex differences truly do matter, then it is essentially impossible that women should not have endured far greater distress than males on average in adapting to that structure. Thus I feel what is really needed at this juncture is a book like this – something that begins to blend the growing science with the already extensive personal experiences of women in medicine. Both are needed to fully realize the potential women offer to medicine and to address those drivers of burnout that affect women differently than men. The reader will no doubt find this book to be satisfying from both a scientific and personal experience perspective and as a road map to more rewarding careers for both women and men in medicine.

Larry Cahill, PhD
Professor, Neurobiology and Behavior
University of California
Irvine, USA

Preface

A Commentary on Gender and Nomenclature

We sit at a very interesting and pivotal time in history when it comes to the understanding of gender. While our awareness of the social construction of gender itself grows, so do our questions about the binary attribution of gender characteristics and the divisions of work and talent based on previous notions of those divisions. Social construction of gender refers to those elements of culture, some that were historically taken as biologically based, that are now being reevaluated and reconfigured. Saying such things as "boys don't cry" or "women should smile more" means participating in those old constructions of gender that do not apply to many of the societies we live in anymore. With increasing frequency, individuals problematize those assumptions.

To acknowledge all of the above is not the same as to say there are no ramifications to being of a certain gender in the world or in professions, and this book provides ample evidence that being a woman and a doctor in this time and place presents unique challenges and risks for burnout, the very subject discussed in these pages. But how do we conduct these discussions in an increasingly diverse environment regarding the understanding of gender and gender relations? How do we focus on the challenges to be dealt with if we do not agree on the language that preambles the discussions about them in the first place?

First of all, we acknowledge that we are in a social environment in flux. That means not all members of particular groups, what linguists like myself call "speech communities," are in agreement with or at the same stage of understanding of social phenomena at any given point in time. We conduct research in highly cross-cultural environments, and understandings of gender are a part of our cultural considerations. Because this volume is collaborative and the editors wanted to respect the style and point of view of each contributing author, every effort was made to maintain the original stance of the writer. This has repercussions, for example, for nomenclature. What do we call a woman who is a physician? Is she a "female doctor"? Perhaps a "woman doctor"? How do those choices impact the very construction of the phenomena they describe? The expression "man doctor" is virtually absent from academic circles, being that "male doctor" is used almost exclusivey in situations where establishing the gender is part of the argument and thus necessary. On the other hand, "female doctor," some will contend, highlights the biological aspects of womanhood sometimes to the detriment of the social ones.

However, to make decisions about which terms to use to refer to women based on the terms historically used to refer to men would be to replicate the same binary I am trying to dismantle in this text (e.g., women in relation to men, and the absence of everyone else). Finally, the choice I made in this preface to use "a woman and a doctor" or "a woman who is a doctor" is less intuitive and fluent especially when repeated many times, and so it is understandable that it does not always figure in these chapters.

As a result, a decision was made to honor the linguistic choices expressed in each individual chapter. Some of them do indeed speak more closely of the biosocial impact of being female (e.g., pregnancy, post-partum, hormonal profile). Others might focus on the more attitudinal aspects of the construction of womanhood, and might therefore call for different language selections. That is, both sex and gender play a role in issues faced by women physicians, and the editors wanted to leave each author free to make those elections based on their unique outlooks and themes of each chapter. The editors recognize the challenges of editing the work of many authors from different specialties and geographic locations, and that is why a linguist is writing this preface.

Another important issue comes about in these discussions. In writing about women, one must remember to recognize the challenges faced by non-binary, intersex, and transgender individuals and the paucity of research to guide our discussion in that regard. There needs to be much more work on the social political ramifications of a newer understanding of gender as non-binary (i.e., more than two), in a continuum, and potentially fluid, notions that are already very predominant among younger generations and that are making their way to scientific and academic literature more and more. That is, in focusing this volume on the challenges faced by women who are doctors, the authors acknowledge that such a construction does not exist simply in opposition to being a man and a doctor but rather in a much more complex environment of multiple possible gender identities, all of which merit research and attention as well.

As we evolve in our understanding of gender and gender relations, we aspire to also better understand and address the challenges faced by women and underrepresented minorities in medicine, and we hope this volume is a step in that direction.

We want the book to be pertinent and lasting, and the best way to do that is to recognize the limitations of language while celebrating its ever-changing nature and the many possibilities for inquiry, research, and the amelioration of life and work conditions for all.

Patricia Friedrich, PhD
Professor of Sociolinguistics
Arizona State University
Tempe, AZ, USA

Contents

Contributors

Jennifer I. Berliner, MD Heart and Vascular Institute, University of Pittsburgh Medical Center, Pittsburgh, PA, USA

Janis E. Blair, MD Division of Infectious Diseases, Mayo Clinic, Scottsdale, AZ, USA

Mayo Clinic College of Medicine and Science, Rochester, MN, USA

Anita K. Blanchard, MD Medical Education, University of Chicago, Chicago, IL, USA

Janice C. Blanchard, MD, PhD Emergency Medicine, George Washington University, Washington, DC, USA

Molly Carnes, MD, MS Departments of Medicine, Psychiatry, and Industrial & Systems Engineering, University of Wisconsin Hospital and Clinics, Madison, WI, USA

Hilary S. Connery, MD, PhD Division of Alcohol, Drugs and Addiction, McLean Hospital, Belmont, MA; Department of Psychiatry, Harvard Medical School, Boston, MA, USA

Suzanne M. Connolly, MD Department of Dermatology, Mayo Graduate School of Medicine, Scottsdale, AZ, USA

Sallie G. DeGolia, MD, MPH Department of Psychiatry and Behavioral Sciences, Stanford University, Stanford, CA, USA

Pamela Frazier, MD Private Practice in Psychiatry and Psychotherapy, Scottsdale, AZ, USA

Christina Girgis, MD Mental Health Service Line, Edward Hines Jr. VA Hospital, Hines, IL, USA

Shelly F. Greenfield, MD, MPH Division of Women's Mental Health and Division of Alcohol, Drugs and Addiction, McLean Hospital, Belmont, MA; Department of Psychiatry, Harvard Medical School, Boston, MA, USA

Lisa Hardesty, PhD Department of Psychiatry and Psychology, Mayo Clinic Health System, North Mankato, MN, USA

Amber Hertz-Tang, MD, MPH Department of Medicine, University of Wisconsin Hospital and Clinics, Madison, WI, USA

Stephanie Kivi, MD Department of Family Medicine, Mayo Clinic Health System, New Prague, MN, USA

Juliana M. Kling, MD, MPH Women's Health Internal Medicine, Mayo Clinic, Scottsdale, AZ, USA

Pelagia Kouloumberis, MD, MS Department of Neurosurgery, Mayo Clinic, Phoenix, AZ, USA

Jamie R. Litvack, MD Surgery, Washington State University, Pullman, WA, USA

Margaret May, MD Psychiatry & Behavioral Sciences, Palo Alto Veterans Affairs Health Care System, Palo Alto, CA, USA

Jaya Mehta, MD Internal Medicine, Mayo Clinic, Phoenix, AZ, USA

Hannah M. Mishkin, MD, MS Department of Emergency Medicine, Reading Hospital-Tower Health, West Reading, PA, USA

Katherine M. Moore, MD Department of Psychiatry and Psychology, Mayo Clinic, Rochester, MN, USA

Kristine D. Olson, MD, MS Internal Medicine, Yale School of Medicine, Yale New Haven Hospital, New Haven, CT, USA

Kirsten S. Paynter, MD Department of Physical Medicine and Rehabilitation (PM&R), Musculoskeletal Longitudinal Course, Mayo Clinic Alix School of Medicine, Scottsdale, AZ, USA

Neha P. Raukar, MD, MS Department of Emergency Medicine, Mayo Clinic, Rochester, MN, USA

Amanda E. Sedgewick, DO, MS Division of Women's Mental Health and Division of Alcohol, Drugs and Addiction, McLean Hospital, Belmont, MA; Department of Psychiatry, Harvard Medical School, Boston, MA, USA

Elaine L. Stageberg, MD, MHA Department of Psychiatry and Psychology, Mayo Clinic, Rochester, MN, USA

Amy L. Stark, MD Department of Psychiatry, Texas Tech University Health Sciences Center, Amarillo, TX, USA

Chee-Chee Stucky, MD Department of General Surgery, Mayo Clinic, Phoenix, AZ, USA

Eva Elisabeth Weinlander, MD Department of Medicine, Division of Primary Care and Population Health, Stanford University School of Medicine, Palo Alto, CA, USA

Jeannette Wolfe, MD Emergency Medicine, University of Massachusetts Medical School-Baystate, Springfield, MA, USA

Introduction

Editors' Commentary: Future Directions and Opportunities for Further Research

The epidemic of burnout that is affecting physicians, both men and women, creates an opportunity to change the way medicine is currently structured and practiced. Indeed, it will be critical to do so if we want to maintain a profession of people who come into medicine as a calling and remain fulfilled and inspired by the sense of meaning, purpose, and connections with patients and colleagues. Inaction risks the continued loss of our colleagues who leave the profession due to disillusionment, burnout, depression, and, in the extreme, suicide. We cannot ignore the frightening statistics of the burnout and suicide rates that threaten the very core of our profession. Rising costs of doing business and diminishing reimbursements, along with regulatory burdens and the electronic medical record, have saddled doctors with more clerical tasks and less quality time with patient care or unscheduled time to think, be creative, or inspired. Trying to do all that on an antiquated system, which often depended on doctors having a wife at home to cook, clean, and raise the children, has become untenable. The system in place is hierarchical, often inflexible, and too often rewards productivity over outcome or common sense.

The imperative to change our system and culture and how we take care of ourselves is now. Although personal resilience is a key factor in preventing burnout, there comes a tipping point where further efforts and recommendations to improve the personal resilience of physicians becomes counterproductive. By nature and training, physicians in the United States are resilient, have grit and a proven capacity to handle stress and workloads that far exceed usual and customary expectations for most workplaces. Rather than looking to the individual physicians to solve the problem of burnout, the culture of medicine must respond, initiate change, and embrace the changing demographics of our medical schools and the rapidly changing environment in which we practice medicine.

The fact that women are experiencing an even greater level of burnout than men, and that more than half of medical students are now women, further raises the stakes. When women physicians were in the minority, they were reluctant to highlight any differences between the sexes for fear of being further marginalized. They tried to assimilate and not complain and adjust the best they could by "doing and having it all." Indeed, they succeeded in becoming both respected members of the profession and offering other, fresh perspectives on how medicine can be practiced. However, we now realize that these accomplishments have come at a cost to individual women in terms of unacceptable rates of burnout, depression, addiction, and disparities in academic and leadership advancement, income, and a sense of "belonging" in traditionally male-dominated specialties.

Among practicing physicians, the experiences, aspirations, and struggles are likely more similar than different between men and women. However, by acknowledging the differences we can adapt the current system to work better for both sexes. Just as examining and understanding rare and orphan diseases leads to a better understanding of the etiology of the more common and "complex" medical disorders, a close examination of the factors driving women physician burnout promises to benefit both men and women physicians. Identifying the drivers of burnout with attention to gender-specific risks and addressing them through organizational change needs to start at the beginning of a medical career. Through this process, men can become even better allies at work and contribute more equally domestically, provided women positively reinforce such changes. Self-determination theory (Ryan 2000) has become a useful model from which to base strategies and tactics that may foster resilience and wellbeing, and it is increasingly applied to improving the learning environment in medical education (Neufeld 2019). The elements of this model ostensibly fit well with the areas we have identified as needing attention to help women physicians thrive. According to self-determination theory, humans need autonomy (choice), competence (mastery), and social connectedness (relatedness) for optimal motivation, engagement, and well-being. The following are a few examples of potential tactics in each category, each divided by three major domains that impact wellness (Bohman et al. 2017), though many need further research to establish their effectiveness in reducing burnout:

1. *Choice*
   (a) Culture
      (i) Ability to stop the clock for training or tenure in accordance with family planning
      (ii) Equitable, paid parental leave
   (b) Efficiency of practice
      (i) Flexible schedules
      (ii) Telemedicine
   (c) Resiliency
      (i) Reproductive planning
      (ii) Dedicating time to one's most meaningful work or project
2. *Achieving mastery and excellence*
   (a) Culture
      (i) Mentorship and sponsorship
      (ii) Continuing education
      (iii) Supportive learning environments
      (iv) Raised awareness of gender and racial stereotypes and evidence-based interventions that diminish their impact on career advancement
      (v) Shifting reimbursement models to reward outcomes and efficient, quality care over productivity and procedures
      (vi) Resources for managing home (meal prep, errands, home repair assistance, etc.)

    (b) Efficiency of practice
        (i)   Adequate time to see and communicate with patients
        (ii) Sufficient support for clerical tasks from scribes, medical assistants, nursing, etc.
        (iii) Efficient workflows
        (iv) Effective teams
    (c) Resiliency
        (i)   Mindfulness practice
        (ii) Limited alcohol, good nutrition, regular exercise, adequate sleep
        (iii) Schedule positive activities
        (iv) Gratitude practice
3. *Social connectedness*
    (a) Culture
        (i)   Facilitated support groups
        (ii) Staff socials
        (iii) Doctors' lounges
        (iv) Peer mentorship
    (b) Efficiency of practice
        (i)   Team huddles
        (ii) Balint groups, Schwartz rounds, peer support after adverse events, etc.
    (c) Resiliency
        (i)   Quality time with friends and family
        (ii) Recognition and appreciation of colleagues

This book recounts evidence for differences between women and men physicians in their biology; gender stereotypes; sexual harassment; domestic responsibilities and work-life conflicts; career trajectories; financial rewards; patient satisfaction and outcomes; levels of depression, addiction, and suicide; feelings of isolation; and level of support, sponsorship, and mentorship. Importantly, the authors offer a multitude of solutions to the challenges underlying burnout in women physicians. Some solutions are low-hanging fruit that can (and should) be easily implemented now. Others will take time to adapt our culture and systems to the current realities of medical profession. Critically, there is a dearth of good research examining gender differences in medicine and even less research on effective interventions to foster professional fulfillment, racial and gender equity, patient outcomes and satisfaction, and a thriving system of healthcare. May the following chapters spur some of you to take on the task of building this body of work with evidence-based research that addresses and solves the unacceptable inequities and suffering that too often faces doctors who were called to this noble profession. The need for change in medicine is urgent, especially for women in medicine. As a profession, we must demonstrate compassion and provide care for those who have pledged their lives to the care of others.

The editors note that all of the chapters were written before the COVID-19 pandemic. Yet, as we now proof the book amidst the uncertainties, threats, and changes in the system associated with the COVID-19 pandemic, its enormous significance must be acknowledged. This health crisis has brought out the best and worse in many regions and healthcare settings. On the one hand, we have witnessed exacerbation of the gender and racial disparities outlined in the forthcoming chapters, increased emotional and physical stress, and economic hardships that limit resources needed to support healthcare professionals in our efforts to prevent, manage, and treat burnout. Germane to this book, we observed that home care and homeschooling fell disproportionately on the younger women physicians, who otherwise might have used the time for academic pursuits during the shutdown of practices. Likewise, as practices were economically stressed and then quickly ramped amidst cancellations of summer programs for their children and fears of exposing family members to the virus upon returning home from their clinical practice, the risk of emotional exhaustion was particularly high for these same women—especially if leaders did not acknowledge these added challenges. On the other hand, it has provided an opportunity to evaluate the benefit of flexible schedules and telemedicine options, reduced workloads (particularly true in the beginning for many practices) and limited travel, as well as integrating daily walks, home-cooked meals, mindfulness and other resilience strategies into daily life and appreciating things we had previously taken for granted including collegial interactions. Further, it created an incentive for some institutions to ensure psychological and physical safety through enhancing their peer support, wellbeing, and mental health programs. As we confront and emerge from this crisis, may our healthcare institutions not only remain steadfast in their efforts to support medical professionals, but learn and grow from this most difficult and unprecedented era. The topics presented in the forthcoming chapters have become even more relevant. It is critical that we don't lose momentum in the midst of fear and economic hardship, but, rather, appreciate that our main 3 precious resource, i.e., our medical professionals, must be supported now more than ever before.

Scottsdale, AZ, USA   Cynthia M. Stonnington, MD
Scottsdale, AZ, USA   Julia A Files, MD

References

Bohman B, Dyrbye L, Sinsky CA, Linzer M, Olson K, Babbott S, Murphy M, DeVries PP, Hamidi MS, Trockel M. Physician well-being: The reciprocity of practice efficiency, culture of wellness, and personal resilience. NEJM Catalyst. August 7, 2017. https://catalyst.nejm.org/physician-well-being-efficiency-wellness-resilience. Accessed on 4 Mar 2019.

Neufeld A, Malin G. Exploring the relationship between medical student basic psychological need satisfaction, resilience, and well-being: a quantitative study. BMC Med Educ. 2019;19:405.

Ryan R, Deci E. Self-determination theory and the facilitation of intrinsic motivation. Am Psychol. 2000;55(1):68–78.

Part I
How Do Women Physicians Differ from Their Male Counterparts?

Sex, Gender, and Medicine

Jeannette Wolfe

Ironically, I first stumbled down the sex and gender rabbit hole as I was trying to avoid my own emotional burnout. The following pages include an amalgam of opinions, facts, and reflections about that journey along with a little peppering of advice that I wish someone had shared with me earlier in my own career. I share with you my story as an emergency medicine physician working in one of the highest acuity departments in the United States, in hope that it will help you make better sense of your own and to remind you that it is truly possible to re-energize your career and rediscover your purpose and passion. I wish you safe travels.

In retrospect, when I was struggling with issues at work there were a lot of factors, personal and professional, that were likely contributing. The one that was holding center court, however, was conflict. If we define conflict as a mismatch between two parties' expectations, emergency departments – with their sick patients, scared families, and overwhelmed staff – have it in spades. My personal Achilles' heel, however, was dealing with unhappy consulting physicians from other departments. Now, if you are an emergency medicine physician, this sort of comes

J. Wolfe (✉)
Emergency Medicine, University of Massachusetts Medical School-Baystate, Springfield, MA, USA
e-mail: jeannette.wolfe@baystatehealth.org

with the job (even if it is something in which most of us receive very little actual training) and clearly, I have witnessed many of my EM colleagues similarly struggle through some difficult interactions. What was striking to me, however, was how we managed the aftermath of those arguments. Most of my colleagues, and at the time they were almost all men, seemed to bounce back much more quickly – a harsh interaction in the trauma room at the beginning of a shift did not necessarily preclude a friendly chat about powder skiing conditions before the end of it. Meanwhile, I'd just get stuck and would literally spend *hours* after a shift methodically replaying challenging interactions and crafting up new "perfect" responses. Responses that would, naturally, reflect my innate intelligence, wit, and professionalism and make it crystal clear that in the future they'd better think twice about messing with me. Unfortunately, this tortuous ritual was usually followed by a few days of low-level dread as I grew increasingly anxious as to how my next encounter with that individual would unfold. In retrospect, the whole process was simply *exhausting*, especially because it seemed to repeat itself every couple of weeks.

The turning point came one night when I was working with another EM physician, whom I had just witnessed get into a really heated conversation with a surgical colleague, and I asked him what he thought was the most difficult thing about the shift. Expecting that he would say that argument, he answered "The toner in the printer didn't work." My immediate thought was "Really?!! You two came close to blows and you are stuck on *ink*!!". At that moment, I realized that although he and I were technically doing the same job, how we were actually *perceiving* that job was totally different. As I assumed that something was probably wrong with me *personally*, I figured out that if I wanted to stay in EM over the long haul, I had some major work to do and so I started reading – a lot. During that process, I serendipitously stumbled upon two books, *Same Words Different Language* by business CEO Barbara Annis and Dr. Leonard Sax's *Why Gender Matters* [1, 2]. These books formally introduced to me the concept that biological sex influences how we physiologically frame the world.

In retrospect, my first impression of those books was simply relief. They suggested that at least some of the differences in perception that I had begun to notice were based on scientific data and rooted in actual chromosomal, hormonal, and environmental differences. I wasn't an alien; I was simply just *not a guy*. Ultimately admitting this simple truth that men and women are fundamentally different and that *that is ok* has changed how I communicate and take care of patients. In addition, it has sparked a deep curiosity to further explore these differences to better understand their extent and the circumstances in which they are relevant.

In many instances, men and women quite literally "sense" the world differently. Take hearing for example. Due to subtle anatomical differences in the male and female larynx and vocal cords, female voices are higher pitched and contain a more complex timbre that appears to cause greater cortical activation when heard compared to male voices [3]. (It is theorized that people experiencing auditory hallucinations are more likely to perceive they are hearing a male's voice because it takes less neuronal firing to trigger its perception.) In addition, men have traditionally had about twice the risk of hearing loss compared to women [4]. Although this gap is slowly decreasing (due to both better safety equipment and increased noise exposure to women), when hearing loss does occur, women often lose the ability to hear lower frequency sounds and men higher ones [5]. Practically speaking, this suggests that men and women who are hard of hearing actually hear conversations differently with men missing out on more consonants (heard best in higher frequencies) and women more vowels (lower frequency). These differences may be further amplified because men are less likely to wear hearing aids and women more likely to disclose their hearing loss and coach others on how to best mitigate it like by saying, "Harriet, could you please talk a bit more slowly and into my good right ear" [6].

Similarly, there are huge sex-based differences in our sense of smell. Compared to men, women have *millions* more olfactory bulb neurons and, depending upon the scent, may be able to detect, compared to men, odors diluted up to 1/100,000th times!

[7, 8] So the next time you clean out your son's backpack and catch the whiff of a pair of overripe gym socks before calling him out, consider that he truly might not actually smell them!

As I got more interested in this material, I discovered a handful of psychology articles demonstrating that men and women often have divergent responses to similar stimuli. For example, researchers showed that when stressed, women often appeared to be more in tune to facial expressions of anger and to the physical discomfort of those around them while men became less aware and often more internally focused [9, 10]. Several studies also suggested that compared to women, men seemed to be more willing to let go of grudges and to move forward [11, 12]. This made me begin to consider the possibility that a lot of the guys I worked with simply "sensed" conflict in a different way than I did. It wasn't right, it wasn't wrong, but just like smelling those socks, it was *different.* This was an epiphany because it allowed me to better depersonalize conflict and to recognize some potential sex- and gender-associated gaps that were often unintentionally separating one individual's intentions from another's perceptions. Importantly, once I was able to see those gaps more clearly, I could then start working on ways to deliberately bridge them. Ultimately, this has helped me to better humanize some of the more difficult personalities I have come across over the years and has greatly increased my job satisfaction.

The next milestone on my personal sex and gender discovery journey was meeting Dr. Marianne Legato. Dr. Legato is an old school, no nonsense cardiologist from Colombia University and in the early 1990s she was approached by the American Heart Association to study sex differences in cardiac disease. Her initial reply, reflecting the view of most doctors and scientists at the time, was something akin to "Why on earth would you want to pay me to study that! A vessel is a vessel, it doesn't matter who it is plugged into." Reluctantly she agreed to participate, and soon she was surprised to discover totally unexpected sex-based differences in myocardial physiology and pathophysiology. This, in turn, made her curious about what other clinically relevant information was being overlooked and ultimately reshaped her career. During the past 25 years Dr. Legato has become the pioneer and inexhaustible champion of the world of Sex- and Gender-Based Medicine (SGBM). She has edited its premier textbook, started several journals, and opened a foundation supporting its research [13, 14]. Perhaps most inspiring to me, however, is Dr. Legato's continued thirst for learning. Now well into her 80s, she can deliver an off the cuff lecture on genomics and the critical importance of considering the variable of biological sex in stem cell policy and technology. Essentially, being introduced to Dr. Legato and hearing about her work motivated me to start looking at ways in which biological sex and gender were impacting medicine.

My next step was serendipitously connecting with other physicians within emergency medicine who were already doing work in sex and gender. In retrospect, it's funny how we navigate through life. Sometimes we spend a great deal of time meticulously researching and ruminating over "best" options and "big" decisions, yet often we are as heavily influenced by relatively happenstance interactions. In my case, it was a phone call. About 10 years into my academic career, I decided to give up my focus on traditional EM research and with that I let my membership to our academic society (SAEM, the Society of Academic Emergency Medicine) lapse. Honestly, there wasn't a lot of love lost because at the time my image of the society was a bunch of gray-haired white guys in nice blue suits rushing around doing seemingly quite important things that rarely involved me. Years later, someone from SAEM approached me to give a talk on gender differences in communication at their national meeting. The sort of funny thing about this is that I would likely have turned it down had I known at the time that SAEM gave no financial support to speakers and that my conference fee would actually be jacked up because I was no longer a member. But I gave the lecture and a couple of weeks later, Dr. Stephanie Abbuhl – one of the executive members of a new SAEM group, the Academy for Women in Academic Emergency Medicine – called me out of the blue and asked me to consider joining their academy. I was a bit wary as I was not entirely clear how it might align with my current path and if I'm honest, I wasn't sure I wanted to spend the money on the SAEM membership fee.

In retrospect, that phone call taught me two important lessons. One, never underestimate the power of a simple invitation – for the right person at the right time, it can truly be a game changer. And two, there is great value in allowing a little space and mental marination before saying yes or no to a new opportunity. Today, I occasionally do consulting with Barbara Annis and her company Gender Intelligence Group (yes, she is the author of that book that so inspired me and over the years – after only a *little* email stalking on my part – we have become good friends). During her workshops, companies will often bring up a perceived gender difference in an employee's willingness to jump into a new professional opportunity. For example, consider the following scenario: you are a boss and have a great promotion to offer one of your employees with just one hitch, they will need to relocate. You have two equally qualified candidates, a man and a woman, and you are meeting with them individually to gauge their interest. First, you talk with the guy and he responds with an enthusiastic "Alright!!!"; a few hours later you chat with the woman and her initial "Ah um wow, thanks" seems comparatively pretty lukewarm. Unchecked, it is easy to see how you might start honing in on your male candidate because he seems more interested and ready to commit. What might be going on here is that the male employee is focusing on the end point – a promotion – and might truly believe that he will be able to figure out any potentially sticky details about a big move on the run. While the female employee may be fixating more on the *process* associated with taking that new position and may more readily appreciate potential logistical barriers. Knowing this, a better approach (and one that was actually used by a European telecommunications company at one of the workshops) might be to give both employees a general description of the job along with an expectation that they will have several weeks to think about it before any further discussion. Ultimately such a strategy might prevent a re-relocation for that male employee (after all, who knew the new location had no elite high school swim clubs), while it might also give that female candidate adequate time to start imagining the real possibility of a change and to explore logistical solutions. The bottom line, when possible, it helps to give yourself a little space to be able to subtly shift from a "no because" to a "maybe if" mindset when making bigger life decisions.

Ok, so my decision about whether or not to pony up an academic membership fee was clearly far less dramatic than taking a job across the country, and ultimately, I chose to rejoin SAEM and join AWAEM. In retrospect, it was clearly one of the best professional decisions I have made because it connected me to a network of women who were eager to collaborate and support each other. Additionally, within AWAEM, I found a smaller group of physicians who were way ahead of me on the EM sex and gender bandwagon and who graciously let me join their posse. This was really important, because up to that point most of what I was doing was by myself so it was a relief to meet a group of women who not only saw the clinical relevance of the inclusion of sex and gender in academic medicine but who could also help me weather some of the inevitable controversial storms associated with it.

Before we go further, let's pause and go over some basic definitions. Although the terms biological sex and gender often get interchanged in the popular press and even, rather annoyingly, by editors of some scientific journals, they are not the same (for an excellent reference of correct sex- and gender-based medical terminology, please see Dr. Tracy Madsen's recent review paper [15]). Essentially, biological sex refers to our innate package of chromosomes and hormones. For most of us, this is a binary grouping in that we are either born with an XX or XY pair of sex chromosomes. And for hormones, although we all are exposed to testosterone, estrogen, and progesterone, their ratios are vastly different depending upon our chromosomal sex. When talking about hormones it's crucial to understand that timing is everything and that the same hormones can have totally different effects depending upon *when* the brain is exposed to them. Specifically, there are two critical periods – prenatal and pubertal – that the hormonal cocktail our brain imbibes leaves behind permanent or so-called "organizational" effects. Exposure to these very same hormones, outside these critical periods, causes only "activational" or temporary changes in brain function. Vastly oversimplified, our organizational hormones help us develop the series of railroads that connect different areas of brain; activational ones influence which tracks get switched on at any particular moment.

To better explore the interrelation and yet subtle differences between activational and organizational hormones, let's consider a few examples. A large amount of prenatal testosterone increases an individual's preference to engage in certain types of more physical play; this is true whether you are a human or a monkey [16]. This is an organizational effect in that the amount of prenatal testosterone we are exposed to sets us up, right out of the gates (or the uterus) with certain patterns of neural networks. On the other hand, if you take a grown man who is an avid sports fan and test his testosterone levels as he watches his favorite team crush their opponent in a high-stakes playoff game, you will likely see an "activational" surge in his testosterone triggered by the sense of competition.

So you might ask: Does a transient little blip of testosterone really matter? Well, yes, no, and maybe; *it all depends upon the context*. The *potential* downstream influence of hormones on behavior is nicely shown by the work of Dr. John Coates. Dr. Coates is a neuroscientist with a really interesting backstory. He took a major pay cut and left the world of high-stakes trading to study the influence of hormones on decision making [17]. His team found that during competitive situations, men (who in general have about 10× the testosterone level of females) often get a surge of testosterone and that this may change the way that they appraise risk such that they become more comfortable with taking risks. Quite importantly, this occurs totally under their conscious radar. Furthermore, his research suggests that for many males "winning" something, like a tennis set or a stock trade, triggers a positive feedback loop that leads to more testosterone release [18].

Ok, when we talk about hormones whether it is cortisol, estrogen, or testosterone, it's helpful to think about their influence on behavior based on an inverted U-shaped curve. Depending upon the specific context, a little surge might be helpful, but too much and watch out! For example, a slight increase in testosterone might be totally beneficial to a young male animal because it may nudge him a little outside his typical comfort zone and give him access to new resources such as food or a mate. Unchecked, however, a continued influx can push that animal way past his contextual sweet spot and into an area that is statistically more risky. For example, they might start scavenging too close to predators or expending too much energy trying to patrol an overly large territory. Dr. Coates believes that young men in the trading floors are susceptible to some of these same testosterone fluctuations and that their physiology likely plays a role in the stability of world markets. In fact, he believes that the collapses of several major financial institutions were likely triggered by the faulty decision making of young men riding out the tail end of their massive winner's streak [19, 20].

This whole area of discovery changed the way I think about our neurobiology and its effect on our behavior. Just staying with testosterone, think about the potential influence of this in our own professional worlds. Could shuffles for dominance in the trauma room between different "medical tribes" be inadvertently triggering testosteronal surges that subtly shift the quality of decision making from a "what" is right to a "who" is right scenario? Is it impacting diagnostic anchoring? By the way, this is just considering a natural testosterone flux. What about the long-term effects of the 3.8 billion dollar *exogenous* testosterone industry that aggressively markets supra-therapeutic doses of testosterone to men who usually lack an actual medical indication to take it? [21] Importantly, these same types of questions readily apply to other hormones too. There are studies suggesting that patients who are chronically stressed or who are taking long-term corticosteroids may actually become more *risk adverse* and it is well known that high levels of progesterone can stimulate excessive rumination [22, 23]. Currently there are far more questions than answers, but this data underscores the value to me of neuro-diverse teams and their potential ability to help check and balance individual member's physiological blind spots.

Now let's move on to gender. Gender is based on how an individual perceives themselves within the context of societal expectations and norms and, unlike the more binary biological sex classification, represents a spectrum. Lab rats have a sex, not a gender. In the research world, it's ideal when a sex and gender difference is discovered if researchers can determine if their results are reflective of a difference in biological sex or in a culturally influenced construct – i.e., gender. For example, in 2018 the Cleveland Clinic published mortality outcome data before and after changes in their ST elevation MI (STEMI) protocols [24]. Their new guideline included four specific components: formalized trigger of cath lab, assigned team roles, transport to open room in cath lab, and radial versus femoral access. Before the protocol the 30-day mortality was 10.7% versus 4.6% for women and men, respectively; after it was 6.5% to 3.3%. Notably, there was not a significant decrease in mortality for men but the *absolute mortality difference* in women fell more than 4%! Now, we know from other data that there are several biological sex differences in cardiac disease that can contribute to this mortality difference such that women who smoke and have diabetes or depression have greater risk of coronary artery disease compared to matched men. Women are also more vulnerable to getting microvascular disease and are overrepresented in the subgroup of patients who present without chest pain [25, 26]. The Cleveland Clinic study nicely shows, however, that an individual's *gender* is also associated with the chance that they will die from their heart attack and suggests that there was simply *something* different in how men and women were evaluated and treated before the protocol. Unfortunately, hunting down the "why" in the gender bucket can be much trickier because these gender differences are often the *sum* of a bunch of ill-defined and difficult to quantify individual touchpoints such as potential subtle differences in triage, high acuity room placement, and time until initial EKG. These differences can be further confounded if women present atypically or describe their pain in an overly expressive manner because that presentation clashes with the mental model that so many of us were taught that associates STEMI with stoic older men who look gray and ashen.

Of course, the above discussion is further complicated by the fact that what is a sex vs a gender difference, in reality, is often hard to define. As a recent obstetrical study shows, the influence of gender starts *before* birth. This study examined pregnant European women's risk preferences after they underwent prenatal ultrasounds. They found that couples who found out they were having a girl became more risk adverse compared to couples having a boy or to those who did not find out their baby's sex. The suggested implication of this study is that knowing a baby's sex not only changes a pregnant woman's perception and decision making; it might also impact fetal development because any physiological shift, such as a cortisol spike, in the mom can have a downstream effect to the fetus. Furthermore, if these differences in risk tolerance continue after birth, babies that get cuddled a little longer or thrown up into the air a little higher will have slightly different brains as these subtly different experiences will physically alter their synapse connections and axonal myelinization patterns via neuroplasticity. So, the belief that we can make a clean vertical line that nicely separates our biology from social constructs is often unrealistic and far more often that line is tipped over with the influence of biological sex *smearing* over to that of gender. In reality, there is actually a little ironic twist to that prenatal ultrasound study – as testosterone delays lung development, infant mortality in developed countries is actually far higher in males! This leads us back to the delicate gap between data and perception.

In retrospect, I should have anticipated that studying sex and gender would be associated with a lot of baggage. As a western trained physician who was baptized by the holy grail of data, I naively believed that once there was more data showing clinically important sex- and gender-based differences, we as a medical community would quickly pivot and adapt to the new evidence. Needless to say, it didn't quite happen this way. Many researchers and physicians struggle to admit that men and women, on average, are simply different. Although they may embrace the emerging world of precision medicine, they still have trouble believing that the first step in getting there is the consideration of whether an individual has an XX or an XY chromosomal pair. I initially found this disconnect puzzling like: don't people *want* to practice up-to-date medicine? SGBM benefits the outcome of both sexes. Yes, it allows us to double-check the validity of all the practices that we developed on male scientific models and simply cut and pasted over to females. However, SGBM also helps us optimize the health of males because when we deliberately study outcomes in both males and females we often find processes in which females have a natural advantage – such as having a better immunological response to most vaccines. Once discovered, this allows us the opportunity to go back to the lab to try and figure out why such a difference occurs which can then lead to new therapies that specifically target and benefit men. So, if SGBM helps women and it helps men, what the heck is the hang up?

In hindsight, I believe the reluctance of the medical community to fully embrace SGBM is because, as previously noted, the components of sex and gender can be difficult to pull apart; hence, they often just get lumped together. This is problematic because the biological sex as a separate variable angle, especially when it can be tied to an objectively measured physiological difference, is not that controversial. In fact, we already have the framework for a similar variable – age – which could be used as a model. Sometimes, *depending upon the context*, age matters; other times it doesn't. Have a sprained ankle? Probably don't care if you are 18 or 50. Have chest pain? Well, that's a different story. Quite bluntly, I believe the problem in getting SGBM more mainstream is dealing with the albatross of gender.

Gender quickly gets problematic because it is deeply interwoven with implicit bias. Most of us have a sense that implicit bias still exists *somewhere* but we deeply *want to believe* it is not an issue that personally affects us or the assumed gender-blind, merit-based professional communities in which we work. When papers are published suggesting otherwise and show that gender appears to still influence patient care, medical training, evaluations, and promotions, this can feel threatening and difficult to accept [21, 27, 28]. A recent study by Handley nicely demonstrates this issue [29]. They started by asking participants to read the abstract from another actual study that revealed implicit bias (specifically, the study showed that abstracts from a national conference were rated higher if the first author was a male) and then doctored up its *result* section for their study. Half of their study participants got the original abstract with its original conclusions while the other half got the original abstract with modified conclusions that showed *no perceived differences* in findings related to the author's gender. They then asked their study participants to comment upon the *quality* of the study's methodological design. They found that male science professors rated the quality of the research as being better in the abstracts showing no gender differences.

Recently, I came across an interesting little MRI study that suggests what might be going on at a neurobiological level when we are given data that challenges a deeply held belief. This 2017 study by Kaplan looked at another area which easily trips most of us up – politics [30]. In this study researchers put individuals with strong political convictions into an MRI machine. Next, they bombarded them with contradictory information about their political party and then reevaluated the strength of their convictions. The authors were interested in the MRIs of individuals who had objective scores before and after the scan that stayed consistent (i.e., they went into and out of the scanner with their same strong convictions). When correlating BOLD signal with belief change, they found two interesting things. One, the lower the belief change, the less activity in the area in the brain (left orbital prefrontal context) that often chews over the validity of new information. And two, the amygdala and insula, areas that are often associated with concern of physical harm and threats, showed more activity with less belief change. I believe that this study highlights the sense of distress that many of us feel when we are confronted with new information that contradicts a deeply held view and reveals why we are vulnerable to prematurely dismissing that information prior to any real objective consideration. This made me realize that if I truly wanted to move the needle on this controversial sex and gender stuff, I not only needed to know the science; I needed to anticipate and manage its *perception* and to consciously work to *create safe spaces* where the material can be openly explored in a curious, nonjudgmental fashion.

There was one more unanticipated roadblock in my new venture, and that was reality of public backlash. There are a lot of people who have strong and often quite differing opinions about any research concerning sex and gender. I think the group that was most surprising to me, however, was the one consisting of a handful of neuroscientists and psychologists who appear to sincerely believe that most sex-based differences are inconsequential and are concerned that most research only reinforces preconceived stereotypes and justifies discrimination [31, 32]. Although I agree that we must carefully analyze and appropriately message results so that they are not overblown, I worry about this trajectory. First, because there are clear sex differences in many mental health and neurological diseases: Alzheimer's, Parkinson's, autism, anxiety and mood disorders, and sociopathy, to name just a few. Second, I'm concerned that fear of public criticism might stall other researchers from adopting the analysis of sex and gender into their own academic work. For example, a recent peer-reviewed paper discussing a mathematical theory about the greater male variability hypothesis (which contends that sex-based evolutionary differences in reproductive strategies lead to a greater *range of variability* in many traits and behaviors in males compared to females) was pulled *after* its online publication [33]. An editorial by the primary author implied its removal wasn't triggered due to any methodological issues, rather from complaint letters sent to the journal stating concerns that the study might be misinterpreted and used to inappropriately discourage women from entering math-oriented fields. Undoubtedly, this was a controversial paper; pulling it, however, sniffs a little too much of academic censorship to me. As the study is no longer available, it cannot be openly analyzed and vetted on social media and this only feeds into additional conjecture. On the same note, last year when I interviewed Dr. Anne Litwin about her qualitative research on the unique challenges women can face when working together, she shared with me that she was actively discouraged from pursuing the topic. The feedback was of concern that if any of her results portrayed professional women in an unfavorable light, they might be used as ammunition to prevent the advancement of women in the future [34]. Wow.

So, in summary, we now know (a) that there are real and important sex- and gender-based differences and (b) they can often be very hard to openly discuss. How do we move past this Catch-22? Well, I think it starts with a deep breath and a sincere acknowledgment that discussing this material can be truly challenging and that unchecked it can viscerally trigger lots of different groups in lots of different ways. Next, we need to objectively identify shared goals. Here's the short list that I'd hope most of us can agree upon: (1) practice up-to-date science, (2) optimize the physical and mental health of all of our patients and ourselves, and (3) maximize the effectiveness of our teams. Having this list handy can help refocus a conversation if and when it starts to veer off track. At the end of the day, the message I want others to take home is that men and women are not the same and that it is okay to talk about it. Many of the ways in which we are different are undoubtedly inconsequential, however *not all of them*. As the Cleveland Clinic STEMI study shows, it is time we approach this tough material in a curious and respectful way because if we continue to dance around it, we are short-changing ourselves, our patients, and our teams [22].

I'd like to conclude by suggesting some different frameworks to approach sex and gender differences. First, when we can, it is helpful to break apart biological sex differences from gender ones because the interventions used to mitigate them are often quite different. When we are talking about biological sex, we are usually focused on potential physiological or pathophysiological differences that may interact with the result of a test, drug, or intervention. For example, because women's hearts are smaller than men's and because women have increased microvascular pathology, women with acute coronary syndrome may have a negative conventional troponin due to a smaller troponin leak and may benefit from being tested by a high sensitivity troponin with a sex-based cutoff value [35]. Adjusting for identified *biological sex* differences will likely focus on *technological* tweaks such as adjusting "normal" lab values, modifying drug dosing, or changing imaging protocols.

Tackling gender-based health inequities, however, will likely require a different approach as here we are not dealing so much with an objective physiological difference but a more nuanced cultural one. A good start to fixing these disparities is to remind colleagues that gender-based implicit bias, just like decision or distraction fatigue, is unconscious and unintentional. And just like those heuristic blind spots, if left unchecked, implicit bias can lead to flawed decision making, inadvertent patient harm, and initially subtle but cumulatively marked, professional inequities. Unlike biological sex differences, attenuating gender-based disparities is often about modifying systems to catch and mitigate unconscious human bias. These include things like: widespread educational training about the negative impact of implicit bias, modification of an electronic record that automatically *defaults* patients *in* to specific evidence-based guidelines, and an organizational commitment to transparently review its demographic statistics on retention, salary, and promotion.

Another conceptual framework I have found extremely helpful in approaching sex- and gender-based differences is one developed by McCarthy et al. [36]. They break differences into three big categories. The first category is represented by two separate circles, one for males, the other females. Almost everything that falls into this category is a biological difference based on reproductive organs. For example, if you have ovaries or XX chromosomes, you go into the female circle, and if you have XY chromosomes and testicles, the male one (though in reality, even this categorization is not quite so neat as there are people born *intersexed* who have an unanticipated glitch in their hormonal, chromosomal, or anatomical development and don't easily fit into either grouping).

The next category comprises of overlapping circles and looks at the mean differences in large groups of men and women with the degree of overlap depending upon the specific trait or behavior being evaluated. Of note for many characteristics, there are significant overlaps between men and women and some researchers use this to say: if the vast majority of men and women look the same here, why do we care about their differences? My response is: What is the downside of better understanding how the people outside the overlapping regions might be thinking or behaving, especially if it is different from my own reactions? For example, in 2016 Sparato and a team at University of Pittsburgh surveyed burnout rates and the use of different types of coping mechanisms in internal medicine residents [37]. Their data showed that twice the number of women reported being burned out compared to men (30% vs. 15%). They also found that although both men and women used acceptance, positive reframing, and self-distraction, men were more likely to use humor and women self-blame and that women were also more likely to seek outside help. I believe in recognizing such differences, researchers can use them to develop new approaches better tailored to the different needs of different residents.

The third category, which personally I find the most interesting, consists of sex convergence and divergence. Convergence challenges the assumption that just because men and women are "doing" the same thing, that the why and how *behind* that doing is also the same. One of my favorite examples of this is a neuroscience paper by Seo [38]. What they did is have men and women record neutral and anxiety-provoking stories from their own past (stories which evoked similar levels of objectively tested "anxious feelings") and then listen to them in an MRI machine as the researchers scanned them. They revealed several differences, but the most interesting one was that the sensation of being "anxious" in men was associated with less firing in the executive functioning areas of the brain while in women it was associated with *more firing*. They extrapolate this to suggest that anxious men may be more vulnerable to acts of impulsivity while anxious women to excessive rumination and suggest that cognitive behavioral therapy in men may be beneficial because it increases executive control function while mindfulness may work better in women because it dampens frontal lobe hyperactivity.

The concept of convergence brings up the possibility that if men and women use different wiring patterns in their brains to sense similar emotions or do similar tasks that there might be different ways to optimize learning new skills. For example, in a recent review done by surgical educators brainstorming on ways to increase gender diversity in surgery, it was suggested that there may be overall differences in gender-based group preferences in how to learn new procedures [39]. For instance it was suggested that when teaching something like suturing that women might prefer an extended period of hands-on coaching while men, a period of solo trial and error with the ability to loop back afterward with questions. Importantly, the message to educators was that both learning styles are acceptable and that one way is not better.

Finally, we are down to divergence. Here, men and women start off in a similar state, but their behavioral response then splits apart after being exposed to the same stimuli. One of my favorite papers from last year, which I fondly call the pet-the-puppy study, emphasizes this point. This is a quirky little study by Sherman that examines the potential for sex-based differences in affiliative behavior, or in English, they wanted to know if men and women seek out physical contact under the same conditions [40]. Because the authors recognized that hugging another adult in public could be heavily influenced by societal or "gendered" expectations, they substituted humans with dogs. The setup was that agility dogs who had just completed a competitive course were videotaped with their trainers while waiting for their official score (though most of the trainers already had a good sense about whether or not their dogs would be advancing). The study examined how much physical contact the trainer made with their dog. The results showed a divergence in *context* of behavior. Men pet their dog more when they anticipated celebration, women elimination. The authors suggest this supports the idea that men are more likely to seek out affiliation in victory while women for comfort after defeat. Coming back full circle, the concept of divergency gives me better insight as to what was going on during those early days in my career when my colleagues and I were recovering so differently to similar difficult interactions.

As we conclude this chapter, I hope this has helped you begin to see the subtle and often not so subtle influence that sex and gender can play in both patient care and our professional development. By skirting away from frankly talking about and earnestly researching sex and gender differences, we have inadvertently hurt our patients and shortchanged ourselves. The traditional medical model has not worked for many of us because we are not the traditional male doctor nor do we treat just the traditional male patient for which the system was inadvertently created. Fortunately, there are opportunities to move forward. As we now have significant data surrounding the existence of important sex- and gender-based differences in both science and professional development, the next step is targeting interventions at both the individual and organizational level via a combination of education, incentives, and accountabilities to facilitate and track real change. As discussed in the chapter, authentic buy-in to such interventions is key and is likely to be more successful if change drivers recognize and deliberately manage anticipated "perceptions" surrounding the more controversial aspects of this material and consider partnering with enlightened male influencers to increase their leverage in facilitating change.

Finally, I'd like to share one more insight. I started down this sex and gender rabbit hole in a desperate search to figure out how to better manage and recover from the professional conflict that was crippling me. Although the literature I discovered certainly provided me with additional tools to manage difficult conversations and improve patient care, ultimately, it did something far greater. The process of discovery got me *re-energized* in both my professional and personal life. In retrospect, I started developing, totally inadvertently, certain habits that can help attenuate burnout: finding a passion, diving into it deeply, connecting it to a greater good, taking new risks, finding like-minded allies, teaching others, celebrating accomplishments, and spotlighting gratitude.

As you start on your own journey toward wellness and renewal, I encourage you to be more mindful about the material to which you naturally gravitate and to allow yourself the time to explore it more deeply. It may be just the spark you need to better illuminate the path in front of you. Be well, Jeannette.

References

1. Annis A. Same words, different language. London: Piatkus Books; 2003.
2. Sax L. Why gender matters: what parents and teachers need to know about the emerging science of sex differences. Double Day. 2005.
3. Weston PSJ, Hunter MD, Sokhi DS, Wilkinson ID, Woodruff PWR. NeuroImage discrimination of voice gender in the human auditory cortex. NeuroImage. 2015;105:208–14. https://doi.org/10.1016/j.neuroimage.2014.10.056.
4. Hoffman HJ, Dobie RA, Losonczy KG, Themann CL, Flamme GA. Declining prevalence of hearing loss in US adults aged 20 to 69 years. JAMA Otolaryngol Head Neck Surg. 2017;143(3):274–85. https://doi.org/10.1001/jamaoto.2016.3527.

5. Homans NC, Metselaar RM, Dingemanse JG, Van Der Schroeff MP, Brocaar MP, Wieringa MH, et al. Prevalence of age-related hearing loss, including sex differences, in older adults in a large Cohort study. Larygnoscope. 2017;127:725–30. https://doi.org/10.1002/lary.26150.

6. West JS, Low JCM, Stankovic KM. Revealing hearing loss: a survey of how people verbally disclose their hearing loss. Ear Hear. 2016;37: 194–205.

7. Oliveira-Pinto AV, Santos RM, Coutinho RA, Oliveira LM, Santos GB, et al. Sexual dimorphism in the human olfactory bulb: females have more neurons and glial cells than males. PLoS One. 2014;9(11):e111733. https://doi.org/10.1371/journal.pone.0111733.

8. Dalton P, Doolittle N, Breslin PAS. Gender-specific induction of enhanced sensitivity to odors. Nat Neurosci. 2002;5:199. Retrieved from https://doi.org/10.1038/nn803

9. Tomova L, von Dawans B, Heinrichs M, Silani G, Lamm C. Is stress affecting our ability to tune into others? Evidence for gender differences in the effects of stress on self-other distinction. Psychoneuroendocrinology. 2014;43:95–104. https://doi.org/10.1016/j.psyneuen.2014.02.006.

10. Mather M, Lighthall NR, Nga L, Gorlick MA. Sex differences in how stress affects brain activity during face viewing. Neuroreport. 2010;21(14):933–7. https://doi.org/10.1097/WNR.0b013e32833ddd92.

11. Koski SE. Behavior: warriors shaking hands. Curr Biol. 2016;26(16):R760–2. https://doi.org/10.1016/j.cub.2016.06.058.

12. Dorrough AR. A cross-national analysis of sex differences in prisoner' s dilemma games and Andreas Gl o. Br J Soc Psychol. 2019;58:225–40. https://doi.org/10.1111/bjso.12287.

13. Legato M. Principles of gender-specific medicine. Gender in the genomic era. 3rd ed. Amsterdam: Academic; 2017.

14. Dr. Marianne J Legato. Accessed 7 Mar 2019. https://gendermed.org/dr-legato/.

15. Madsen T, Bourjeily G, Hasnain M, et al. Sex- and gender-based medicine: the need for precise terminology 1 2. Gender Genome. 2017;1(3):122–8. https://doi.org/10.1089/gg.2017.0005.

16. Hassett JM, Siebert ER, Wallen K. Sex differences in rhesus monkey toy preferences parallel those of children. Horm Behav. 2008 Aug;54(3):359–64. https://doi.org/10.1016/j.yhbeh.2008.03.008. Epub 2008 Mar 25.

17. Wolfe J (host). Influence of testosterone and cortisol on decision making with Dr. John Coates. Sex and Why podcast August 8, 2018. https://www.sexandwhy.com/sex-why-episode-8-influence-of-testosterone-and-cortisol-on-decision-making/. Accessed 10 Mar 2019.

18. Page L, Coates J. Winner and loser effects in human competitions. Evidence from equally matched tennis players. Evol Hum Behav. 2017;38:530. https://doi.org/10.1016/j.evolhumbehav.2017.02.003.

19. Coates JM, Herbert J. Endogenous steroids and financial risk taking on a London trading floor. Proc Natl Acad Sci U S A. 2008;105(16):6167–72. https://doi.org/10.1073/pnas.0704025105.

20. Coates J, Gurnell M. Combining field work and laboratory work in the study of financial risk-taking. Horm Behav. 2017;92:13–9. https://doi.org/10.1016/j.yhbeh.2017.01.008.
21. Annual testosterone drug revenue in the US in 2013 (in billion UA dollars). https://www.statista.com/statistics/320301/predicted-annual-testosterone-drug-revenues-in-the-us/. Accessed 12 Marfv 2019.
22. Kandasamy N, Hardy B, Page L, et al. Cortisol shifts financial risk preferences. Proc Natl Acad Sci U S A. 2014;111(9):3608–13. https://doi.org/10.1073/pnas.1317908111.
23. Ferree NK, Kamat R, Cahill L. Influences of menstrual cycle position and sex hormone levels on spontaneous intrusive recollections following emotional stimuli. Conscious Cogn. 2011;20(4):1154–62.
24. Huded CP, Johnson M, Kravitz K, et al. 4-step protocol for disparities in STEMI care and outcomes in women. JACC. 2018;71(19). https://doi.org/10.1016/j.jacc.2018.02.039.
25. Mehta LS, Beckie TM, Devon HA, et al. Acute myocardial infarction in women a scientific statement from the American Heart Association. Circulation. 2016;133(9):916. https://doi.org/10.1161/CIR.0000000000000351.
26. Wolfe J (host). Sex differences in heart disease with Dr. Basmah Safdar. Sex and Why Podcast. https://www.sexandwhy.com/episode-4-sex-differences-in-heart-disease/.
27. Mueller AS, Jenkins TM, Osborne M, Dayal A, O'Connor DM, Arora VM. Gender differences in attending physicians' feedback to residents: a qualitative analysis. J Grad Med Educ. 2017;9(5):577–85. https://doi.org/10.4300/JGME-D-17-00126.1.
28. Witteman HO, Hendricks M, Straus S, Tannenbaum C. Articles are gender gaps due to evaluations of the applicant or the science? A natural experiment at a national funding agency. Lancet. 2019;393(10171):531–40. https://doi.org/10.1016/S0140-6736(18)32611-4.
29. Handley IM, Brown ER, Moss-Racusin CA, Smith JL. Quality of evidence revealing subtle gender biases in science is in the eye of the beholder. Proc Natl Acad Sci U S A. 2015;112(43):13201–6. https://doi.org/10.1073/pnas.1510649112.
30. Kaplan JT, Gimbel SI, Harris S, Ahluwalia R, Jacks JZ, Devine PG, et al. Neural correlates of maintaining one's political beliefs in the face of counterevidence. Sci Rep. 2016;6:39589. https://doi.org/10.1038/srep39589.
31. Joel D, Berman Z, Tavor I, Wexler N, Gaber O, Stein Y, et al. Sex beyond the genitalia: the human brain mosaic submission PDF. Proc Natl Acad Sci U S A. 2015;112:15468. https://doi.org/10.1073/pnas.1509654112.
32. Joel D, Fine C. Can we finally stop talking about "Male" and "Female" Brains? Dec 3, 2018 NY Times. https://www.nytimes.com/2018/12/03/opinion/male-female-brains-mosaic.html. Accessed 10 Mar 2019.

33. Hill T. Academic activists send a published paper down the memory whole. Sept 7, 2018 Quillette. https://quillette.com/2018/09/07/academic-activists-send-a-published-paper-down-the-memory-hole/. Accessed 10 Mar 2019.
34. Wolfe J (host). New Rules for Women with Dr. Anne Litwin. Sex and Why Podcast Feb 21, 2018. https://www.sexandwhy.com/episode-6-new-rules-for-women/. Accessed 10 Mar 2019.
35. Shah ASV, Griffiths M, Lee KK, Mcallister DA, Hunter AL, Ferry AV, et al. High sensitivity cardiac troponin and the under-diagnosis of myocardial infarction in women: prospective cohort study. BMJ. 2015;350:g7873. https://doi.org/10.1136/bmj.g7873.
36. McCarthy MM, Arnold AP, Ball GF, Blaustein JD, De Vries GJ. Sex differences in the brain: the not so inconvenient truth. J Neurosci. 2012;32:2241–7.
37. Spataro BM, Tilstra SA, Rubio DM, Mcneil MA. The toxicity of self-blame: sex differences in burnout and coping. J Women's Health. 2016;25(11):1147–52. https://doi.org/10.1089/jwh.2015.5604.
38. Seo D, Ahluwalia A, Potenza MN, Sinha R. Gender differences in neural correlates of stress-induced anxiety. J Neurosci Res. 2017;125:115–25. https://doi.org/10.1002/jnr.23926.
39. Ali A, Subhi Y, Ringsted C, Konge L. Gender differences in the acquisition of surgical skills: a systematic review. Surg Endosc. 2015;29(11):3065–73. https://doi.org/10.1007/s00464-015-4092-2.
40. Sherman GD, Rice LK, Jin ES, Jones AC, Josephs RA. Sex differences in cortisol's regulation of affiliative behavior. Horm Behav. 2017;92:20–8. https://doi.org/10.1016/j.yhbeh.2016.12.005.

Patient Satisfaction and Outcomes

2

Jennifer I. Berliner

Patient Satisfaction Scores, Patient Outcomes, and Burnout

The available literature indicates that patient satisfaction assessments play a complex role for women physicians, in part due to expectations of a subset of their patients that appears to be gendered [1]. There is also a growing concern that patient satisfaction scores may increase both male and female physician burnout and result in physician job dissatisfaction, attrition, and inappropriate patient care [2, 3]. The available, albeit limited, literature generally endorses better outcomes for patients of female physicians compared to male physicians in various settings [4–8]. Women physicians are more likely to demonstrate patient-centered skills, spend more time with their patients [9, 10], adhere to guidelines, and provide preventive care [5, 11–17]. Although data has suggested that these practice patterns may result in improved patient outcomes and stronger relationships with patients leading to an increase in professional fulfillment, the additional time and burden may increase the risk of burnout. Once a physician experi-

J. I. Berliner (✉)
Heart and Vascular Institute, University of Pittsburgh Medical Center, Pittsburgh, PA, USA
e-mail: berlinerji@upmc.edu

© Springer Nature Switzerland AG 2020
C. M. Stonnington, J. A. Files (eds.), *Burnout in Women Physicians*,
https://doi.org/10.1007/978-3-030-44459-4_2

ences burnout, the chances of medical errors are greatly increased
[18, 19], which negatively impacts patient satisfaction and
outcomes. It is therefore imperative to (1) recognize those physician qualities and behaviors that improve outcomes and add value
and (2) further examine whether patient satisfaction scores are the
best way to assess good quality care.

Patient Satisfaction Scores

Patient satisfaction has become a chief focus within healthcare
organizations over the past decade. This is, in part, a response to
both the Patient Protection and Affordable Care Act of 2010,
which mandated that the patient experience and satisfaction
become essential components of healthcare quality assessments,
and the Centers for Medicare and Medicaid Services (CMS)
announcement that future payments would be heavily impacted
by the assessment of healthcare quality and value [20]. As a result,
patient satisfaction scores are currently considered a major quality indicator. Administrators of healthcare systems commonly
rely on patient satisfaction scores to both judge the success of the
physicians they employ as well as a metric to compare their performance to other healthcare organizations.

Patient satisfaction scores have been directly related to clinical outcomes, patient retention, patient doctor relationships,
and medical malpractice claims [21–24]. Jha and colleagues
examined whether a hospital's performance on the Hospital
Consumer Assessment of Healthcare Providers and Systems
(HCAHPS) survey was related to its performance on clinical
care quality indicators. Hospitals with a higher level of patient
satisfaction provided clinical care which was higher in quality
for all conditions examined including acute myocardial infarction, congestive heart failure, surgery, and pneumonia. Another
observational study compared clinical performance, patient satisfaction, and 30-day risk-standardized readmission rates for
acute myocardial infarction, heart failure, and pneumonia. This
study confirmed the relationship between higher overall patient

satisfaction with lower 30-day risk-standardized hospital readmission rates after adjusting for clinical quality from an organizational perspective [25].

It is, however, imperative to recognize the obvious limitations of relying on patient-reported data in isolation. Importantly, patient-reported impressions of quality of care do not always align with medical personnel's impression of the same encounters [26]. Patients typically focus on the entire patient experience. This includes, but is not restricted to, the care provided during the visit. In fact, one study found that high patient satisfaction was associated with a higher probability of an inpatient visit, greater healthcare expenditures, and higher mortality [2]. This highlights the essential need to employ processes that evaluate both the actual medical care provided and the patient experience. Medical care outcomes, both positive and negative, must remain paramount in the evaluation of healthcare organizations. Furthermore, there is data to suggest that the utilization of patient satisfaction surveys may result in physician job dissatisfaction, attrition, and inappropriate patient care due to fear of a bad evaluation [3]. Further research is needed to confirm that patient satisfaction scores, particularly when not accounting for appropriate nuance, add positive value to the evaluation of healthcare organizations and the providers overall.

Given the emphasis that healthcare organizations place on patient satisfaction scores, there is a significant amount of research being performed to help understand the factors that define patient satisfaction and may affect scores for individual physicians. Patient satisfaction scores are influenced both by patient characteristics and physician behaviors. Four factors have been identified as being integral in defining patient satisfaction: *the patient's personal preference, the patient's expectation, the response tendency of the patient due to personal characteristics, and the quality of care received* [27].

Research has demonstrated an association between race and gender concordance, physician age, and patient satisfaction scores [28, 29]. The relationship between race concordance and higher patient ratings of care seems to be independent of patient-centered communication, suggesting that patient and physician attitudes may mediate this relationship. There is also a significant amount of research evaluating the relationship between physician gender and patient satisfaction. Investigations have focused on whether there is a relationship between a physician's gender and patient satisfaction as well as the impact of physician and patient gender concordance on patient satisfaction. The remainder of this chapter will review the current literature and explore the relationship between patient satisfaction scores, patient outcomes, and physician gender.

Physician-Patient Communication

Women physicians with higher patient satisfaction scores are thought to incorporate stronger emphasis on patient-centered skills. These practice skills include being more attentive, providing more information and displaying more sympathy [9]. When comparing gender differences in physician-patient communication of pediatricians, women physicians typically spend more time with their patients than their male counterparts [10]. Women physicians engaged in more social exchange, more encouragement, reassurance, and information gathering with the children. This study observed that children were more satisfied with physicians of the same gender while parents were more satisfied with the women physicians [30]. Some, but not all studies, found that women obstetrics-gynecology patients preferred a female physician [31, 32]. One group of investigators videotaped primary care providers to further study whether differences exist in outpatient clinic encounters between male and female primary care physicians [12]. Although they did not demonstrate a statistically significant difference in the total time spent with patients, they did observe that female physicians engaged in more preventive services and communicated differently with their patients. This concept has been reinforced in several clinical trials. In one study involving gynecologists, after controlling for patient-centered communication, no significant gender differences remained; i.e., patient-centered communication drove patient satisfaction more than the physician's gender. However, women physicians tended to use that style of communication more than their male counterparts. The authors encouraged further research on how to improve such communication skills for all physicians [33].

Gender Concordance and Patient Satisfaction Scores

A preference for gender concordance, a woman patient's preference to be cared for by women physicians, has been repeatedly demonstrated. This has been verified in studies evaluating women's choices of general practitioners [34–37], consultations for women's health problems [38], gynecological care [39], and emergency medicine [40]. A meta-analysis performed by Janssen et al. found that many women prefer to see a woman obstetrician-gynecologist, especially when a physical examination is required [31, 32, 41–46]. There are many theories to explain the reason women prefer to be seen by women physicians. The obvious one is that women feel more comfortable with women, especially when the examination involves a detailed physical examination. In addition to the ease of undergoing a physical examination by someone of the same gender, investigators have found that gender concordance encourages improved communication, patient satisfaction, and fosters a more trusting relationship between a patient and his or her physician [10, 33, 47–49].

The association between women physicians and high patient satisfaction scores is not a universal finding. Interestingly, notwithstanding the overwhelming evidence that women prefer to be seen by physicians of the same sex, the relationship becomes less clear when evaluating patient satisfaction scores. In one multicenter study, the gender of the physician treating patients in an emergency room was not a significant factor in Press Ganey Evaluations by patients [50]. Another study performed by Schmittdiel et al. found that in their population, women who chose female doctors were the least satisfied for four out of five measures of satisfaction. This study evaluated a random sample of HMO members and categorized them into four dyads: female patients of female physicians, male patients of female physicians, female patients of male physicians, or male patients of male physicians. They further stratified patients on whether they had chosen or been assigned to their physician. Of all of the divisions, male patients of female physicians were the most satisfied. Female patients were more likely to have chosen their physician to be a female physician. Despite this, female patients who chose a female physician were the least satisfied patients. Of note, preventive care and health promotion practices were comparable for male and female physicians. These differences were not seen among patients who had been assigned to their physicians and were not due to differences in any of the measured aspects of health values or beliefs. This study suggests that female patients who choose their physician may have higher expectations which are difficult for physicians to fulfill [1]. In fact, when men and women physicians portrayed the same high patient-centered narrative, there was a stronger positive effect on satisfaction and evaluations for men than women physicians. This supports the idea that while higher verbal patient-centered behavior by male physicians is a marker of clinical competence, these same behaviors are considered expected behaviors for women physicians and translated into less significant effects on satisfaction and evaluations for women physicians [51]. In fact, there is evidence that male physicians may get more credit when they demonstrate the same degree of patient-centered care as female physicians [52]. (See Chap. 5 for more on gender stereotypes.)

In a small study published by Garcia et al., the authors further explored the relationship between gender concordance and patient satisfaction. The populations of patients included in this study were African American, Caucasian, and Latino adults, who received their outpatient care in university-based primary care clinics in Northern California. This study found that women in all English-proficient groups described gender concordance as important to their relationships with primary care physicians. However, Spanish-speaking patients uniformly preferred Spanish-speaking physicians [53]. This study further underscores that gender concordance may represent only one of many patient satisfiers that contribute to the complex relationship between physician preference and patient satisfaction.

Outcomes of Female Physicians

In addition to discrepancies in patient satisfaction scores based on the sex of the provider, a significant amount of attention is focused on differences in both medical and surgical healthcare outcomes based on physician gender. The following section will review and summarize the available research.

In addition to being more likely to participate in patient-centered communication, the literature indicates that women physicians are more likely to adhere to clinical guidelines and provide preventive care [5, 11–17]. Gender concordance has been linked to medical decision making, achievement of diabetes and hypertension treatment goals, and receipt of preventive counseling. Women physicians appear to reach the treatment goal for blood pressure, HbA1c levels in women patients, and cholesterol levels in all patients more often than men physicians [54–56]. A study performed by Schmittdiel et al. investigated the relationship between outcomes of risk factor modification based upon physician gender. They monitored control of HbA1c levels, LDL-C levels, and systolic blood pressure. The results demonstrated that women patients of women physicians had better HbA1c control. Although in the general population, women patients have lower levels of LDL-C and blood pressure control than patients who are men, women patients of women providers have better LDL-C and systolic blood pressure and were more likely to receive treatment intensification of all three cardiovascular disease risk factors than women patients of men primary care providers, indicating a link between gender concordance and clinical outcomes. Furthermore, women physicians were more likely than their men counterparts to intensify hyperlipidemia and hypertension therapy for their patients [4].

Similar findings have been demonstrated when evaluating the influence of physician gender and adherence to guideline-recommended treatment of chronic heart failure in patients in eastern Germany. Guideline-recommended medication use and achievement of target doses have been observed to be higher in patients treated by women physicians. Furthermore, although there was no difference in treatment for men or women patients cared for by women physicians, physicians who are men used significantly less medication and lower doses in women patients. In a multivariate analysis, female physician gender was an independent predictor of beta-blocker prescription [5].

Although research supports the idea that women physicians focus on patient-centered communication and medical care that is more likely to adhere to clinical guidelines and recommended preventive care, does this behavior translate into better clinical outcomes for patients of women physicians? This question was addressed in a study performed by Tsugawa and colleagues [6]. The investigators analyzed a random sample of hospitalized patients greater or equal to 65 years old who were treated for a medical condition by a general internist and receive Medicare fee-for-service benefits. They examined the relationship between physician sex and 30-day mortality and readmission rates after adjusting for patient, physician, and hospital characteristics. They found that patients treated by women internists had lower mortality and readmission rates compared to patients treated by internists who are men. These findings suggest that previously documented differences in practice patterns between men and women may translate into different patient outcomes. Similarly, Dahrouge et al. evaluated quality of care based on physician gender in family medicine practitioners in Ontario, Canada. They observed that patients of women physicians were more likely to receive recommended cancer screening and diabetes management. They had fewer emergency room visits and hospitalizations. Complex patients were also noted to visit the emergency room less if their physicians were women[7].

The findings of the above study were verified by authors of another study, who evaluated survival rates following acute myocardial infarctions based on the gender of the treating emergency department physician. A higher mortality was noted among women patients treated by men physicians. Men and women patients experience similar outcomes when treated by women physicians, suggesting that unique challenges arise when physicians who are men treat women patients. Even more interesting, they found that men physicians with more exposure to women patients and women physicians have more success treating women patients [57].

Studies evaluating outcomes based on physician gender have also been performed in procedure-based medical subspecialties and surgical specialties. Mehrotra and colleagues performed a retrospective cohort study in which they evaluated physician performance on adenoma detection rate after risk adjusting for differences in patient population and procedure indication. They noted that women physicians detected roughly 10% more adenomas than men physicians, supporting that women physicians had higher performance in adenoma detection [8].

Comparison studies evaluating postoperative outcomes based on the surgeon's gender have also demonstrated small, statistically significant differences in outcomes. A population-based, retrospective matched cohort study evaluated the outcomes of patients undergoing 25 surgical procedures. Patients were matched by age, sex, comorbidity, surgeon volume, surgeon age, and hospital. Fewer patients treated by women surgeons died, were readmitted to the hospital, or had complications within 30 days than those treated by men surgeons. A stratified analysis by patient, physician, and hospital characteristics did not significantly modify the effect of surgeon sex on outcome. They did find that improved postoperative outcomes for patients treated by women surgeons were restricted to patients who have had elective operations, which might reflect better patient selection for surgery [58].

In conclusion, the available research suggests a positive relationship between patient satisfaction and patient outcomes for patients cared for by women physicians. Overall, women patients prefer to receive medical care from women physicians. Positive patient satisfaction and outcomes appear to be driven by patient-centered communication, preventative care, and adherence to clinical guidelines. The small amount of literature available suggests that women patients of women physicians may have better outcomes. Future research to further elucidate these relationships is warranted. The available data supports the value of patient satisfaction scores on a global level; however the possible role of patient satisfaction scores in contributing to physician burnout should be explored further. If a causative relationship between patient satisfaction scores and physician burnout is realized, healthcare organizations may benefit from focusing on value and outcome rather than patient satisfaction scores. Women physicians will benefit from research regarding strategies that accommodate and support their positive doctor-patient relationships and outcomes to foster professional fulfillment while not increasing physician burnout. Ultimately, both our physicians and our patients will benefit from healthcare delivery that leverages the skills necessary to create high-quality patient experiences and the best possible outcomes for our patients in the most supportive environments for our physicians. Ideally, our healthcare systems and practices should accommodate for and reward those behaviors, rather than make it harder on doctors who take that extra time and care to meet the needs of the patient.

References

1. Schmittdiel J, Grumbach K, Selby JV, Quesenberry CP Jr. Effect of physician and patient gender concordance on patient satisfaction and preventive care practices. J Gen Intern Med. 2000;15(11):761–9.
2. Fenton JJ, Jerant AF, Bertakis KD, Franks P. The cost of satisfaction: a national study of patient satisfaction, health care utilization, expenditures, and mortality. Arch Intern Med. 2012;172(5):405–11.
3. Zgierska A, Rabago D, Miller MM. Impact of patient satisfaction ratings on physicians and clinical care. Patient Prefer Adherence. 2014;8:437–46.
4. Schmittdiel JA, Traylor A, Uratsu CS, Mangione CM, Ferrara A, Subramanian U. The association of patient-physician gender concordance with cardiovascular disease risk factor control and treatment in diabetes. J Womens Health (Larchmt). 2009;18(12):2065–70.
5. Baumhakel M, Muller U, Bohm M. Influence of gender of physicians and patients on guideline-recommended treatment of chronic heart failure in a cross-sectional study. Eur J Heart Fail. 2009;11(3):299–303.
6. Tsugawa Y, Jena AB, Figueroa JF, Orav EJ, Blumenthal DM, Jha AK. Comparison of hospital mortality and readmission rates for medicare patients treated by male vs female physicians. JAMA Intern Med. 2017;177(2):206–13.
7. Dahrouge S, Seale E, Hogg W, Russell G, Younger J, Muggah E, et al. A comprehensive assessment of family physician gender and quality of care: a cross-sectional analysis in Ontario, Canada. Med Care. 2016;54(3):277–86.
8. Mehrotra A, Morris M, Gourevitch RA, Carrell DS, Leffler DA, Rose S, et al. Physician characteristics associated with higher adenoma detection rate. Gastrointest Endosc. 2018;87(3):778–86. e5.

9. Meeuwesen L, Schaap C, van der Staak C. Verbal analysis of doctor-patient communication. Soc Sci Med. 1991;32(10):1143–50.

10. Roter DL, Hall JA, Aoki Y. Physician gender effects in medical communication: a meta-analytic review. JAMA. 2002;288(6):756–64.

11. Franks P, Bertakis KD. Physician gender, patient gender, and primary care. J Womens Health (Larchmt). 2003;12(1):73–80.

12. Bertakis KD, Helms LJ, Callahan EJ, Azari R, Robbins JA. The influence of gender on physician practice style. Med Care. 1995;33(4):407–16.

13. Lurie N, Slater J, McGovern P, Ekstrum J, Quam L, Margolis K. Preventive care for women. Does the sex of the physician matter? N Engl J Med. 1993;329(7):478–82.

14. Henderson JT, Weisman CS. Physician gender effects on preventive screening and counseling: an analysis of male and female patients' health care experiences. Med Care. 2001;39(12):1281–92.

15. Andersen MR, Urban N. Physician gender and screening: do patient differences account for differences in mammography use? Women Health. 1997;26(1):29–39.

16. Frank E, Harvey LK. Prevention advice rates of women and men physicians. Arch Fam Med. 1996;5(4):215–9.

17. Franks P, Clancy CM. Physician gender bias in clinical decisionmaking: screening for cancer in primary care. Med Care. 1993;31(3):213–8.

18. Tawfik DS, Profit J, Morgenthaler TI, Satele DV, Sinsky CA, Dyrbye LN, et al. Physician burnout, well-being, and work unit safety grades in relationship to reported medical errors. Mayo Clin Proc. 2018;93(11):1571–80.

19. Panagioti M, Geraghty K, Johnson J, Zhou A, Panagopoulou E, Chew-Graham C, et al. Association between physician burnout and patient safety, professionalism, and patient satisfaction: a systematic review and meta-analysis. JAMA Intern Med. 2018;178(10):1317–30.

20. Rogo-Gupta LJ, Haunschild C, Altamirano J, Maldonado YA, Fassiotto M. Physician gender is associated with press Ganey patient satisfaction scores in outpatient gynecology. Womens Health Issues. 2018;28(3):281–5.

21. Prakash B. Patient satisfaction. J Cutan Aesthet Surg. 2010;3(3):151–5.

22. Fitzpatrick R. Satisfaction with health care. In: Fitzpatrick R, editor. The experience of illness. London: Tavistock; 1984. p. 154–75.

23. Jha AK, Orav EJ, Zheng J, Epstein AM. Patients' perception of hospital care in the United States. N Engl J Med. 2008;359(18):1921–31.

24. Glickman SW, Boulding W, Manary M, Staelin R, Roe MT, Wolosin RJ, et al. Patient satisfaction and its relationship with clinical quality and inpatient mortality in acute myocardial infarction. Circ Cardiovasc Qual Outcomes. 2010;3(2):188–95.

25. Boulding W, Glickman SW, Manary MP, Schulman KA, Staelin R. Relationship between patient satisfaction with inpatient care and hospital readmission within 30 days. Am J Manag Care. 2011;17(1):41–8.

26. Robbins A. The problem with satisfied patients. The Atlantic. Available at: https://www.theatlantic.com/health/archive/2015/04/the-problem-with-satisfied-patients/390684/. 2015.

27. Coulter A, Fitzpatrick R, Cornwell J. The point of care. Measures of patients' experience in hospital: purpose, methods and uses. The King's Fund. Available at: https://www.researchgate.net/publication/230687403. July 2009.

28. Cooper LA, Roter DL, Johnson RL, Ford DE, Steinwachs DM, Powe NR. Patient-centered communication, ratings of care, and concordance of patient and physician race. Ann Intern Med. 2003;139(11):907–15.

29. Hall JA, Irish JT, Roter DL, Ehrlich CM, Miller LH. Satisfaction, gender, and communication in medical visits. Med Care. 1994;32(12):1216–31.

30. Bernzweig J, Takayama JI, Phibbs C, Lewis C, Pantell RH. Gender differences in physician-patient communication. Evidence from pediatric visits. Arch Pediatr Adolesc Med. 1997;151(6):586–91.

31. Johnson AM, Schnatz PF, Kelsey AM, Ohannessian CM. Do women prefer care from female or male obstetrician-gynecologists? A study of patient gender preference. J Am Osteopath Assoc. 2005;105(8):369–79.

32. Janssen SM, Lagro-Janssen AL. Physician's gender, communication style, patient preferences and patient satisfaction in gynecology and obstetrics: a systematic review. Patient Educ Couns. 2012;89(2):221–6.

33. Christen RN, Alder J, Bitzer J. Gender differences in physicians' communicative skills and their influence on patient satisfaction in gynaecological outpatient consultations. Soc Sci Med. 2008;66(7):1474–83.

34. Phillips D, Brooks F. Women patients' preferences for female or male GPs. Fam Pract. 1998;15(6):543–7.

35. Ahmad F, Gupta H, Rawlins J, Stewart DE. Preferences for gender of family physician among Canadian European-descent and South-Asian immigrant women. Fam Pract. 2002;19(2):146–53.

36. Raji YR, Raji OR, Bello TB, Ekore JO. Effects of gender on patient's satisfaction with physician care and communication skills in a tertiary hospital in Nigeria. IFE PsychologIA. 2018;26(2):62–71.

37. Bertakis KD, Franks P, Azari R. Effects of physician gender on patient satisfaction. J Am Med Womens Assoc (1972). 2003;58(2):69–75.

38. van den Brink-Muinen A, de Bakker DH, Bensing JM. Consultations for women's health problems: factors influencing women's choice of sex of general practitioner. Br J Gen Pract. 1994;44(382):205–10.

39. Schmittdiel J, Selby JV, Grumbach K, Quesenberry CP Jr. Women's provider preferences for basic gynecology care in a large health maintenance organization. J Womens Health Gend Based Med. 1999;8(6):825–33.

40. Derose KP, Hays RD, McCaffrey DF, Baker DW. Does physician gender affect satisfaction of men and women visiting the emergency department? J Gen Intern Med. 2001;16(4):218–26.

41. Schnatz PF, Johnson AM, O'Sullivan DM. Qualities and attributes desired in menopause clinicians. Maturitas. 2007;56(2):184–9.

42. Mavis B, Vasilenko P, Schnuth R, Marshall J, Jeffs MC. Female patients' preferences related to interpersonal communications, clinical competence, and gender when selecting a physician. Acad Med. 2005;80(12):1159–65.

43. Fisher WA, Bryan A, Dervaitis KL, Silcox J, Kohn H. It ain't necessarily so: most women do not strongly prefer female obstetrician-gynaecologists. J Obstet Gynaecol Can. 2002;24(11):885–8.

44. Ekeroma A, Harillal M. Women's choice in the gender and ethnicity of her obstetrician and gynaecologist. Aust N Z J Obstet Gynaecol. 2003;43(5):354–9.

45. Makam A, Mallappa Saroja CS, Edwards G. Do women seeking care from obstetrician-gynaecologists prefer to see a female or a male doctor? Arch Gynecol Obstet. 2010;281(3):443–7.

46. Baskett TF. What women want: don't call us clients,and we prefer female doctors. J Obstet Gynaecol Can. 2002;24(7):572–4.

47. Gross R, McNeill R, Davis P, Lay-Yee R, Jatrana S, Crampton P. The association of gender concordance and primary care physicians' perceptions of their patients. Women Health. 2008;48(2):123–44.

48. van Dulmen AM, Bensing JM. Gender differences in gynecologist communication. Women Health. 2000;30(3):49–61.

49. Roter DL, Hall JA. Physician gender and patient-centered communication: a critical review of empirical research. Annu Rev Public Health. 2004;25:497–519.

50. Milano A, Dalawari P, McGregor AJ, Meloy PG, Kalantari A, Kirby SE, et al. Emergency department evaluation of patient satisfaction. Does physician gender impact Press Ganey scores? A multicenter study. Am J Emerg Med. 2018;36(9):1708–9.

51. Hall JA, Roter DL, Blanch-Hartigan D, Mast MS, Pitegoff CA. How patient-centered do female physicians need to be? Analogue patients' satisfaction with male and female physicians' identical behaviors. Health Commun. 2015;30(9):894–900.

52. Hall JA, Gulbrandsen P, Dahl FA. Physician gender, physician patient-centered behavior, and patient satisfaction: a study in three practice settings within a hospital. Patient Educ Couns. 2014;95(3):313–8.

53. Garcia JA, Paterniti DA, Romano PS, Kravitz RL. Patient preferences for physician characteristics in university-based primary care clinics. Ethn Dis. 2003;13(2):259–67.

54. Journath G, Hellenius ML, Manhem K, Kjellgren KI, Nilsson PM, Hyper-Q Study Group S. Association of physician's sex with risk factor control in treated hypertensive patients from Swedish primary healthcare. J Hypertens. 2008;26(10):2050–6.

55. Berthold HK, Gouni-Berthold I, Bestehorn KP, Bohm M, Krone W. Physician gender is associated with the quality of type 2 diabetes care. J Intern Med. 2008;264(4):340–50.

56. Flocke SA, Gilchrist V. Physician and patient gender concordance and the delivery of comprehensive clinical preventive services. Med Care. 2005;43(5):486–92.
57. Greenwood BN, Carnahan S, Huang L. Patient-physician gender concordance and increased mortality among female heart attack patients. Proc Natl Acad Sci U S A. 2018;115(34):8569–74.
58. Wallis CJ, Ravi B, Coburn N, Nam RK, Detsky AS, Satkunasivam R. Comparison of postoperative outcomes among patients treated by male and female surgeons: a population based matched cohort study. BMJ. 2017;359:j4366.

Rates of Burnout, Depression, Suicide, and Substance Use Disorders

3

Elaine L. Stageberg, Amy L. Stark, and Katherine M. Moore

Vignette

J is a 51-year-old partnered, mother of two teenage children, female cardiologist who has been practicing as an academic physician at the same institution since finishing fellowship nearly 20 years ago. She's finding that with increasing frequency, she's finishing the day feeling "completely exhausted," wondering if her contributions to the department have been recognized and valued. Her partner, B, has commented that J's wine consumption has increased from about once monthly to several times per week and it seems that J *needs* the wine in order to relax at the end of the day. After arriving home after 6 pm most nights, J manages to spend a few minutes catching up with her teenagers

E. L. Stageberg · K. M. Moore (✉)
Department of Psychiatry and Psychology, Mayo Clinic, Rochester, MN, USA
e-mail: Stageberg.elaine@mayo.edu; Moore.katherine@mayo.edu

A. L. Stark
Department of Psychiatry, Texas Tech University Health Sciences Center, Amarillo, TX, USA
e-mail: Amy.stark@ttuhsc.edu

© Springer Nature Switzerland AG 2020
C. M. Stonnington, J. A. Files (eds.), *Burnout in Women Physicians*, https://doi.org/10.1007/978-3-030-44459-4_3

before they are out of the house to do their own activities—she feels like it's never enough—before returning to emails to prepare for her role on various professional committees or to charting to catch up on patient care and documentation issues. Her elderly mother, who lives nearly 800 miles away, is needing more care and support as she ages, complicated by the fact that her father passed away 2 years ago and now there are no family members close to assist her mother. J feels some resentment that her career has tied her to this city so far from her mother but the thought of researching a cross-country move is more than she can handle on any given day, and she's hopeful that a promotion to vice chair of the department may be coming soon anyway. J wonders if she should schedule a visit with her doctor to discuss the possibility that her frequent tearfulness and lack of interest in activities that she used to enjoy, such as knitting, cooking, or running, are depression, but she also fears the possibility that a psychiatric diagnosis or treatment could negatively impact her medical license.

Introduction

Definition

Burnout is a clinical constellation of symptoms of emotional and psychological job-related stress. While there is no one complete, standardized, and accepted definition, burnout is commonly characterized as a combination of "emotional exhaustion, depersonalization, and low personal accomplishment caused by the chronic stress of medical practice" [1]. This chapter will explore the epidemiology of burnout and its connection with depression, suicide, and addiction, specifically in women physicians. It remains challenging to adequately describe the epidemiological indicators of physician burnout, with a wide range of study methodology, definitions, and outcomes reported in the literature. Although challenging to study from an epidemiological perspective—likely related to the lack of one consistent definition and under-report due to stigma or fear of professional repercussions—the majority of physicians are likely to personally describe some or all symptoms of burnout during their training or career, with estimates for trainees and early career physicians at 51–60% [2]. These personal symptoms have long reaching effect and result in negative consequences in the medical system: higher rates of burnout correlate to higher rates of errors, longer recovery times for patients, and lower patient satisfaction [3].

Importance of Epidemiological Data

In "The inevitability of physician burnout: Implications for interventions," published in the inaugural edition of the peer-reviewed journal "Burnout Research" in April 2014, Montgomery writes, "The increasingly high levels of job burnout observed among physicians globally is set to continue as fewer resources and tighter budgets ratchet up the personal and professional pressure" [4]. He also states, "burnout is the inevitable consequence of the way that medical education is organized and the subsequent maladaptive behaviors that are reinforced in healthcare organizations via the hidden curriculum" [4]. He describes a hidden curriculum that erodes professionalism and increases cynicism and postulates that once these maladaptive behaviors become entrenched, it is challenging, and at times even impossible, to reframe and retrain physicians. This underscores the urgent need to standardize the definition and to thoroughly understand the epidemiology of burnout in order to design studies and interventions that aim to address this burgeoning problem.

Correlations of Burnout with Depression, Substance Use Disorders, and Suicide

Although burnout, depression, and substance use disorder are separate clinical entities, the three are related in that burnout can increase risk for depression or addiction and conversely a diagnosis of depression or addiction can increase risk for burnout. Interestingly, as will be discussed in this chapter, female physicians may be at risk for rates of depression and addiction greater than their counterparts in the general population [5].

Epidemiology of Burnout in Women Physicians

Understanding Variability in the Data

Studies on the epidemiology of burnout are widely variable due to marked variation in the definition or clinical criteria for burnout, variations in the assessment of burnout, study and data quality, and difficulty in determining associations of burnout as related to age, sex, geography, time, or medical specialty [6]. A Google search of "epidemiology of burnout" will produce results in which the vast majority of search results are related to physicians, nurses, and other healthcare professionals. Although burnout is not exclusive to the healthcare professions, there appears to be a particular problem with burnout among healthcare professionals as compared to other professions today.

The Maslach Burnout Inventory

Unlike major depressive disorder or substance use disorders, burnout is not currently included in the Diagnostic and Statistical Manual of Psychiatry – DSM-5. Burnout is, however, included in the ICD-10 under the subcategory of problems related to life management difficulty (Z73). In order to more fully describe the symptoms of burnout, the Maslach Burnout Inventory (MBI) was developed in 1981 by Christina Maslach and Susan Jackson to serve as a standardized and validated tool for the assessment of burnout. Maslach characterized burnout as a triad of emotional exhaustion, depersonalization, and low personal accomplishment. The MBI is a 22-item assessment using scales to examine levels of emotional exhaustion, depersonalization, personal accomplishment, cynicism, and professional efficacy [1].

In addition to the MBI, there are a number of publicly available tools that can be used to assess symptoms of burnout. These include, but are not limited to, the Astudillo and Mendinueta Burnout Questionnaire [7], the Modified Compassion Satisfaction and Fatigue Test [8], the Copenhagen Burnout Inventory [9], the Hamburg Burnout Inventory [10], and the Pines and Aronson

Burnout Measure [11]. Combining such a large number of readily available screening tools with an unstandardized, and at times nebulous, definition of burnout makes a complete characterization of the epidemiology of burnout a difficult, if not herculean task.

One of the most comprehensive examinations of burnout in physicians comes from the systematic review completed by Lisa Rotenstein, MD, MBA, and colleagues and published in JAMA in 2018. In this article, the authors reviewed 182 studies related to burnout prevalence published between 1991 and 2018, involving 109,628 individuals. They note that despite an ongoing wide variability in the definition and description of burnout, 85.7% of all studies used the MBI as part of the burnout assessment. Among those using the MBI, the most commonly used version was the MBI-Human Services Survey, which is designed for people working in human services jobs, such as physicians [6].

Unsurprisingly, given the aforementioned challenges, the prevalence reported in the studies analyzed in the Rotenstein meta-analysis ranges from 0% to 80.5%. Estimates for emotional exhaustion were 0% to 86.2%, for depersonalization 0% to 89.9%, and for diminished sense of personal accomplishment 0% to 87.1%. Furthermore, all these values varied based on discordant cutoff scores chosen to be used with the MBI.

Several studies used the more stringent MBI cutoff scores for burnout of at least 27 on the emotional exhaustion scale, at least 10 on the depersonalization scale, and a score of no greater than 33 on the personal accomplishment scale [12]. These studies estimated a physician burnout prevalence of 2.6–11.8%. With such strict criteria for defining burnout, these studies were likely to have captured all of those physicians who definitively experienced burnout and yet may have missed those who experienced burnout but not at the level captured with these criteria. In other words, these studies can be thought of as having the highest specificity for burnout in physicians. These strict criteria may not serve the profession well in clinical practice or in identifying those physicians experiencing burnout and in need of assistance [12]. When relaxing the criteria to include *either* a high emotional exhaustion score *or* a high depersonalization score, that number increased from 2.6% nearly tenfold to 24.1% [12].

A separate study by Shanafelt and colleagues estimated the prevalence to be even higher—with this study concluding the prevalence of burnout in physicians to be 48.8%, much higher than other workers assessed in the same study, whose prevalence of burnout was 28.4% [2].

Systems of Care and Personal Factors That Contribute to Burnout

In this section, we will explore the data that demonstrates that female physicians are at higher risk for burnout than their male counterparts across both the lifespan and the training/career span.

Physicians Versus Other Professionals

It appears that the phenomenon of burnout occurs more commonly in medicine than among other professions. In a "Letter to the Editor" accompanying their study regarding rates of burnout in physicians in the years from 2001 until 2017, Shanafelt and colleagues specifically compare the rates of burnout in physicians to others in fields with commensurate levels of education (doctorate or professional degrees such as JD, PhD). The letter noted that when compared to other groups of professionals, physicians worked more hours per week and were more likely to experience burnout, even when adjusted for age, sex, relationship status, and hours worked per week [13].

Risk Factors for Physician Burnout

Several studies have revealed specific risk factors that are associated with an increased likelihood of burnout. Based on an extensive literature search, Amoafo and colleagues [14] found that younger age, female sex, not being married, long working hours, and low reported job satisfaction to be consistently predictive of burnout syndrome. Likewise, a subsequent systematic review found the demographic factors of age, gender, marital status, specialty, and job position to be drivers of burnout, as well as the organizational factors of workload, interpersonal demands, job insecurity, and lack of resources [15].

In one cross-sectional study that specifically examined resident physicians in a developing country (Lebanon), residents were placed into two categories based on the MBI-HSS – "high" versus "not high" [16]. Risk factors for high scores on burnout included female gender, working more than 30 hours in one shift or 80 hours per workweek, or experiencing a major stressor in life. In a Hungarian study of trainees and general practitioners using the MBI-HSS, it was found that residents experienced a significantly higher level of burnout than general practitioners. Additionally, the study highlighted differences that exist between male and female respondents. Males were more likely to report higher levels of depersonalization than females and more likely to report a sense of low personal accomplishment. Females were more likely to report burnout associated with dependent care, with evidence showing a direct correlation with increased number of children and incidence of burnout. Additionally, the number of patients in a practice, which was used as a surrogate for workload, was associated with depersonalization in females. Overall, the study showed that females were more likely to report emotional exhaustion while males were more likely to report depersonalization and reduced personal accomplishment [17].

The data reporting on gender disparity for physician burnout is mixed, ranging from no difference [18] to more than double the rates for women physicians [19]. The variability in data likely relates to differences in specialties [20], measures used [6], cutoff scores [12], and whether burnout rates were adjusted for other mediating factors [21]. Overall, the burnout rates do appear to be significantly higher for women physicians compared to their male counterparts [22], potentially attributable to gender differences in roles and responsibilities, disparities in early career, work satisfaction, and levels of depression, past-traumatic events, implicit bias, and harassment. One study shows that women physicians experience double the rate of burnout (30% vs. 15%) and emotional exhaustion (22% vs. 9%) as men [19].

Roles and Responsibilities

Female medical students and physicians traditionally carry more responsibility related to family life in addition to their careers. They often are expected to continue to fulfill traditional female roles in marriage, childbearing and childrearing, and family caregiving while working to advance their careers [23]. The additional roles, responsibilities, and stressors added to the female physician place her at increased risk for continued development of maladaptive coping, like substance use. In a survey-based study of physician recipients of K08 or K23 awards through the National Institutes of Health, it was found that women were more likely than men to have a spouse or domestic partner (hereafter referred to as "partner") who was employed full-time outside of the home (85.6% vs. 44.9%) and even after adjusting for work hours, partner employment, and other factors including number and age of children, women worked 8.5 hours per week more than their men counterparts on domestic activities [24]. These studies underscore the importance of not only examining the well-being of female medical students and physicians across the life and career span, but in working to elucidate and understand the unique attributes, risk factors, and potential interventions most likely to be helpful at each stage.

Learner and Early Career Physicians

A comprehensive survey of medical students, residents, and early career physicians conducted in 2011–2012 via the American Medical Association Physician Masterfile (the first national study of its kind) revealed alarming data about the prevalence of burnout, depression, suicidal ideation, and fatigue. Burnout prevalence will be discussed here, and sections later in the chapter will be dedicated to the remaining topics. In this survey, 51.4% of early career physicians, 60.3% of residents, and 55.9% of medical students had scores on the MBI consistent with burnout. All groups studied were more likely to experience burnout than population control samples [2]. In this study, female respondents demonstrated statistically significant higher rates of high fatigue and positive screening for depression as compared to their male counterparts. However, the study did not demonstrate statistically significant gender differences for burnout or recent suicidal ideation [2]. Romani and Ashkar describe a concerning trend of burnout throughout the career span with 31–49.6% of medical students reporting burnout, 50–75% of residents, and 45.8% of practicing physicians [25], indicating that burnout remains a part of the medical profession regardless of training or practicing level.

Work Satisfaction

Physician burnout is not only a concern for the affected individual but also represents a concern for the healthcare system as a whole. With a large percentage of physicians reporting burnout, there is also a large percentage of physicians who feel dissatisfaction in their jobs. In a survey of 181 female neurologists in the United States completed in a closed Facebook group for this population, 42.6% reported experiencing burnout using the Mini-Z survey, a self-report questionnaire created by Mark Linzer, which rates burnout on a five-point Likert scale [26]. And 35.4% reported feeling neutral or dissatisfied toward their job. Here too, as in the previously mentioned Hungarian study, this study showed that for females with three or more children, less than one-third report that they would become a physician again. While most respondents were not considering a reduction of their clinical hours in the future, it is difficult to imagine that a healthcare system with nearly one-third of its female physicians feeling merely neutral or even dissatisfied with their jobs is functioning optimally. Undoubtedly, this is an area of concern and for future investigation for administrators, public health officials, regulatory bodies, the government, and others, to ensure a healthy and robust healthcare system is functioning in the United States. The authors conclude "burnout among women neurologist is important issue leading to personal dissatisfaction, suboptimal patient care, and threats to the future Neurology work force. There is an unmet need to address gender specific factors leading to burnout…" [27]. A similar survey-based study completed by Shanafelt et al. in June 2008 using surveys emailed to members of the American College of Surgeons with 61 broad-ranging questions and the participants blinded to study hypotheses was the most comprehensive and largest study of its kind—with nearly 8000 surgeons responding. Respondents were thought to be generalizable to the overall population of surgeons in the United States, with 13% of respondents being female, roughly correlated to the 8% of female surgeons in the country. Alarmingly, 40% of respondents met criteria for burnout—an amount that the authors felt was similar to colleagues in other specialties. Higher-risk correlates were found relating to younger age, compensation based exclusively on productivity, working more hours per week, and more nights per week on call. Of the respondents, 30% screened positive for depression. Fortunately, 70% of respondents reported that they would choose a career as a physician and surgeon again, although only 50% would recommend the career path to their children. The authors did not comment on gender-related issues in the article [28].

Epidemiology of Depression in Women Physicians

Relationship of Burnout and Depression

The relationship between burnout and clinically diagnosable major depressive disorder cannot be denied—with some speculating that burnout is a form of depression. In the aforementioned study by Dyrbye et al., it was found that 40% of early career physicians, 50.8% of resident physicians, and 58.2% of medical students screened positive for depression, rates very similar to the previously discussed rates of burnout reported in the same survey. As symptoms of depression—depressed mood, anhedonia, physical symptoms, guilt, hopelessness, appetite and sleep changes, and suicidal ideation—are related to the symptoms described on the common burnout scales—emotional exhaustion, depersonalization, and lack of personal accomplishment, it is easy to see how the two would be closely correlated. A study completed by Maslach et al. in 2001 found that patients with burnout symptoms demonstrated no statistical difference in depressive symptoms versus those with a diagnosed depressive disorder [29], demonstrating that burnout and depression are indeed related.

Considerable scientific inquiry has been spent on this topic as well, indicating the desire by researchers to understand the relationship between burnout and depression. In a meta-analysis of some 92 studies examining the overlap of burnout and depression, Bianchi opens the article by simply stating, "The overlap of burnout and depression has been debated since the birth of the burnout construct in the 1970s." [30]. One potential difference between burnout and depression is that burnout is job and situation specific whereas depression is thought to be more pervasive. In many of the early articles describing burnout, language similar to major depressive disorder was used, such as hopeless, helpless, and anhedonia. It is inevitable to see that burnout substantially overlaps with depressive symptoms and that a history of depressive symptoms predisposes one to an increased risk of developing of burnout and vice versa. The authors note that based on review of the 92 studies considered, "the evidence for the singularity of the burnout phenomenon is inconsistent." They rightfully point out that the difficulty in describing the relationship between burnout and clinical depression has created a major limitation in the current knowledge and to barrier to any future conclusions about the possibility of the burnout-depression overlap. While no specific recommendation is given regarding the inclusion of burnout in the Diagnostic and Statistical Manual for psychiatrists, the authors do speculate that perhaps the lack of scientific rigor in the development of the MBI, which is now used as the gold standard school in burnout research, may have confounded the problem of distinguishing burnout from depression. Additionally, they recommend that "systemic clinical observation" be used to determine if there is indeed a singularity in burnout and if another diagnostic category is needed [30]. At the least, pairing any screening for burnout with existing, evidence-based screening tools for depression, anxiety, and substance use disorders could reduce confounding psychiatric diagnoses and the present of burnout [31].

Rates of Physician Depression

The Consensus Statement on "Confronting Depression and Suicide in Physicians" published in 2003 by Center et al. stated "depression is as common in physicians as in the general population," citing evidence from Ford et al. that surveyed male graduates of a medical school and finding the prevalence to be 12.8%, which matches the 12% lifetime prevalence in the general population found by Blazer et al. For females, they cited the Women Physicians' Health Study and found the lifetime prevalence of depression to be 19.5%, which again matched the lifetime prevalence in the nationally representative study published by Blazer et al. [32].

Contrary to the idea that the prevalence of depression is the same for physicians as the general population is information obtained from a survey study completed by Guille et al. in 2010. This study found that depression may be more prevalent in physicians in training versus the general young adult population or graduate students, based on the use of a screening, but nondiagnostic, tool [5]. This survey was sent to 1394 interns across 19 hospitals and completed by 740 (58%). In these responses, 42.5% screened positive for depression using the Patient Health Questionnaire (PHQ-9), with a cutoff score of ≥10. These numbers are similar to those found in a meta-analysis completed by Mata et al. based on 31 cross-sectional studies and 23 longitudinal studies from 1963 to 2015 examining prevalence estimates of depression or depressive symptoms in 17,560 resident physicians. The meta-analysis revealed a summary estimate of prevalence at 28.8%, with a range from 20.9% to 43.3%, the authors noting that most of these studies used self-reported questionnaires with varying sensitivity and specificity estimates [33]. When examined over time, the 54 studies revealed an average increase of 0.5% per calendar year in the studied years of 1963–2015 in the prevalence of depression or depressive symptoms. Perhaps this indicates a true increase or perhaps it is indicating increased awareness of the problem, but regardless demonstrates the swift attention that needs to be given to this growing concern [33].

Epidemiology of Suicide in Women Physicians

Physician Death via Suicide

In an article regarding physician suicide published by Iannelli and colleagues in 2014 in the journal *General Hospital Psychiatry*, the authors open their article by quoting Rupinder Legha, who published "A History of Physician Suicide in America": "The problem of physician suicide is not solely a matter of whether it takes place at a rate higher than the general public. That a professional caregiver can fall ill and not receive adequate care and support, despite being surrounded by other caregivers, begs for a thoughtful assessment to determine why it happens at all." At 300 reported deaths per year, approximately one physician per day dies via completed suicide [32].

It is with this lens that we will remember our physician colleagues who have died via suicide and take steps to prevent future deaths. This significant loss serves as the basis for seeking to improve our understanding of the epidemiology of burnout and its consequences in physicians, as described in this section of the chapter.

The increased risk for death via suicide in physician populations has been known and studied for some time, and it is well established that "the rate of suicide is higher among physicians than the general population" [34]. Here we will examine studies regarding the epidemiology of physician death via suicide beginning from a historical perspective then focusing specifically on women physicians.

Suicide Rates Among Physicians

Using data from the National Violent Death Reporting System from 2003 to 2008, Gold and colleagues examined 31,636 deaths via suicide, 203 of whom were identified as physicians. Physicians and residents were included, but medical students and physician assistants were excluded. Because of the information available in the database, the officers were able to study a number of characteristics of the sample population. Results of this study revealed that physicians who died via suicide were more likely to be older and more likely to be married than those in other occupations, but there was no significant difference in a current diagnosed mental health disorder or current depressed mood. It showed that physicians were significantly less likely to have a substance use disorder, including alcohol use disorder. It was found that physicians were more likely to use lethal means such as antipsychotics, benzodiazepines, or barbiturates in overdose than nonphysicians. Most strikingly, physicians were much less likely to have had a recent crisis or trigger leading to suicide, but rather much more likely to have occupational concerns contributing to the suicide, indicating that research regarding burnout and burnout prevention is of utmost importance for the health of the profession as a whole. Alarmingly, based on therapeutic drug levels filed in blood samples, it was found that although physicians had a greater likelihood of having a known mental illness, there was not a greater likelihood of having antidepressant pharmacotherapy in the blood samples, indicating that physicians receive lower rates of care than the general population, despite their seemingly greater access to medical settings. The authors conclude "the results of this study paint a picture of the typical physician suicide victim that is substantially different from that of the nonphysician suicide victim in several important ways." Sadly, the authors also note in the study that it is speculated that the rate of physician suicide is actually higher than reported due to possible deliberate miscoding of cause of death on physician death certificates.

Lindeman et al. published a systematic review of 14 studies of physician suicide worldwide from 1963 to 1991 and found that there exists a statistically significant increase in relative risk for death via suicide in physicians versus the general population—with males ranging from 1.1 to 3.4 and females, alarmingly, ranging from 2.5 to 5.7 [35].

In 2000, Hawton and colleagues examined the risk of suicide in National Health Service physicians between 1979 and 1995. They found that the suicide rate among the study population was

19 per 100,000 person years of risk. Compared to females in the general population, there was an increased risk for death via suicide for female physicians, but a significantly decreased risk for male physicians compared to males in the general population [36]. There was no significant difference in suicide risk based on age for either females or males. They did find a difference in suicide risk based on specialty—with community health, anesthesia, psychiatry, and general practice having an increased risk versus the other specialties. They concluded their study by stating "the excess risk of suicide in female doctors in the NHS workforce is an important pattern….especially so in light of increasing numbers of women coming into medicine. Further work is required…" [36].

Suicide Rates Among Medical Trainees

Physician death via suicide also impacts trainees, who are at a challenging time in their personal and professional growth. A recent study examined the overall cause of death in resident physicians in the United States between 2000 and 2014 and found similarly concerning data. In this study, Yaghmour et al. used information obtained from the National Death Index to determine the cause of death for deceased residents. From 2000 to 2014, 324 residents were reported as having died out of the sample size of 381,614 residents. The second leading cause of death among residents was suicide at 66 deaths, with neoplastic diseases being the leading cause at 80 deaths [37]. They were able to carry the study further to specifically identify that the periods of greatest risk for resident death via suicide were early in training: the first quarter of the academic year and after the winter holiday season. The findings from this study provide training programs and accrediting bodies with information that could be used to produce targeted interventions for when residents are most vulnerable. This study unfortunately demonstrates the continued concern for death via suicide in physician populations. Two positive notes from this study are that "resident death occurs significantly less frequently than in the age- and gender-matched general population" and that suicide in medical trainees is a preventable cause of death, and the risk can be mitigated with a concerted focus of efforts to support the residents.

A study examining medical students and young doctors in their first postgraduate year of training in Norway revealed a prevalence of suicidal ideation of 14% during both the last year of medical school and the first postgraduate year of training, an overall lifetime prevalence of suicidal ideation at 43%, exceedingly high when compared to an estimated rate of 4.8% for the general US population. Of those 43% with suicidal ideation, 8% advance to planning a suicide attempt, and 1.4% advance to making an attempt. Overall, the author notes that while suicidal ideation was rather high, actual attempt of suicide remained low. The authors note that there were differences in the predictors of suicidal ideation between medical students and first-year trainee. Lack of control and personality traits were important factors during medical school, and job stress and working hours were independent predictors during the first year of postgraduate training. The authors identified interruptions during work and time pressure as the most significant factors of job stress related to suicidal ideation, providing some evidence for the basis of interventions to help young doctors with burnout and suicidal ideation. The authors did not find a significant difference in risk for suicidal ideation, planning, or attempts based on gender [38].

In a study examining physicians who might be at higher risk for death via suicide, clinicians who were referred to the Vanderbilt Comprehensive Assessment Program for a fitness for duty assessment (due to a variety of behavioral health concerns) from 2001 to 2009 were sampled. The authors were able to describe a number of correlations to attempted or completed suicide. This study was based on a convenience sample of 141 physicians for whom follow-up data was available. Of these physicians, seven were known to have attempted suicide and five were known to have died by suicide. Two of these deaths via suicide occurred in the first month after the assessment of fitness for duty. The authors note that these deaths represent an "alarmingly high" suicide death rate among physicians who are undergoing fitness for duty assessment; at 3.5%, the rate is 175 times higher than the general population of 0.02%. In terms of past psychiatric history, 57% of the physicians with attempted or completed suicide reported a history of past mental health issues, while only 16% of the physicians without attempted or completed suicide reported the same. In terms of practice variables, 71% of the physicians with attempted or completed suicide were in solo practice versus 31% of the physicians without attempted or completed suicide. As part of the fitness for duty assessment, personality assessments were given, including the Minnesota Multiphasic Personality Inventory and the Beck Depression Inventory, with no clinically or statistically significant differences between the two groups. Four of the five physicians who died via suicide had a substance use disorder, with four of these physicians having a benzodiazepine use disorder, three having alcohol use disorder, and two with a diagnosis of opioid use disorder. It was noted that three of the five physicians who died by suicide were under investigation by authorities or medical boards for improper prescribing of controlled substances. Two had a diagnosis of bipolar disorder and one had a diagnosis of major depressive disorder. Six of the seven physicians who attempted suicide were diagnosed with either traits of a personality disorder or met criteria for a personality disorder via personality assessment. Interestingly, the authors note that "every physician with subsequent suicidal behavior received recommendations for formal treatment following evaluation…compared to 66% in the remainder" [39]. Coupled with the alarmingly high rate of completed suicide in the physicians referred for fitness for duty evaluation, the fact that all physicians who went on to attempt or complete suicide were referred for formal treatment indicates that such an assessment should raise serious concerns about the health and safety of the physician undergoing the assessment. The authors state "we need better strategies to identify pre suicidal physicians and improved attention and treatment and rehabilitation."

Suicide Rates Among Women Physicians

It has been challenging to define risk for female physicians and suicide based on limited number of female physicians in suicide studies. The risk for death via suicide does appear to vary significantly for male versus female physicians and is different for physicians based on gender than in the general population based on gender. In the general population, males have an estimated fourfold greater suicide rate compared to females. However, a meta-analysis by Schernhammer and Colditz [40] identified a much higher risk of suicide among female physicians than among the general population. The suicide rate ratio was 2.27 (95% CI = 1.90–2.73). This compared to an overall suicide rate ratio of 1.41 (95% CI = 1.21–1.65) for male physicians, consistent with a modestly higher risk of suicide in male physicians than in the general population. The findings were based on 24 rate ratios for male physicians and 13 suicide rate ratios for female physicians. Interestingly, female physicians have a lower rate of attempted suicide, but a higher rate of completed suicide versus females in the general population [32].

Epidemiology of Substance Use Disorders in Women Physicians

Relationship of Burnout, to Substance Use and Suicide

Substance use disorders (SUD) appear to be a risk factor for the development of burnout, depression, suicidal ideation, and completion in physicians. Notably, the relationship between SUD and burnout appears to be bidirectional. A longitudinal cohort study completed with medical students in 1992 revealed that while social-relational deficits or narcissistic personality styles were predictors of risky alcohol use, so too were social support deficits and patient care-related stressors. In essence, it appears that although substance use disorders can increase one's risk of burnout, burnout in turn can increase one's risk of substance use disorders [23]. SUDs are a common complicating factor to the development of not only burnout, but of psychiatric disorders and suicide in both the general population and in physicians. To date, there is an abundance of research of SUD in the general population and a smaller amount related to gender-specific studies and to physicians with SUD. Unfortunately, there is little published about female physicians with SUD. Examining the similarities and differences that female physicians have with the general female population and their male physician counterparts may help to explain some of the data that is available to date. With this in mind, we will first examine the epidemiology of SUD in women, then in physicians, and, finally, in women physicians. Because of the dearth of research available specifically regarding the female physician with SUD, much of what is discussed here will be qualitative or generally descriptive of this subpopulation.

SUD in women have been increasing across all classes of intoxicants since the 1960s, and a decreased age at the onset of use has also been observed [41, 42]. This increased use has served to shrink the gender gap traditionally seen in SUD. In the 1980s there was a 5:1 male-to-female ratio, which in the new millennium has tightened to 3:1, with an estimated lifetime prevalence of SUD in North American women of 5–8% [42, 43]. A well-described phenomenon called "telescoping" highlights the gender-specific relationship that women have with SUD: women have repeatedly shown an accelerated progression from the initiation of use to the onset of dependence compared with men [41–44]. Telescoping can be clearly identified in multiple classes of substances and may contribute to a more severe pathological presentation (compared with men) when a woman initially seeks treatment. Women appear to be more likely to use substances of abuse to self-medicate physical or psychiatric ailments than men who more commonly use substances recreationally for pleasure. Additionally, relapses are more likely to be related to stress or negative emotions [41, 42]. In general, women are less likely to enter treatment. However, once engaged in treatment, gender is not a predictor of treatment retention, completion, or success [42].

There are measurable biological differences in men and women with SUD. As noted above, women have a higher propensity to return to use in the context of negative affect. This may be related to dysregulation of the hypothalamus-pituitary axis (HPA) resulting in greater emotional intensity at lower levels of HPA arousal [42]. Women are more likely to incur alcohol-related liver impairments more quickly and with less consumption than men. They are also more likely to develop cirrhosis [43, 44]. There are also documented gender-specific differences in response to medication-assisted treatment for opioid use disorder with women showing a greater response to buprenorphine as opposed to methadone when compared to men. This was demonstrated by significantly fewer positive urine drug screens and fewer occurrences of self-reported return to use [42].

Women with SUD are also significantly more likely than men to have psychiatric comorbidity and a substantially higher risk for suicide [9, 42]. Interestingly though, the prognosis for women with comorbid SUD and psychiatric illness is better than for women with SUD alone. Perhaps this is due to the fact that more women do use substances to self-medicate other problems, and when the primary pathology (an affective or anxiety disorder) is appropriately treated, the SUD is more likely to remit. Post-traumatic stress disorder (PTSD) is more common in all patients with SUD, but in women seeking treatment, reported rates of physical or sexual abuse have been shockingly high, ranging from 55% to 99% [42]. Not only are women more likely to have a trauma history, but they are more likely to have relapses related to trauma symptoms [41].

In 1992, Hughes and colleagues conducted a mailed, anonymous, self-report survey of 9600 physicians of various specialties and career stages. This resulting study, Prevalence of Substance Use Among US Physicians (PSUS), is the first to examine the prevalence of substance use in this population. The questionnaire examined the self-reported use of 13 illicit substances including, but not limited to, alcohol, benzodiazepines, opioids, marijuana, cocaine, and heroin, assessing the use of respondents over a lifetime, in the past year, and past month. It also asked if respondents either had been given or felt they had diagnoses of substance use or dependence and if treatment was received.

PSUS provided a wealth of data about a distinctive pattern of substance use in physicians. As compared to the general population, physicians are more likely to identify alcohol as their drug of choice and much less likely to use illicit street drugs. Misuse of prescription medications was more likely to be identified as "self-treatment" as opposed to recreational. Since the publication of

PSUS in 1992, this has been an area of increased interest and study, particularly in light of the strong association of SUD with burnout, depression, and suicidal ideation.

Several studies in the late 2000s described similar rates of substance use in physicians as in the general population [45–47]. However, a more recent study suggests that physician substance use has increased beyond that of the general population with a respective prevalence of 15.4 and 12.6 [48]. Some specialities appear to be at greater risk for development of SUD with anesthesia, emergency medicine, and psychiatry topping the list [45]. There is some good news, though. Physicians who enter treatment experience rates of success that are significantly higher than that of the general population with some studies quoting as high as 96% success rate [45–47]. Physicians have unparalleled access to intensive treatment and aftercare programs. This may contribute to the significantly lower relapse rate seen in physicians with SUD (19%): a third as much as the general population [49].

Rates of Substance Use Disorders

Female physicians with SUD have some traits in common with females in the general population and other traits in common with their male physician colleagues. However, they represent a unique entity with many features related to their use—defying what is seen in the broader groups to which they belong.

As with all physicians, it is difficult to identify who may develop SUD even with some known risk factors. However, there does appear to be some risk factors that are gender-specific, like having a prior psychiatric illness or a childhood history of trauma. Of course, risk factors that are known to affect the general population, such as a family history of SUD, also continue to have a bearing on this subpopulation. Like women in the general population, female physicians with SUD are more likely than males to identify sedative/hypnotic medications as their drug of choice [50]. Unlike females in the general population, alcohol use disorder is more commonly observed in females physicians than in male physicians [49]. Female physicians come to clinical attention more often with a complaint related to physical illness or emotional disturbance as opposed to seeking treatment for a primary SUD; they also remain less likely than their male counterparts to enter treatment. As with the general population, though, there are no gender differences between physicians in treatment completion following enrollment. However, female physicians have been shown to have a quicker time to relapse than males.

The area of SUD in female physicians is in desperate need of continued study. It is unclear if female physicians are best treated in a setting geared toward healthcare professionals (which have largely been designed around the needs of men) or in a women's only treatment center (which may not identify and address some of the psychosocial issues related to their profession). However, it is known that female physicians are at a higher risk than either of the broader populations to which they belong for suicidal behaviors. Female physicians are twice as likely as male physicians to endorse past or current suicidal ideation, nine times as likely to endorse a past suicide attempt, and more than four times as likely to report having made an attempt while intoxicated [50]. Female physicians with SUD should be regarded as a high-risk population and should be carefully assessed for any psychiatric comorbidity and suicidality.

Barriers to Care

Efforts have been underway for many years to minimize physician suicide. In 2002, the American Foundation for Suicide Prevention planning group met in Philadelphia, Pennsylvania, to examine physician depression, suicide, and barriers to treatment. Their work was published by Center et al. in "Confronting Depression and Suicide in Physicians: A Consensus Statement," by the American Medical Association in 2003. Unfortunately, they reported that there exists little to no data regarding physician use of mental health services. They did note that for medical students with depression, only 22% sought and utilized services and for medical students with suicidal ideation, only 42% received treatment [32].

In the aforementioned study completed by Guille et al. of intern physicians who screened positive for depression using the PHQ-9, only 22.7% reported receiving some type of treatment, either pharmacotherapy or psychotherapy, during their intern year [5]. In this survey, barriers to care identified included lack of time, preference to manage the problem on their own, lack of convenient access, and confidentiality concerns. The authors reported that compared to interns who did receive mental health treatment, those who did not were significantly less likely to believe that mental health treatment would work [5].

In a study examining the perceptions of medical students reasons for not seeking care often mirrored barriers for the general population: lack of time (48%), lack of confidentiality (37%), stigma (30%), and cost (28%). Notably, medical students identified an additional barrier of fear of documentation in the medical record (24%) [51].

In one positive example of physician-specific care, DuPont and others examined the role of state physician health programs (PHPs) for the treatment of physicians with substance use disorders. They noted that while PHPs do not directly provide substance abuse treatment, they do provide a number of services that is quite different than what is available to the general public. These services include early detection, assessment, evaluation, and referral to residential treatment for 60–90 days. Following treatment, there is close follow-up with random urine monitoring and status reports for employers and licensing boards for approximately 5 years. They note that this is "an intensity, duration, and quality of care that is rarely available in most standard addiction treatments." The outcomes from these intensive services are quite positive with less than 25% of physicians providing a positive urine drug screen during the 5-year monitoring period and 71% of physicians still practicing medicine at 5 years. The authors note that even individuals who participate in court-mandated treatments do not experience the intensity or duration of support nor the positive outcomes that are achieved through the PHP. The authors further note that less than one-third of physicians were formally mandated to participate in the PHP by their state licensing board, while the remainder of physicians participated voluntarily, likely due to safe harbor provided by the PHP from legal, employment, and licensure consequences of substance use disorder. This exemplifies the benefits to physicians (and their patients) of minimizing barriers to care [52].

Barriers to care related to medical licensure are complex, vary by state and situation, and are ever-evolving. While some state licensing boards are removing questions about diagnosis and treatment, and instead choosing to focus on current impairment that affects one's ability to care for patients [53], the majority are not. A national study of almost all (94.1%) medical licensure board applications conducted in 2016 revealed that only one-third of states were asking questions on the initial and renewal applications that were consistent with American Medical Association (AMA), American Psychiatric Association (APA), and Federation of State Medical Boards policies and recommendations [54]. Some states inquire about impairment in the past few years, while others ask about any historical impairment. Furthermore, states vary widely in their use of that information [2]. Several lawsuits have cited the Americans with Disabilities Act (ADA) to claim that use of this information by medical boards is discriminatory, while other lawsuits have held that the ADA does not apply to state licensing boards [32]. In addition to licensing boards, physicians often need to disclose information about their health history to hospitals, credentialing bodies, and malpractice carriers [32].

In the Policy on Physician Impairment, the Federation of State Medical Boards (FSMB) has stated "the diagnosis of an illness does not equate with impairment" and has proposed that physicians have voluntary options for physician health programs and protected confidentiality. They note that encouraging physicians to seek treatment early in the illness would be a more favorable path than waiting until impairment (and potential harm to patients) has occurred [53]. The FSMB quotes the Federation of State Physician Health Programs in their policy, writing "physician illness and impairment exist on a continuum with illness typically predating impairment, often by many years. This is a critically important distinction. Illness is the existence of a disease. Impairment is a functional classification and implies the inability of the person affected by disease to perform specific activities"

[55]. Minimizing barriers to care, including the real or perceived threat of harm to one's medical license and career, would encourage more physicians to seek treatment, thus minimizing the potential that these physicians would eventually become impaired.

To minimize barriers to care, some might suggest that we also address prevention of depression in physicians. In 2010, Beekman et al. published a literature review of existing information about prevention strategies for depression. They noted that there are accepted prevention methods for other illnesses, such as metabolic diseases or cardiovascular disease, and we should impart the same preventive care to those at risk for developing mental illnesses. They included examples such as a brief psychological intervention for people recently diagnosed with cancer, the routine prescription of escitalopram or problem-solving therapy to those with recent stroke, the use of problem-solving therapy in those with macular degeneration, and the use of a nurse-led intervention in those with diabetes or rheumatic disease. In each of these studies except for the psychological intervention for people diagnosed with cancer, the interventions showed reduction in the incidence of depression in the study populations versus control [56]. In a meta-analysis completed by Cuijpers et al. in 2008, it was found that psychological interventions such as cognitive behavioral therapy have been shown to reduce the incidence of depression by 22%, with a number needed to treat of only 22. The authors state succinctly, "prevention may become an important way, in addition to treatment, to reduce the enormous public health burden of depression in the coming years" [57]. One can easily see how a targeted psychological intervention could be applied to medical students, resident physicians, and career physicians, yielding a meaningful impact on the reduction of depression.

References

1. Maslach C, Jackson SE. The measurement of experienced burnout. J Organ Behav. 1981;2(2):99–113.
2. Dyrbye LN, West CP, Satele D, Boone S, Tan L, Sloan J, et al. Burnout among U.S. medical students, residents, and early career physicians relative to the general U.S. population. Acad Med. 2014 Mar;89(3):443–51.

3. Halbesleben JR, Rathert C. Linking physician burnout and patient outcomes: exploring the dyadic relationship between physicians and patients. Health Care Manag Rev. 2008 Jan-Mar;33(1):29–39.

4. Montgomery A. The inevitability of physician burnout: implications for interventions. Burn Res. 2014;1(1):50–6.

5. Guille C, Speller H, Laff R, Epperson CN, Sen S. Utilization and barriers to mental health services among depressed medical interns: a prospective multisite study. J Grad Med Educ. 2010 Jun;2(2):210–4.

6. Rotenstein LS, Torre M, Ramos MA, Rosales RC, Guille C, Sen S, et al. Prevalence of burnout among physicians: a systematic review. JAMA. 2018 Sep 18;320(11):1131–50.

7. Astudillo W, Mendinueta C. Exhaustion syndrome in palliative care. Support Care Cancer. 1996 Nov;4(6):408–15.

8. Figley CR, editor. Treating compassion fatigue. New York: Brunner/Mazel. O B. Hudnall Stamm, Traumatic Stress Research Group, 1995–1999; 1995.

9. Kristensen TS, Borritz M, Villadsen E, Christensen KB. The Copenhagen burnout inventory: a new tool for the assessment of burnout. Work Stress. 2005;19(3):192–207.

10. Burisch M. The Hamburg Burnout Inventory (HBI): Background and Some Early Results. [type of work]. In press 2017.

11. Malach-Pines A. The burnout measure short version (BMS). Int J Stress Manag. 2005;30(1):78–88.

12. Brondt A, Sokolowski I, Olesen F, Vedsted P. Continuing medical education and burnout among Danish GPs. Br J Gen Pract. 2008;58 (546):15–9.

13. Shanafelt TD, Sinsky C, Dyrbye LN, Trockel M, West CP. Burnout among physicians compared with individuals with a professional or doctoral degree in a field outside of medicine. Mayo Clin Proc. 2019;94(3):549–51.

14. Amoafo E, Hanbali N, Patel A, Singh P. What are the significant factors associated with burnout in doctors? Occup Med (Lond). 2015;65(2): 117–21.

15. Azam K, Khan A, Alam MT. Causes and adverse impact of physician burnout: a systematic review. J Coll Physicians Surg Pak. 2017;27(8): 495–501.

16. Ashkar K, Romani M, Musharrafieh U, Chaaya M. Prevalence of burnout syndrome among medical residents: experience of a developing country. Postgrad Med J. 2010;86(1015):266–71.

17. Adam S, Mohos A, Kalabay L, Torzsa P. Potential correlates of burnout among general practitioners and residents in Hungary: the significant role of gender, age, dependant care and experience. BMC Fam Pract. 2018;19(1):193.

18. Fields AI, Cuerdon TT, Brasseux CO, Getson PR, Thompson AE, Orlowski JP, et al. Physician burnout in pediatric critical care medicine. Crit Care Med. 1995;23(8):1425–9.

19. Spataro BM, Tilstra SA, Rubio DM, McNeil MA. The toxicity of self-blame: sex differences in burnout and coping in internal medicine trainees. J Womens Health (Larchmt). 2016;25(11):1147–52.
20. Shanafelt TD, West CP, Sinsky C, Trockel M, Tutty M, Satele DV, et al. Changes in burnout and satisfaction with work-life integration in physicians and the general US working population between 2011 and 2017. Mayo Clin Proc. 2019;94(9):1662–4.
21. Gomez-Baya D, Lucia-Casademunt AM, Salinas-Perez JA. Gender differences in psychological well-being and health problems among European health professionals: analysis of psychological basic needs and job satisfaction. Int J Environ Res Public Health. 2018;15(7).
22. Templeton K, Bernstein CA, Sukhere J, Nora LM, Newman C, Burstin H, et al. Gender-based differences in burnout: issues faced by women physicians (NAM Perspecrives Discussion Paper). Washington, D.C.: National Academy of Medicine; 2019; Available from: https://nam.edu/gender-based-differences-in-burnout-issues-faced-by-women-physicians/.
23. Richman JA. Occupational stress, psychological vulnerability and alcohol-related problems over time in future physicians. Alcohol Clin Exp Res. 1992;16(2):166–71.
24. Jolly S, Griffith KA, DeCastro R, Stewart A, Ubel P, Jagsi R. Gender differences in time spent on parenting and domestic responsibilities by high-achieving young physician-researchers. Ann Intern Med. 2014;160(5):344–53.
25. Romani M, Ashkar K. Burnout among physicians. Libyan J Med. 2014;9(1):23556.
26. Shimotsu ST, Poplau S, Linzer M. Validation of a brief clinician survey to reduce clinician burnout. J Gen Intern Med. 2015;30:S79–80.
27. Moore LR, Ziegler C, Hessler A, Singhal D, LaFaver K. Burnout and career satisfaction in women neurologists in the United States. J Womens Health (Larchmt). 2019;28(4):515–25.
28. Shanafelt TD, Balch CM, Bechamps GJ, Russell T, Dyrbye L, Satele D, et al. Burnout and career satisfaction among American surgeons. Ann Surg. 2009;250(3):463–71.
29. Maslach C, Schaufeli WB, Leiter MP. Job burnout. Annu Rev Psychol. 2001;52:397–422.
30. Bianchi R, Schonfeld IS, Laurent E. Burnout-depression overlap: a review. Clin Psychol Rev. 2015;36:28–41.
31. Oquendo MA, Bernstein CA, Mayer LES. A key differential diagnosis for physicians-major depression or burnout? JAMA Psychiatry. 2019.
32. Center C, Davis M, Detre T, Ford DE, Hansbrough W, Hendin H, et al. Confronting depression and suicide in physicians: a consensus statement. JAMA. 2003;289(23):3161–6.
33. Mata DA, Ramos MA, Bansal N, Khan R, Guille C, Di Angelantonio E, et al. Prevalence of depression and depressive symptoms among resident physicians: a systematic review and meta-analysis. JAMA. 2015;314(22):2373–83.

34. Gold KJ, Sen A, Schwenk TL. Details on suicide among US physicians: data from the National Violent Death Reporting System. Gen Hosp Psychiatry. 2013;35(1):45–9.
35. Lindeman S, Laara E, Hakko H, Lonnqvist J. A systematic review on gender-specific suicide mortality in medical doctors. Br J Psychiatry. 1996;168(3):274–9.
36. Hawton K, Clements A, Sakarovitch C, Simkin S, Deeks JJ. Suicide in doctors: a study of risk according to gender, seniority and specialty in medical practitioners in England and Wales, 1979-1995. J Epidemiol Community Health. 2001;55(5):296–300.
37. Yaghmour NA, Brigham TP, Richter T, Miller RS, Philibert I, Baldwin DC Jr, et al. Causes of death of residents in ACGME-accredited programs 2000 through 2014: implications for the learning environment. Acad Med. 2017;92(7):976–83.
38. Tyssen R, Vaglum P, Gronvold NT, Ekeberg O. Suicidal ideation among medical students and young physicians: a nationwide and prospective study of prevalence and predictors. J Affect Disord. 2001;64(1): 69–79.
39. Iannelli RJ, Finlayson AJ, Brown KP, Neufeld R, Gray R, Dietrich MS, et al. Suicidal behavior among physicians referred for fitness-for-duty evaluation. Gen Hosp Psychiatry. 2014;36(6):732–6.
40. Schernhammer ES, Colditz GA. Suicide rates among physicians: a quantitative and gender assessment (meta-analysis). Am J Psychiatry. 2004;161(12):2295–302.
41. Becker JB, McClellan M, Reed BG. Sociocultural context for sex differences in addiction. Addict Biol. 2016;21(5):1052–9.
42. Greenfield SF, Back SE, Lawson K, Brady KT. Substance abuse in women. Psychiatr Clin North Am. 2010;33(2):339–55.
43. Zilberman ML, Tavares H, Blume SB, el-Guebaly N. Substance use disorders: sex differences and psychiatric comorbidities. Can J Psychiatr. 2003;48(1):5–13.
44. Lal R, Deb KS, Kedia S. Substance use in women: current status and future directions. Indian J Psychiatry. 2015;57(Suppl 2):S275–85.
45. Berge KH, Seppala MD, Schipper AM. Chemical dependency and the physician. Mayo Clin Proc. 2009;84(7):625–31.
46. Knight JR, Sanchez LT, Sherritt L, Bresnahan LR, Fromson JA. Outcomes of a monitoring program for physicians with mental and behavioral health problems. J Psychiatr Pract. 2007;13(1):25–32.
47. McLellan AT, Skipper GS, Campbell M, DuPont RL. Five year outcomes in a cohort study of physicians treated for substance use disorders in the United States. BMJ. 2008;337:a2038.
48. Bryson EO. The opioid epidemic and the current prevalence of substance use disorder in anesthesiologists. Curr Opin Anaesthesiol. 2018; 31(3):388–92.

49. Oreskovich MR, Shanafelt T, Dyrbye LN, Tan L, Sotile W, Satele D, et al. The prevalence of substance use disorders in American physicians. Am J Addict. 2015;24(1):30–8.
50. Wunsch MJ, Knisely JS, Cropsey KL, Campbell ED, Schnoll SH. Women physicians and addiction. J Addict Dis. 2007;26(2):35–43.
51. Plaut SM, Maxwell SA, Seng L, O'Brien JJ, Fairclough GF Jr. Mental health services for medical students: perceptions of students, student affairs deans, and mental health providers. Acad Med. 1993;68(5):360–5.
52. DuPont RL, McLellan AT, Carr G, Gendel M, Skipper GE. How are addicted physicians treated? A national survey of Physician Health Programs. J Subst Abus Treat. 2009;37(1):1–7.
53. Federation of State Medical Boards. Policy on Physician Impairment. Chicago, IL: Federation of State Physician Health Programs; 2011 [cited 2019]; Available from: https://www.fsmb.org/siteassets/advocacy/policies/physician-impairment.pdf.
54. Dyrbye LN, West CP, Sinsky CA, Goeders LE, Satele DV, Shanafelt TD. Medical licensure questions and physician reluctance to seek care for mental health conditions. Mayo Clin Proc. 2017;92(10):1486–93.
55. Federation of State Medical Boards. Physician Health Program Guidelines. Chicago, IL: Federation of State Physician Health Programs, Inc.; 2005 [cited 2019]; Available from: https://www.fsphp.org/2005-fsphp-physician-health-program-guidelines.
56. Beekman AT, Smit F, Stek ML, Reynolds CF 3rd, Cuijpers PC. Preventing depression in high-risk groups. Curr Opin Psychiatry. 2010;23(1):8–11.
57. Cuijpers P, van Straten A, Smit F, Mihalopoulos C, Beekman A. Preventing the onset of depressive disorders: a meta-analytic review of psychological interventions. Am J Psychiatry. 2008;165(10):1272–80.

Domestic Responsibilities and Career Advancement

4

Neha P. Raukar and Hannah M. Mishkin

An Exploration of the Influence of Gender and Domestic Responsibilities on the Trajectory of One's Career

The family unit has historically been based on the male breadwinner model. In this model, the male partner is responsible for the financial well-being of the family by performing *paid* work outside the home. To complement this, the female partner is responsible for the domestic responsibilities performing *unpaid* domestic work in the home [1–3]. This model was based, in part, on the fact

N. P. Raukar (✉)
Department of Emergency Medicine, Mayo Clinic, Rochester, MN, USA
e-mail: Raukar.Neha@mayo.edu

H. M. Mishkin
Department of Emergency Medicine, Reading Hospital-Tower Health, West Reading, PA, USA
e-mail: hannah.mishkin@towerhealth.org

© Springer Nature Switzerland AG 2020
C. M. Stonnington, J. A. Files (eds.), *Burnout in Women Physicians*,
https://doi.org/10.1007/978-3-030-44459-4_4

that historically, men often had greater opportunities for educational advancement and therefore greater opportunities to earn higher incomes. As our society has evolved, more educational and career opportunities have become available to women, including careers that require a significant educational commitment as well as a considerable time commitment. Medicine has been no exception. There has been a substantial increase in the number of women entering the field of medicine with women now making up approximately half of medical school classes in the United States [4, 5].

In addition to the increase in career responsibilities, women continue to take on the majority of traditional domestic responsibilities [6]. The expected equilibration between professional and domestic responsibility has not occurred, leaving women disproportionately responsible for a large amount of unpaid work in the home [3]. The unpaid work includes both household domestic tasks as well as parenting and the management of extended family obligations. "Domestic tasks" include activities such as cooking, cleaning, laundry, home maintenance, yard work, shopping for necessities, errands, and finances. "Parenting" includes meeting physical needs (such as feeding or bathing), as well as meeting psychosocial needs (such as talking or playing with children, driving them to activities, and attending their recitals or sporting events) [3]. Extended family responsibilities that require management include care of elderly family members, organizing family events, and remembering family birthdays as well as holiday coordination.

As more women choose medicine as a career, they are faced with unforeseeable hurdles, likely multifactorial, as they try to advance in academic medicine. A lack of female senior leaders to serve as role models, limited sponsorship from either sex, active gender discrimination, social and family issues, as well as a lack of same-sex mentorship may be contributing factors [1, 7]. The burden of domestic responsibilities is hypothesized to also affect a woman's ability to achieve in academic medicine. All of these factors may play a role in women's choice of medical specialty, creating an uneven distribution within certain specialities [5, 8].

When investigating the reasons for an uneven distribution in the specialties, three dominant themes were identified: lifestyle and career choices, family planning and career trajectory, and the goal of seeking balance. It was found that the timing of maternity leave was a very big challenge as women struggle to plan families and balance a career trajectory [4]. This is due to the inopportune overlaping timing of starting a career in medicine and being biologically suited to have children.

The research shows that women do not have the same success in academic medicine as men, especially early in their careers [3]. Using obtaining a K grant as a marker of academic success [3], married men were more likely to be awarded a grant, and of those, men who had a partner were four times more likely to have a partner who was not working full time (part time or not at all), while the women were more likely to have a full-time working partner. Of the single awardees, women obtained more K awards than their male counterparts. Among those partnered K awardees with children, men spent 12 hours *less* on parenting or domestic tasks per week than women, and in the subgroup where both partners worked full time outside the home, men still spent 9 hours less on parenting or domestic tasks. Interestingly, those awardees who were married or in a domestic partnership without children had more similar patterns of time allocation both at work and at home, suggesting that the differences relate specifically to gender differences in the performance of child care rather than other household tasks [3].

Another marker of academic success is tenured track status. Since the mid-1980s the number of traditional tenured track positions has decreased with the introduction of the clinical track. For medical schools that have a traditional tenured track, 80% had a higher proportion of men than women. The opposite holds true for institutions with a clinical tenured track where women make up the greater proportion of faculty (77%) [9]. When adjusting for years in practice for attending physicians, women were more likely to be on a clinical track rather than a tenured track, despite having the same adjusted number of publications [1].

The pattern of disproportionate domestic responsibility is found in both attending and trainee female physicians [1]. A survey of surgical trainees and faculty found that female surgeons were more likely to be married to a professional who works full time [1, 10] with 31% of male surgeons' domestic partners compared to 100% of female surgeons' domestic partners work-ing full time [1]. For those clinicians with children, women were five times more likely to have to rely on a nanny for child care. When caring for a child who was sick or had to be out of school, women relied on their spouse 25% of the time whereas men relied on their spouse 70% of the time [10]. When it came to other responsibilities, women were more likely to manage plan-ning child care, meals, vacations, and grocery shopping, with financial organizing shared between the sexes [1].

These facts can explain why students and trainees intentionally delay childbearing. Female surgical trainees were found to be more than 2.5 times more likely to delay childbearing until after medical school and more than three times as likely to delay until after residency when compared to their male cohorts [1]. Dyrbye and colleagues found that women were 3x more likely than their male counterparts to report that having a family slowed their careers (57.3% vs. 20.2%; $P = 0.001$) [10].

Women who are partnered have unique additional stressors at work that are not shared by their male counterparts [10]. When attending to family or domestic responsibilities, they are per-ceived as lacking commitment to their career. For example, a woman leaving at 5 pm to tend to her family is perceived differ-ently, and negatively, when compared to a man leaving at 5 pm. Women, even when supported, fear that they project a ste-reotype that they are less committed [11].

The disparate work-life conflicts of women compared to men negatively influences the career trajectory of young women and subsequently contributes to burnout. The increase in domestic responsibilities as they progress along their early career path is a significant contributor to the risk of depression in female train-ees. A survey of medical students in their fourth year of medical school and then 6 months later (when the students were interns in various specialties) found that work-family conflict increased almost 20% from pre-intern year to intern year. As medical stu-dents, there was no significant difference between the sexes, but over time, the work-family conflict increased and disproportion-ately affected women more than men [2]. Furthermore, symp-toms of depression increased in both sexes from pre-intern year to intern year, but increased more for women. Additionally, numerous other studies have demonstrated that female residents in a surgical program are more likely to experience work-home conflict, which also factors into burnout and depression [1, 10, 5, 12]. Overall, when compared to men, female trainees had slightly higher rates of burnout and had lower quality of life scores than men [10].

Why the Gender Disparity?

In an article entitled "Why Do Women Do the Lion's Share of Housework," various factors were found to influence this decision. In 1965, women performed 30 hours of unpaid labor versus 4.9 hours for men. In 1995, those numbers changed to 17.5 hours for women and 10 hours for men. Since then, there has continued to be a decline in the number of women's hours spent on unpaid labor, but no concomitant increase in the number of hours men spend doing unpaid labor.

There are different theories that help explain this disparity. The *gender resource model* refers to the fact that women historically have had less opportunities than men and therefore had less bargaining power in the household. With increasing education, women are able to negotiate less domestic responsibility, but this does not completely address the fact that they still do relatively more. The *time availability model* is similar in that women historically had more time, however, as women have spent more time out of the house working on a career, many educated women still take on the "second shift" of housework and childcare responsibilities when they get home from work. Finally, the influence of gender ideology, where there is an inverse relationship between traditional gender roles and egalitarianism, cannot be discounted. While we are acculturated into relatively fixed male and female roles, there appears to be a trend toward more egalitarian gender roles with each successive generation. The result of these egalitarian attitudes does not necessarily increase the male workload, but rather, decreases the women's.

Traditionally, certain domestic responsibilities were deemed feminine or masculine, and the extent to which one performs certain chores to preserve femininity or masculinity remains a question. However, when men and women have relatively equal professional standing and men continue to perform less domestic labor, other explanations have been entertained. Scholars have described *gendered performance* as an explanation. In this model, men attempt to preserve some presentation of themselves as masculine, and because domestic labor is culturally defined as feminine, not doing it is culturally considered masculine [3, 13].

Finally, there are also structural and cultural norms that influence the way we organize our households with differences noted between liberal and more traditional societies. National level gender inequality tends to dampen individual efforts. For example, a couple may have very egalitarian ideas, but if they are located in a traditional society they are less likely to share domestic responsibilities, suggesting that our surroundings have a significant influence on our behaviors.

Future Direction

A modifiable factor that contributes to depression and burnout is work-family conflict. There are institutions that are attempting to mitigate this in order to alleviate these stressors. A task force at Stanford discovered that their faculty were not using the "flexibility policies in fear of being perceived as less committed" and concluded that a culture change must occur. Stanford established a pilot program entitled Academic Biomedical Career Customization [11]. The primary goal was to alleviate work-life and work-work conflicts while promoting career development. In this program, voluntary participants identified career and personal goals and were given a customized plan for achieving those goals along with resources. Participants completed a self-reflective guide, met with a coach to summarize those goals, and, finally, were assisted in developing a plan for using a combination of available institutional flexibility policies and resources to achieve the combination of professional and personal goals. In this way, the group established a culture change that expected faculty to utilize the flexible policies, rather than feel stigmatized by using them. Incorporated in the model was a "time-banking" system that allowed concrete tracking of "favors" that faculty did for each other and attributed credits to these favors. The value of the favors was designated by the individual groups to identify which activity had the most team value. The credits each faculty member accrued were logged and could be exchanged for personal or professional assistance, such as cleaning services, or help with grant writing or coaching. The results were promising with an increase in job satisfaction in the area of wellness, understanding of professional development opportunities, and institutional support.

To help mitigate burnout and improve retention, creative and flexible strategies and policies need to be implemented, directed at a number of different stressors [1]. Home-life directed interventions (such as on-site daycare, backup childcare, in-house nanny recruitment/referral services) may alleviate these stressors and result in decreased burnout and improved retention and should be considered by academic institutions and hospital healthcare systems [1]. Furthermore, interventions, such as ramp on/off to support a trainee or attending level physicians as they prepare for, and return from, maternity leave, can help alleviate burnout. Home-life directed interventions/resources available to trainees may equalize the gender differences at the training level and can help increase the numbers of female physicians in academic medicine. For a further look at solutions for issues related to domestic responsibilities and burnout among women physicians, see Chap. 7 (Work -Life Conflicts).

References

1. Baptiste D, Fecher AM, Dolejs SC, Yoder J, Schmidt M, Couch MEMD, Ceppa DP. Gender differences in academic surgery, work-life balance, and satisfaction. J Surg Res. 2017;218:99–107.
2. Guille C, Frank E, Zhao Z, Kalmbach DA, Nietert PJ, Mata DA, Sen S. Work-family conflict and the sex difference in depression among training physicians. JAMA Intern Med. 2017;177(12):1766–72.

3. Jolly S, Griffith KA, DeCastro R, Stewart A, Ubel P, Jagsi R. Gender differences in time spent on parenting and domestic responsibilities by high-achieving young physician-researchers. Ann Intern Med. 2014;160:344–53.
4. Mobilos S, Chan M, Brown JB. Women in medicine: the challenge of finding balance. Can Fam Physician. 2008;54:1285–6.e1–5.
5. Riska E. Gender and medical careers. Maturitas. 2011;68:264–7.
6. Ly D, Jena AB. Sex differences in time spent on household activities and care of children among US physicians, 2003–2016. Mayo Clin Proc. 2018;93(10):1484–7.
7. Chapman CH, Hwang WT, Wang X, Deville C. Factors that predict for representation of women in physician graduate medical education. Med Educ Online. 2019;24(1):1624132.
8. DeFazio CR, Cloud SD, Verni CM, Strauss JM, Yun KM, May PR, Lindstrom HA. Women in emergency medicine residency programs: an analysis of data from accreditation Council for Graduate Medical Education–approved Residency Programs. AEM Educ Train. 2017;1(3):175–8.
9. Mayer AP, Blair JE, Ko MG, Hayes SN, Chang Y-HH, Caubet SL, Files JA. Gender Distribution of U.S. Medical School Faculty by Academic Track Type. Acad Med. 2014;89(2):312–7.
10. Drybye LN, Shanafelt TD, Balch CM, Satele D, Sloan J, Freischlag J. Relationship between work-home conflicts and burnout among american surgeons: a comparison by sex. Arch Surg. 2011;146(2):211–7.
11. Fassioto M, Simard C, Sandborg C, Valantine H, Raymond J. An integrated career coaching and time-banking system promoting flexibility, wellness, and success: a Pilot Program at Stanford University School of Medicine. Acad Med. 2018;93:881–7.
12. Strong E, et al. Work–life balance in academic medicine: narratives of physician-researchers and their mentors. J Gen Intern Med. 2013;28(12):1596–603.
13. Lachance-Grzela M, Bouchard G. Why do women do the lion's share of housework? A decade of research. Sex Roles. 2010;63:767–80.

Part II

Drivers of Burnout That Disproportionately Affect Women and Their Potential Solutions

Gender Stereotypes

5

Amber Hertz-Tang and Molly Carnes

Bias at the Table: Trapped Between a Sticky Floor and a Glass Ceiling

Dr. Gadhi is considering applying for the open division head of cardiology position at her institution. She reads the job description:

The ideal candidate for our position is a strong leader with an innovative approach to challenges. This individual should be able to take strategic risks and be confident thriving in a competitive, world-class environment.

While Dr. Gadhi launched an independent research career 15 years ago, published many high-quality papers, and chaired multiple professional committees, she decides to wait to apply. She feels she does not currently meet the qualifications for the position. Perhaps if she undergoes more formal leadership training or gets the prestigious grant she is applying for, she will

A. Hertz-Tang (✉)
Department of Medicine, University of Wisconsin Hospital and Clinics, Madison, WI, USA
e-mail: ahertz@uwhealth.org

M. Carnes
Departments of Medicine, Psychiatry, and Industrial & Systems Engineering, University of Wisconsin Hospital and Clinics, Madison, WI, USA
e-mail: mlcarnes@wisc.edu

© Springer Nature Switzerland AG 2020
C. M. Stonnington, J. A. Files (eds.), *Burnout in Women Physicians*,
https://doi.org/10.1007/978-3-030-44459-4_5

be ready to apply for division head. She volunteers to serve on the search committee instead and is surprised to see that the candidate eventually selected is a man who has less leadership experience and fewer accomplishments than she has. She also discovers that his current salary is substantially higher than hers. Seven years later, Dr. Gadhi decides to retire early, feeling that her career has plateaued and finding her work no longer fulfilling.

The United States of America ranks 49th among all nations in gender parity, mainly due to limited female participation in political and leadership roles according to the 2017 Global Gender Gap Report [1]. While for the past 12 years women have comprised approximately 50% of matriculating medical students, only 24% [2] of full professors, 14% of chairs, and 16% of deans are women [3]. This could be written off as an expected lag in leadership achievement since women only reached equal representations as physicians a decade ago. However, specialties such as obstetrics and gynecology and pediatrics that reached gender parity in residency in the mid-1980s and are now *predominantly* female still lag significantly behind, with women comprising only 30% of major leadership positions while comprising 70–80% of residents [4, 5]. Clearly, there are other forces at work preventing women from attaining leadership positions. Inability to fulfill career aspirations is associated with burnout and physician turnover while attaining meaning in work is protective [6–8].

Women are just as likely as men to have aspirations for leadership positions and to self-assess as having leadership ability [9, 10]. Women and men are also equally effective as leaders and may be more likely than men to demonstrate transformational rather than transactional leadership [11]. There is robust evidence in the business realm that increasing the number of women in leadership positions can improve operational performance, advance innovation, promote group performance, and increase recruiting ability [12–14]. So, if it isn't time lag, decreased interest, or lesser ability to take on leadership, why are women in medicine not attaining leadership roles? Women face subtle and overt biases based on gender stereotypes that delay or impede their ability to achieve professional goals such as a desired leadership position [15, 16]. Failure to attain a desired leadership position or achieve other career aspirations can contribute to burnout and premature attrition from academic medicine or from medical practice completely [6, 17]. In a study from Japan, an organizational climate that scored highly in terms of gender equity had no difference in burnout scores between male and female physicians; however, organizational climates that scored at or below the mean on gender equity had significantly higher rates of burnout in female than male physicians [18]. In a longitudinal study of faculty from a large public university in the United States, a positive department climate was associated with greater academic productivity over time for male and female faculty [19].

Women are less likely than men to be asked to take on a leadership role regardless of their rank [9]. This may stem from an ongoing "think manager-think male phenomenon" first described by Virginia Schein in 1970 [20, 21]. Beliefs about traits and behaviors of men and women are widely shared and derive from long-term exposure to social messages that reinforce gender stereotypes. Simply knowing these stereotypes – even when disavowed – creates implicit (and sometimes explicit) expectations about how men and women *should* and *should not* behave. When men or women behave in ways that violate these expectations, they may experience "backlash" or social disincentives and negative reactions [22]. Women are ascribed communal attributes – helpful, kind, gentle, and nurturing. Men are ascribed agentic attributes – strong, independent, self-confident, decisive, and ambitious. However, many of the qualities we use to describe leaders are also traits attributed to men [23, 24]. If women adhere to female gender expectations and behave communally, they risk being seen as lacking the skills expected of a leader. Conversely, if a woman leads with the agentic behaviors expected of a leader, she may experience backlash from both men and women for acting in competition with expected gender norms [25]. Fortunately, a transformational leadership style combines both agentic and communal behaviors and is the most effective type of leadership [11].

In the scenario above, Dr. Gadhi is considering applying for a leadership position. Upon reading the job description, she encounters language ascribing the position with agentic traits. She doesn't identify as a "risk-taker" despite having developed an independent area of research. She doesn't identify as a "strong" leader despite having served as chair on multiple professional committees. It is worth emphasizing that even had Dr. Gadhi applied for the position, the men and women serving on the committee are also influenced by the gendered wording which can unintentionally prime male gender stereotypes and activate their own implicit biases. Filtered through stereotyped assumptions they may be less likely to choose her for the position than a male applicant for similar reasons [26, 27]. The job description could have been worded without agentic terms such as the following:

Candidates for our position must have demonstrated leadership experience; for example, served in leadership roles in professional and national organizations; collaboratively built research, education, and/or clinical program; and supported the career development of a diverse cadre of people including women and ethnic/racial minorities.

This job description removes unnecessary and abstract descriptors such as "world-class" and gendered terms such as "strong", "risk," and "competitive" [28, 29]. It is also more specific in how one could demonstrate leadership. Using more communal terms such as "serve", "collaborate," and "supported" is more likely to draw female candidates [30] and hopefully those that practice transformational leadership. Using research by Gaucher, Friesen, and Kay on gendered terms and job applications [27] online tools have been developed to help those writing job descriptions to review the language they use for gendered terms. One example is the website "gender-decoder.katmatfield.com." Pasting the first job description above yields a "strongly masculine-coded" job ad whereas the revised job description yields a "neutral" job ad. Tools like this have not yet to our knowledge been validated to lead to increased gender diversity in leadership or decrease burnout rates among female physicians but they may be used by both sides of the hiring table to reflect on how implicit bias may be impacting their decisions.

The wording of a job description with male gendered descriptors for high-status or leadership positions is really only an external manifestation of implicit gender bias, and selection of gender neutral and less abstract descriptors is certainly not the final solution to gender equality in leadership. Research shows that evaluators require greater proof of competence in terms of more scholarly work and awards from women than they do from men [15]. Sadly this applies to more than just the hiring process but also in promotion, career mentorship, and grant approval and renewal [31, 32]. However, it is possible to reduce and even overcome implicit bias in evaluation in addition to removing abstract agentic descriptors. Women are evaluated lower (and more stereotypically female) when they make up less than 25% of the applicant pool than when they make up 33% of the applicant pool so ensuring that at least 33% of candidates for a position are female may help reduce gender bias in evaluation [33]. Informing evaluators of research showing that women are equally competent leaders can be effective as can asking evaluators to acknowledge and reflect on their susceptibility to bias [33, 34]. Finally, institutional leaders need to reflect on the current structure of leadership in medicine, especially academic medicine. If women continue to feel marginalized, isolated, and invisible [35], academic medicine will miss out on their vital contributions. The academic hierarchy itself impairs upward mobility of potentially transformational leaders, especially women with women of color being most disadvantaged [36–38]. Valuing a collaborative and transparent approach to leadership may help increase the number of effective, transformational leaders throughout academic medicine, enable more women to achieve leadership positions, and simultaneously help address systemic burnout [39, 40].

This section has discussed how gender biases based on stereotypes conspire to prevent women from obtaining leadership positions, securing resources, and having a voice to effect change. The result can be unfulfilled career aspirations, burnout, and a disproportionate loss of women from the workforce. Since women may be more likely than men to practice collaborative and transformational leadership, achieving gender parity in leadership positions benefits more than individual women [41, 42] and may be vital to the innovation and success of our health organizations.

Bias at the Bedside: "Lady Doctors" Face Gendered Expectations with Staff and Patients

Dr. Padilla is running late again. Her last encounter went over by 20 min, as her young female patient needed cervical cancer screening and disclosed a history of remote sexual assault. Her next patient, Mr. Brown, is an elderly man with many comorbidities including severe depression and anxiety; he has frequently told her he prefers "lady doctors" because he finds they listen better and don't rush him out. Dr. Padilla does her best to be empathetic and listen to her patients' concerns, but this is causing her to spend many hours after clinic working on clinic notes and managing her electronic in-basket to the point she is not spending as much time with her family as she would like. She is struggling to find joy in her work and is strongly considering cutting back her clinic time, knowing this will mean shuffling some of her more complex patients who prefer to see a female physician to her male colleagues.

Panel Composition

Dr. Padilla is experiencing a situation not uncommon to many female primary care providers. Female physicians, especially those in primary care, are more likely to see patients with mental health diagnoses and complex psychosocial problems [43]. A review of 26 studies conducted in mostly primary care settings concluded that both male and female patients talk more often and are more likely to bring up psychosocial issues during visits with female physicians [44]. This added complexity increased the encounter duration by 10% compared to encounters with male physicians. The resulting increased time pressure and emotional burden for female physicians may impact female physician satisfaction and increase risk for burnout [45]. Some practices have begun altering compensation practices to account for this variation so that panel size and compensation is adjusted based on patient gender as well as age [46].

Gender Bias and Satisfaction Surveys

Medical schools are dedicating more time to instructing students on patient-centered techniques of communication, both verbal and nonverbal. Students learn to ask open-ended questions, to make eye contact, and to use appropriate and empathetic touch. What is not taught is how gender affects a patient's expectations in their interactions with physicians.

Female physicians are more likely than male physicians to engage in patient-centered communication techniques such as: partnership building with patients, positive nonverbal communication, and open-ended questions [44]. In one large observational study, female physicians conducted more preventive screening and had better patient outcomes in terms of hospital mortality and readmission rates [47]. Despite this, most studies report no difference in patient satisfaction scores between male and female physicians [48]. This may be because patients attribute the patient-centered behaviors of their female physicians to their gender rather than to their professional competence, in line with stereotyped assumptions that women are warmer and more relationship -oriented than men. One study found that while both male and female medical students who behaved in a patient-centered manner were perceived as more compassionate, patient-centeredness was perceived as an aspect of competence only for male students [49]. Patients may interpret good communication skills differently in female and male physicians due to different expectations created by gender stereotypes. Good communication skills may be expected in female physicians simply because they are women, while in male physicians, good communication skills are equated with a competence that must be learned. In this study with medical students, the gender difference was moderated by informing patients that patient-centeredness is a dimension of physician competence [49].

Gender bias in patient satisfaction surveys has been demonstrated among practicing physicians and is most apparent when a female patient is seen by a female doctor [48, 50]. Extrapolating from the study in medical students, it is possible that this gender bias may be overcome by educating patients both during the clinic visit and on patient satisfaction surveys that patient-centeredness is a dimension of physician competence. Because gender is a diffuse status cue whereby men are imbued with higher status than women, [51] women benefit far more than men from external conferral of status. Thus, posting pictures with information about the training and accomplishments of the female physicians in a clinic might enhance patients' perception of their competence [25]. The Affordable Care Act of 2010 includes patient satisfaction as a factor in payments to healthcare organizations. If those organizations tie physician reimbursement to patient satisfaction, it is important to understand how female physicians can get "credit" for their patient-centeredness. Data on patient satisfaction and physician reimbursement should also be closely examined because linking salary to a process that is systematically biased against women in institutions that receive federal funding could be in violation of Title VII and VI of the Civil Rights Act of 1964 [52].

As described previously, because the gender stereotype of women includes communal behaviors like "nurturing" and "compassionate," patients expect these gender congruent behaviors from their female physicians. If female physicians do not exhibit these behaviors, they may be more harshly penalized in patient satisfactions scores than similarly behaving male physicians. For example, in an experimental study female patients were more likely to be satisfied with their visit if their female physician was "caring" and were less satisfied if the female physician was not "caring" whereas patient satisfaction was not affected by whether a male physician was "caring" [53]. Patients were also more likely to describe a female physician as "dominating" for modeling the same behaviors as a male physician such as speaking more often, asking questions, speaking loudly, or frowning [54]. Additionally, patients were more likely to describe a female physician as "dominating" for behaviors such as multitasking or looking at the electronic medical record during the patient encounter than they were for male physicians doing the same behaviors [54]. This is supported by Ridgeway who discusses that since there is a cultural conception that female gender is associated with lower status and decreased competence in male-typed work, women who assert authority in traditionally male-dominated contexts violate expectations about their presumed status and encounter social backlash impairing their likability and potentially their influence [55]. However, women can mitigate this backlash by combining assertive behaviors with positive social "softeners" such as smiling and leaning forward [55, 56]. Many health organizations are attempting to intervene on burnout by implementing electronic health record efficiency training to help physicians use their time during clinic visits more efficiently and to finish documentation during the clinic visit rather than during "pajama time" in the evenings. This research suggests that female physicians who attempt to use their time efficiently during the encounter by multitasking or looking at the electronic medical record may be more likely to be penalized in patient satisfaction scores than male physicians for exhibiting assertive behaviors that violate their status expectations.

This is an excellent example of how interventions aimed at improving physician burnout must take gender expectations into account to ensure they do not heighten burnout or widen compensation disparities.

Gender Bias, Occupational Segregation, and Stereotype Threat

Historically, nurses were expected to defer to the authority of the physician. Recognizing the significant patient safety implications in this approach, the nursing and physician professions have worked to flatten this medical hierarchy with a goal of improving care [57]. Positive and effective communication practices are associated with higher-quality care and research is being performed to understand how gender may play a role in communication practices between nurses and physicians [58].

Until Title IX in 1972 allowed women access to medical education, both fields were inversely gender segregated with considerable power differential. The relationship between physician and nurse was historically structured as a continuation of social male-female gender roles where female nurses provided the emotional and nurturing care to the patient while following orders provided by the predominantly male physicians [59]. While the number of female physicians has increased over the past few decades to nearly 50%, the percentage of female nurses has remained relatively unchanged at 90% [60]. It is notable that the movement for interprofessional practice and efforts to flatten the medical hierarchy have occurred in parallel to the increasing numbers of female physicians entering the workforce [59, 61]; however, issues of gender and status within nurse-physician interactions are complex.

While we do not know of studies at this time that look specifically at the impact on burnout, multiple studies have looked at how this gender segregation may impact work satisfaction and interpersonal work relationships, which are drivers of burnout [62]. For example, a study of female nurses' perceptions in nurse-physician interactions found that compared to male physicians there was a higher expectation for female physicians to carry out tasks, decreased likelihood to help female physicians, and increased likelihood to resent female physicians for behaviors (such as failure to dispose of sharps). However, this study also showed that female nurses felt more comfortable approaching female physicians regarding safety concerns for patients [63].

Another qualitative study of female nurses and physicians in the United States reiterated that nurses felt female physicians were less likely to ask for assistance and more likely to do tasks on their own. Nurses frequently reported resenting when female residents displayed authority or felt dismissed by the resident. However, most nurses reported that their relationships with female physicians were more positive than their relationships with male physicians [64]. In a study of internal medicine residents, both male and female residents noted that female residents needed to pay more attention to the "tone" in which they communicated with nurses and 30% of female residents and no male resident ranked gender as the number one barrier to effecting patient care [65].

Survey and interview-based studies in the United States and Norway of female physicians interacting with nursing staff reveal that female physicians describe feeling more pressure than their male colleagues to be friendly and egalitarian and to make social overtures when communicating with nursing staff [59, 66]. Additionally, female physicians feel less supported than their male colleagues and more likely to have their medical decision-making questioned [59, 66].

These studies suggest that nurses are more comfortable communicating with female physicians and potentially more hostile when female physicians display authority [59, 64]. This is supported in experimental studies showing that women are less liked and judged less suitable as an employer if they are successful in male sex-typed jobs, however they can overcome these negative perceptions by emphasizing their communal traits such as valuing employee concerns, relationship-building, or even just disclosing that they have children [67].

Occupational segregation may be contributing to burnout in women in more ways than through decreased support or strained work relationships between physicians and staff, however. Occupational segregation may also feed into gendered beliefs about performance. Stereotype threat is the concept that repeated encounters with a negative stereotype can erode confidence, impair performance, and lead to disengagement.

Many aspects of the health care environment would be predicted to cause stereotype threat in female physicians including: the existence of sexism and harassment, social backlash in voicing opinions or disagreeing, and occupational segregation [68]. In a study where raters were asked to describe attributes that would be necessary for success in a particular occupation, raters were more likely to cite communal traits including nurturing, gentleness, and kindness if the occupation had more than 75% women but if the occupation had more than 75% men, raters were more likely to cite agentic traits including aggression, dominance, and competitiveness [69]. This suggests that women working in a primarily male field may be exposed to, and possess within themselves, predetermined beliefs that they may lack what is necessary for success. Occupational segregation is rampant in healthcare. Nurses, social workers, physical therapists, and occupational therapists are all much more likely to be female than male. This reinforces the concept that women are expected to be in subordinate positions while men are expected to be leaders. Anecdotally, most female physicians have at least one story where a patient or staff member has mistaken them for the nurse and the male medical student for the attending physician.

However, it may be possible to counteract the effects of stereotype threat with strategies including: promoting awareness about stereotype threat, clearly differentiating roles (e.g., I have noted great reduction in identity mistakes since our institution introduced ID badges that clearly display "Physician" in large font), targeting at least 50% of invited speakers to be female, displaying pictures and publicly recognizing successful female physicians, prioritizing building leadership efficacy in female physicians, and striving to increase women in leadership positions [68].

One could argue that occupational segregation and stereotype threat should be transient problems in medicine as more women continue to enter the field such that they are no longer minorities in their institution. However, the increasing number of female physicians appears to be more concentrated in a few discrete fields and gender segregation is still very evident within medical specialties. As an example, the percentage of women entering specialties such as pediatrics and obstetrics and gynecology (63% and 57% in 2017, respectively) has increased more rapidly than in specialties such as urology or orthopedics (8.7% and 6.6% in 2017, respectively) [70]. Over 40% of female physicians are in primary care specialties including family medicine, pediatrics, and internal medicine while only 20% of male physicians are in these specialties; the remaining 80% of men are more evenly divided among all the various specialties [70]. While the rate of burnout is very high across all medical specialties, specialty choice has been identified as a risk factor for burnout [71]. Specialties with more direct patient care, such as family medicine, internal medicine, and emergency medicine, are associated with higher risk of burnout [71].

There are many possible reasons as to why and how occupational segregation is occurring within medicine specialties. Women are more likely to identify time for family, long-term patient relationships, and a desire to provide a needed service as reasons to choose a specialty and are less likely to choose a specialty based on financial considerations than men [72]. Perhaps some women choose to enter specialties more associated with these values. It is often suggested that women may avoid specialties associated with unpredictable schedules or that are heavily procedural; however, obstetrics and gynecology is a surgical specialty infamous for its unpredictable schedule and it is second only to pediatrics in terms of highest percentage of women. Conversely, diagnostic radiology is associated with a more predictable lifestyle; however, women only made up 25.6% of diagnostic radiologists in 2017 [70].

Another possibility is that women are subtly being directed into specific specialties that implicitly align with gender expectations. Heilman has demonstrated that just the knowledge that a women is successful at male sex-typed work increased negative perceptions of her compared to her male colleagues and made her less desirable as a boss. Interestingly, if the women was successful at female or gender neutral sex-typed work, there was not an increase in negative perceptions [73]. So perhaps, female medical students are choosing specialties that align with stereotyped assumptions that they will be communal and relational and where they would suffer less social backlash than by choosing and succeeding in more male-dominated higher -salaried technical specialties. Additionally, by entering specialties with a higher female presence, women would be decreasing their exposure to stereotype threat. These would be interesting areas of future research.

Some specialties, such as endocrinology, are seeing the composition of male to female change not as much attributable to an increase in female physicians as due to a decrease in the number of men entering that specialty [74]. Pelley et al. point out that as an occupation becomes female predominant, salary decreases across the occupation for all genders. This jeopardizes the entire field as it becomes less desirable for both male and female physicians as well as decreasing career satisfaction, which is a risk factor for burnout [75].

Dispelling gendered stereotypes such as men are more associated with procedures or "intensive" specialties while women are associated with more nurturing specialties such as primary care or obstetrics has to begin early in medical school. Female medical students are more likely to take on leadership roles in small groups after a statement describing the importance of these roles under "safe" conditions [68]. Potentially increasing female medical students' exposure to procedures in a safe environment such as a simulation center may also have an effect.

In summary, patients and staff may have different expectations and perceptions in their interactions with female physicians as compared to male physicians. These gender biases may be reflected in workload, patient relationships as measured by patient satisfaction scores, and support at work all of which may drive burnout in female physicians. Additionally, occupational gender segregation and stereotype threat may impact female physicians in terms of salary, career satisfaction, and specialty choice. Educating patients and staff about gender bias by including informational statements on patient satisfaction surveys, training modules, and wall postings may be a step in mitigating its effect, but definitive research in this area is lacking. Interventions that improve transparency and accountability in salary calculations have been successful in achieving gender pay equity in other fields, but may not be applicable across medical specialties or subspecialties [76]. Stereotype threat for female physicians, which may be triggered when performing in male-stereotyped domains such as leadership or highly technical fields, can be decreased by increasing awareness of this phenomenon. This needs to be in conjunction with ubiquitous affirmations that research confirms gender (or race) has no influence on the ability to perform any relevant role within science or medicine. Other actions might include exposure throughout medical training and practice to multiple diverse physicians across the gender spectrum in the belief that "if you see it, you can be it," leadership programs that include research on gender stereotypes and how to mitigate their influence, training faculty to avoid giving feedback that reinforces gender stereotypes, and addressing hiring and promotional practices as discussed in the first section "Bias at the Table."

Bias at Home: Parental Leave Is Leaving Both Men and Women Behind

Dr. Liu and his wife had twin girls 1 year ago. Unfortunately, due to complications during pregnancy, his daughters had required extensive medical care and frequent doctor's appointments. While his institution had only offered 1 week of paid paternity leave, he had been able to extend his time with accrued sick leave and vacation. The head of his division was initially supportive and even shared her struggles balancing family with work. When he had requested more unpaid time off through the Family Medical Leave Act (FMLA) to provide support for his daughters' ongoing healthcare needs, his division head agreed; however, she also suggested he consider looking for a more flexible position given the change in his life circumstances. Two of Dr. Liu's female colleagues had taken extended time for maternity leave and one had used it to care for her elderly father. Rather than Dr. Liu taking time off as originally intended, his wife, who was a pediatrician in private practice in the community, decided to switch to part time and Dr. Liu continued full time as a physician-scientist in his department.

In 1993, the United States passed the Family Medical Leave Act with the intent of helping employees balance the demands of the workplace with the needs of their family while minimizing discrimination on basis of gender and promoting equality for men and women. FMLA allows 12 weeks of unpaid job protection, making it one of the least generous policies among industrialized nations [77]. The United States is also one of the only countries that does not allocate maternity or parental leave through a national policy [77]. As an example, in Australia women receive 12 months of paid leave while fathers and partners receive 2 weeks. Switzerland does not have any statutory paternity leave while mothers can receive 14 weeks of paid leave. While these policies are well-intended to promote breastfeeding and to provide financial support to women after childbearing, they also reinforce traditional gender roles of women as primary caregivers and stigmatize women as inadequate mothers if they choose to return to work sooner. Multiple studies have demonstrated the importance of including partners in parental leave policies both for the benefit of families and to promote gender parity in the workforce including higher female employment and less gender stereotyping at work [78–80]. Additionally, studies have shown paid parental leave leads to better outcomes for children which has led the American Academy of Pediatrics to support policies for paid parental leave [81–83]. Interestingly, while physician organizations have come out in favor of policies for paid parental leave, many hospitals and academic institutions do not offer these policies to their faculty and residents. A study that reviewed leave policies among 12 US medical schools found schools offered a mean of 8.6 weeks of paid support with a range of 6–16 weeks. Additionally some schools extended this benefit only to "primary caregivers" or failed to include fathers or partners in their policy [78].

Even when leave policies include fathers and partners, the frequency at which fathers and partners actually take leave worldwide can be as low as 2% [80, 84]. In Japan, men and partners are given 30 weeks of paid paternity leave, one of the most generous policies in the world; however, only 3% of men request leave [85]. Men are just as likely as women to report family-work conflict and to report increased personal satisfaction with family-friendly policies such as avoiding late-night meetings [86]. So it seems unlikely that men are not using leave policies purely out of personal preference. An experimental study in Japan demonstrated that while men reported a strong desire to use paternity leave, they overestimated the strength of negative attitudes of others toward the use of paternity leave and so were less willing to use paternity for fear of social backlash and professional repercussions [85]. Another experimental study in the United States demonstrated that men who asked for family leave were perceived as poor workers and were less likely to receive recommendations for leadership roles, promotions, or high-profile projects. They were also more likely to be perceived as weak, emotional, and insecure and were more likely to be penalized with salary reductions and decreased responsibilities or to be encouraged to go work for a different organization. This study also showed that black male workers were more penalized than white male workers and that female employers were more likely to perceive male workers who asked for leave as poor workers than did male employers [86]. One conclusion from this study is that while women are more likely to use FMLA policies, they may be more likely to judge men negatively for doing so. When women participate in the stigmatization against men using family leave, the burden of care needs ironically may fall more heavily on women and further reinforces the stereotype of women as caregivers. This then increases work-life conflict and decreases partner support, both of which are risk factors for burnout [71, 87]. A survey of female physicians in Massachusetts found that women who worked full-time reported better career satisfaction than those that worked part-time and there was no difference in satisfaction with family life between the two groups. More importantly however, this study showed that women who worked their preferred number of hours, be it part time or full time, reported better job role quality, schedule fit, life satisfaction, marital role quality, and lower rates of burnout. Therefore, imposing part-time work on women who do not want may also be harmful [88].

While part-time employment may be detrimental to female physicians' academic career advancement [88], the negative perceptions associated with men asking for family leave do not appear to extend to women. Another experimental study confirmed that men who took family leave received lower performance evaluations compared to those who did not, but found no difference in performance evaluations of women who asked for family leave compared to women who did not. This implicit bias occurred despite all participants explicitly endorsing egalitarian role attitudes [89].

Paid parental leave policies that offer benefits based on a ratio of the individual's earnings rather than a flat allowance may also increase utilization of leave by men [77]. Policies that pay at least 50% of previous earnings have higher utilization by men than policies that pay a lower percentage or a flat allowance [77]. This may be due to the persistent gender gap in earnings seen worldwide. Men often earn more than their partners, resulting in a greater loss of income if men use family leave than if women do [90]. California's enactment of a paid parental leave policy that offered a 55% wage replacement rate increased the utilization of leave by fathers 46% while only increasing leave take by mothers by 13% [79]. Several countries have enacted maternity time maximums and paternity time minimums or "use it or lose it" policies [90]. This has increased the utilization of paternity leave in several countries. Germany implemented a 2-month paternity minimum where if it was not used it could not be transferred to the mother and saw an increase in fathers using parental leave from 4% to 34% subsequently [80].

In this section, we have discussed how gender stereotypes associating men with the role of "breadwinner" and women with the role of "caregiver" may be discouraging men from participating in caregiving roles by decreasing their utilization of family leave policies for fear of negative professional and social consequences. Perceived as contrary to male gender stereotypes, men who take leave may be perceived as weak, "unmanly," and poor workers. As in the case of Dr. Liu, this stigma prevents men from being more involved in caregiving and forces women to take on the majority of caregiving responsibilities to the detriment of their career advancement [80, 91, 92]. These practices exacerbate gender pay gaps and reinforce a male leadership bias by affirming that high-status members of the organization do not take family leave. This situation illustrates how social norms transcend policies even when the policies are well intended or appear to be equitable. It is imperative for the benefit of all workers and their families to reduce the stigma against men taking advantage of flexible leave policies. To do this, male and female leaders must encourage all individuals on their team – but particularly men – to access leave policies when appropriate, vocally support any man who chooses to do so, and ensure that this action incurs no professional penalties. Normalize male paternity leave with such actions as openly displaying pictures of male physicians on leave with their kids; stating in positive terms in meetings who is on, planning to take, or returning from paternity leave; and using some of the strategies to combat microaggressions in response to statements that question the commitment, "manhood," or competence of men who access flexible leave policies [93]. Improve financial benefits so that families can afford to use leave policies and ensure leave policies do not differentiate based on gender, recognizing that families should have the choice regarding caregiving roles.

Bias and Burnout: Putting It Together

This chapter has discussed how gender stereotypes lead to pervasive biases that disadvantage female (and sometimes male) physicians throughout their careers and contribute to multiple drivers of burnout. Because the stereotypes that give rise to gender bias are deeply embedded in the culture of medicine, only a systems approach will be successful in attaining goals of well-being, professional fulfillment, and equitable access to resources for female physicians. Interventions at individual and institutional levels are required for cultural change. For individual physicians, patients, and administrators, training must go beyond increasing awareness of how gender stereotypes influence evaluation of oneself and others, decision-making, and interpersonal interactions. These limited approaches can backfire and increase bias [94, 95]. Effective interventions arm motivated individuals with evidence-based strategies that can be practiced [96]. Since gendered expectations can have unintended and unwanted consequences, interventions aimed at addressing burnout may risk increasing burnout of female physicians. The effects of any intervention must be evaluated on both male and female physicians separately. Finally, all members of the medical community need to recognize that gender bias imposes constraints on individuals across the gender spectrum and that when physicians are able to achieve their full potential every member of a healthcare organization benefits, including patients.

References

1. World Economic Forum. World Economic Forum Gender Gap Index 2017. Available from: http://www3.weforum.org/docs/WEF_GGGR_2017.
2. Association of american medical colleges. U.S. Medical School Faculty 2017. Available from: https://www.aamc.org/data/facultyroster/reports/.
3. Association of american medical colleges. The state of women in academic medicine: the pipeline and pathways to leadership, 2015–2016. 2015. Available from: https://www.aamc.org/members/gwims/statistics/489870/stats16.html.

4. Hofler LG, Hacker MR, Dodge LE, Schutzberg R, Ricciotti HA. Comparison of women in department leadership in obstetrics and gynecology with those in other specialties. Obstet Gynecol. 2016; 127(3):442–7.

5. Craig LB, Buery-Joyner SD, Bliss S, Everett EN, Forstein DA, Graziano SC, et al. To the point: gender differences in the obstetrics and gynecology clerkship. Am J Obstet Gynecol. 2018;219(5):430–5.

6. Levine RB, Lin F, Kern DE, Wright SM, Carrese J. Stories from early-career women physicians who have left academic medicine: a qualitative study at a single institution. Acad Med. 2011;86(6):752–8.

7. Dyrbye LN, Trockel M, Frank E, Olson K, Linzer M, Lemaire J, et al. Development of a research agenda to identify evidence-based strategies to improve physician wellness and reduce burnout. Ann Intern Med. 2017;166(10):743–4.

8. Shanafelt TD, West CP, Sloan JA, Novotny PJ, Poland GA, Menaker R, et al. Career fit and burnout among academic faculty. Arch Intern Med. 2009;169(10):990–5.

9. Wright AL, Schwindt LA, Bassford TL, Reyna VF, Shisslak CM, St Germain PA, et al. Gender differences in academic advancement: patterns, causes, and potential solutions in one US College of Medicine. Acad Med. 2003;78(5):500–8.

10. Pololi LH, Civian JT, Brennan RT, Dottolo AL, Krupat E. Experiencing the culture of academic medicine: gender matters, a national study. J Gen Intern Med. 2013;28(2):201–7.

11. Eagly AH, Johannesen-Schmidt MC, van Engen ML. Transformational, transactional, and laissez-faire leadership styles: a meta-analysis comparing women and men. Psychol Bull. 2003;129(4):569–91.

12. Innovation by design: the case for investing in women. Anita Borg Institute; 2014.

13. Women matter time to accelerate. McKinsey&Company; 2017.

14. International Finance Corporation. Investing in women: new evidence for the business case. 2017.

15. Institute of Medicine. Beyond Bias and barriers: fulfilling the potential of women in academic science and engineering. Washington, D.C.: The National Academies Press; 2007.

16. Heilman ME. Gender stereotypes and workplace bias. Res Organ Behav. 2012;32:113–35.

17. Pololi LH, Krupat E, Civian JT, Ash AS, Brennan RT. Why are a quarter of faculty considering leaving academic medicine? A study of their perceptions of institutional culture and intentions to leave at 26 representative U.S. medical schools. Acad Med. 2012;87(7):859–69.

18. Taka F, Nomura K, Horie S, Takemoto K, Takeuchi M, Takenoshita S, et al. Organizational climate with gender equity and burnout among university academics in Japan. Ind Health. 2016;54(6):480–7.

19. Sheridan J, Savoy JN, Kaatz A, Lee YG, Filut A, Carnes M. Write more articles, get more grants: The impact of department climate on faculty research productivity. J Womens Health (Larchmt). 2017;26(5):587–96.

20. Schein VE, Mueller R, Lituchy T, Liu J. Think manager--think male: a global phenomenon? J Organ Behav. 1996;17(1):33–41.
21. Schein VE. The relationship between sex role stereotypes and requisite management characteristics. J Appl Psychol. 1973;57(2):95.
22. Amanatullah ET, Tinsley CH. Punishing female negotiators for asserting too much...or not enough: exploring why advocacy moderates backlash against assertive female negotiators. Organ Behav Hum Decis Process. 2013;120:110–22.
23. Eagly AH, Karau SJ. Role congruity theory of prejudice toward female leaders. Psychol Rev. 2002;109(3):573–98.
24. Carnes M, Bartels CM, Kaatz A, Kolehmainen C. Why is John more likely to become department chair than Jennifer? Trans Am Clin Climatol Assoc. 2015;126:197–214.
25. Amanatullah ETT, C. H. Ask and Ye shall receive? How gender and status moderte negotiation success. Negot Confl Manag Res. 2013;6(4):253–72.
26. Marchant A, Bhattacharya A, Carnes M. Can the language of tenure criteria influence women's academic advancement? J Womens Health (2002). 2007;16(7):998–1003.
27. Gaucher D, Friesen J, Kay AC. Evidence that gendered wording in job advertisements exists and sustaine gender inequality. J Pers Soc Psychol. 2011;101(1):109–28.
28. Rubini M, Menegatti M. Hindering women's careers in academia: gender linguistic bias in personnel selection. J Lang Soc Psychol. 2014;33(6): 632–50.
29. Wigboldus DH, Semin GR, Spears R. Communicating expectancies about others. Eur J Soc Psychol. 2006;36(6):815–24.
30. Born MP, Taris TW. The impact of the wording of employment advertisements on students' inclination to apply for a job. J Soc Psychol. 2010;150(5):485–502.
31. Carnes M, Bland C. Viewpoint: a challenge to academic health centers and the National Institutes of Health to prevent unintended gender bias in the selection of clinical and translational science award leaders. Acad Med. 2007;82(2):202–6.
32. Kolehmainen C, Carnes M. Who resembles a scientific leader-Jack or Jill? How implicit bias could influence research grant funding. Circulation. 2018;137(8):769–70.
33. Isaac CLB, Carnes M. Interventions that affect gender bias in hiring: a systematic review. Acad Med. 2009;84(10):1440–6.
34. Kaatz A, Gutierrez B, Carnes M. Threats to objectivity in peer review: the case of gender. Trends Pharmacol Sci. 2014;35(8):371–3.
35. Pololi LH, Jones SJ. Women faculty: an analysis of their experiences in academic medicine and their coping strategies. Gend Med. 2010;7(5): 438–50.
36. Carr PL, Szalacha L, Barnett R, Caswell C, Inui T. A "ton of feathers": gender discrimination in academic medical careers and how to manage it. J Womens Health (2002). 2003;12(10):1009–18.

37. Ginther DK, Kahn S, Schaffer WT. Gender, race/ethnicity, and National Institutes of Health R01 research awards: is there evidence of a double bind for women of color? Acad Med. 2016;91(8):1098–107.

38. Carnes M, Bland C. A challenge to academic health centers and the National Institutes of Health to prevent unintended gender bias in the selection of clinical and translational science award leaders. Acad Med. 2007;82(2):202–6.

39. Shanafelt TD, Gorringe G, Menaker R, Storz KA, Reeves D, Buskirk SJ, et al. Impact of organizational leadership on physician burnout and satisfaction. Mayo Clin Proc. 2015;90(4):432–40.

40. Conrad P, Carr P, Knight S, Renfrew MR, Dunn MB, Pololi L. Hierarchy as a barrier to advancement for women in academic medicine. J Womens Health (Larchmt). 2010;19(4):799–805.

41. Konrad AM, Cannings K, Goldberg CB. Asymmetrical demography effects on psychological climate for gender diversity: differential effects of leader gender and work unit gender composition among Swedish doctors. Hum Relat. 2010;63(11):1661–85.

42. Sugimoto CR, Ahn YY, Smith E, Macaluso B, Lariviere V. Factors affecting sex-related reporting in medical research: a cross-disciplinary bibliometric analysis. Lancet. 2019;393(10171):550–9.

43. McMurray JE, Linzer M, Konrad TR, Douglas J, Shugerman R, Nelson K. The work lives of women physicians results from the physician work life study. The SGIM Career Satisfaction Study Group. J Gen Intern Med. 2000;15(6):372–80.

44. Roter DL, Hall JA. Physician gender and patient-centered communication: a critical review of empirical research. Annu Rev Public Health. 2004;25:497–519.

45. Linzer M, Harwood E. Gendered expectations: do they contribute to high burnout among female physicians? J Gen Intern Med. 2018;33(6):963–5.

46. Trowbridge E, Bartels CM, Koslov S, Kamnetz S, Pandhi N. Development and impact of a novel academic primary care compensation model. J Gen Intern Med. 2015;30(12):1865–70.

47. Tsugawa Y, Jena AB, Figueroa JF, Orav EJ, Blumenthal DM, Jha AK. Comparison of hospital mortality and readmission rates for medicare patients treated by male vs female physicians. JAMA Intern Med. 2017;177(2):206–13.

48. Brosseau L, Wells GA, Tugwell P, Egan M, Dubouloz CJ, Casimiro L, et al. Ottawa Panel evidence-based clinical practice guidelines for the management of osteoarthritis in adults who are obese or overweight. Phys Ther. 2011;91(6):843–61.

49. Blanch-Hartigan D, Hall JA, Roter DL, Frankel RM. Gender bias in patients' perceptions of patient-centered behaviors. Patient Educ Couns. 2010;80(3):315–20.

50. Rogo-Gupta LJ, Haunschild C, Altamirano J, Maldonado YA, Fassiotto M. Physician gender is associated with press Ganey patient satisfaction scores in outpatient gynecology. Womens Health Issues. 2018;28(3):281–5.

51. Ridgeway CL, Bourg C, Eagly AH, Beall AE, Sternberg RJ. Gender as status: An expectation states theory approach. In: The psychology of gender. 2nd ed. New York: Guilford Press; 2004. p. 217–41.

52. Pub. L. 88-352, 78 Stat. 241 (1964).

53. Schmid Mast M, Hall JA, Roter DL. Disentangling physician sex and physician communication style: their effects on patient satisfaction in a virtual medical visit. Patient Educ Couns. 2007;68(1):16–22.

54. Schmid Mast M, Hall JA, Cronauer CK, Cousin G. Perceived dominance in physicians: are female physicians under scrutiny? Patient Educ Couns. 2011;83(2):174–9.

55. Ridgeway CL. Gender, status, and leadership. J Soc Issues. 2001;57(4):637–55.

56. Carli LL, LaFleur SL, Loeber CC. Nonverbal behavior, gender, and influence. J Pers Soc Psychol. 1995;68(6):1030–41.

57. Page A, Institute of Medicine (U.S.). Committee on the Work Environment for Nurses and Patient Safety. Keeping patients safe : transforming the work environment of nurses. Washington, D.C.: National Academies Press; 2004. xxi, 462 pages p.

58. Stimpfel AW, Rosen JE, McHugh MD. Understanding the role of the professional practice environment on quality of care in Magnet(R) and non-Magnet hospitals. J Nurs Adm. 2014;44(1):10–6.

59. Gjerberg E, Kjolsrod L. The doctor-nurse relationship: how easy is it to be a female doctor co-operating with a female nurse? Soc Sci Med. 2001;52(2):189–202.

60. Smiley R. The 2017 National Nursing Workforce Survey. J Nurs Regul. 2017;9(3):s1–s88.

61. Heru AM. Pink-collar medicine: women and the future of medicine. Gend Issues. 2005;22(1):20–35.

62. West CP, Dyrbye LN, Shanafelt TD. Physician burnout: contributors, consequences and solutions. J Intern Med. 2018;283:516.

63. Zelek B, Phillips SP. Gender and power: nurses and doctors in Canada. Int J Equity Health. 2003;2(1):1.

64. Glenn T, Rhea J, Wheeless L. Interpersonal communication satisfaction and biologic sex: nurse-physician relationships. Commun Res Rep. 1997;14:24–32.

65. Bartels C, Goetz S, Ward E, Carnes M. Internal medicine residents' perceived ability to direct patient care: impact of gender and experience. J Women's Health. 2008;17(10):1615–21.

66. Wear D, Keck-McNulty C. Attitudes of female nurses and female residents toward each other: a qualitative study in one U.S. teaching hospital. Acad Med. 2004;79(4):291–301.

67. Heilman ME, Okimoto TG. Why are women penalized for success at male tasks?: the implied communality deficit. J Appl Psychol. 2007;92(1):81–92.

68. Burgess DJ, Joseph A, van Ryn M, Carnes M. Does stereotype threat affect women in academic medicine? Acad Med. 2012;87(4):506–12.

69. Cejka MA, Eagly AH. Gender-stereotypic images of occupations correspond to the sex segregation of employment. Pers Soc Psychol Bull (Online). 1999;25(4):413–23.

70. American Medical Association Physician Masterfile. Active physicians by sex and specialty. 2018. Available from: www.aamc.org/data/workforce/reports/492560/1-3-chart.html.

71. Shanafelt TD, Hasan O, Dyrbye LN, Sinsky C, Satele D, Sloan J, et al. Changes in burnout and satisfaction with work-life balance in physicians and the general US working population between 2011 and 2014. Mayo Clin Proc. 2015;90(12):1600–13.

72. West CP, Drefahl MM, Popkave C, Kolars JC. Internal medicine resident self-report of factors associated with career decisions. J Gen Intern Med. 2009;24(8):946–9.

73. Heilman ME, Wallen A, Fuxhs D, Tamkins M. Penalties for success: reactions to women who succeed at male tasks. J Appl Psychol. 2004;89:416–27.

74. Pelley E, Danoff A, Cooper DS, Becker C. Female physicians and the future of endocrinology. J Clin Endocrinol Metab. 2016;101(1):16–22.

75. Leigh JP, Tancredi DJ, Kravitz RL. Physician career satisfaction within specialties. BMC Health Serv Res. 2009;9:166.

76. Castilla EJ. Accounting for the gap: a firm study manipulating organizational accountability and transparency in pay decisions. Organ Sci. 2015;26(2):311–33.

77. Adema W, Clarke C, Frey V. Paid parental leave: lessons from OECD countries and selected U.S. States. OECD Social, Employment and Migration Working Papers. 2015;172.

78. Riano NS, Linos E, Accurso EC, Sung D, Linos E, Simard JF, et al. Paid family and childbearing leave policies at top US medical schools. JAMA. 2018;319(6):611–4.

79. Bartel A, Rossin-Slater M, Ruhm CJ, Stearns J, Waldfogel J, National Bureau of Economic Research. Paid family leave, fathers' leave-taking, and leave-sharing in dual-earner households. Cambridge, MA: National Bureau of Economic Research; 2015. Available from: http://www.nber.org/papers/w21747.

80. Horvth LK, Grether T, Wiese BS. Fathers' realizations of parental leave plans: leadership responsibility as help or hindrance? Sex Roles. 2018;79(3–4):163–75.

81. Burtle A, Bezruchka S. Population health and paid parental leave: what the United States can learn from two decades of research. Healthcare (Basel). 2016;4(2):30.

82. Klevens J, Luo F, Xu L, Peterson C, Latzman NE. Paid family leave's effect on hospital admissions for pediatric abusive head trauma. Inj Prev. 2016;22(6):442–5.

83. Leading Pediatric Groups Call for Congressional Action on Paid Family Leave [press release]. 2/7/2017. 2017.

84. Almqvist A-L. Why most Swedish fathers and few French fathers use paid parental leave: an exploratory qualitative study of parents. Fathering. 2008;6(2):192–200.
85. Miyajima T, Yamaguchi H. I want to but I won't: pluraslistic ignroance inhibits intentions to take paternigy leave in Japan. Front Psychol. 2017;8:1508.
86. Rudman LA, Mescher K. Penalizing men who request a family leave: is flexibility stigma a femininity stigma? J Soc Issues. 2013;69(2): 322–40.
87. Schueller-Weidekamm C, Kautzky-Willer A. Challenges of work-life balance for women physicians/mothers working in leadership positions. Gend Med. 2012;9(4):244–50.
88. Carr PL, Gareis KC, Barnett RC. Characteristics and outcomes for women physicians who work reduced hours. J Womens Health (Larchmt). 2003;12(4):399–405.
89. Butler A, Skattebo A. What is acceptable for women may not be for men: the effect of family conflicts with work on job-performance ratings. J Occup Organ Psychol. 2004;77:553–64.
90. Ray R, Gornick JC, Schmitt J. Parental leave policies in 21 countries. Assessing generosity and gender equality. Washington: Center For Economic and Policy Research; 2008.
91. Jolly S, Griffith KA, DeCastro R, Stewart A, Ubel P, Jagsi R. Gender differences in time spent on parenting and domestic responsibilities by high-achieving young physician-researchers. Ann Intern Med. 2014;160(5):344–53.
92. Carr PL, Raj A, Kaplan SE, Terrin N, Breeze JL, Freund KM. Gender differences in academic medicine: retention, rank, and leadership comparisons from the National Faculty Survey. Acad Med. 2018;93(11): 1694–9.
93. Fine E, SJ, Bell CF, Carnes M, Neimeko CJ, Romero M. Teaching academics about microaggressions: a workshop model adaptable to various audiences. Understanding Interventions J. 2018;9:271.
94. Duguid MM, Thomas-Hunt MC. Condoning stereotyping? How awareness of stereotyping prevalence impacts expression of stereotypes. J Appl Psychol. 2015;100(2):343–59.
95. Moss-Racusin CA, Pietri ES, Hennes EP, Dovidio JF, Brescoll VL, Roussos G, et al. Reducing STEM gender bias with VIDS (video interventions for diversity in STEM). J Exp Psychol Appl. 2018;24(2): 236–60.
96. Carnes M, Devine PG, Baier Manwell L, Byars-Winston A, Fine E, Ford CE, et al. The effect of an intervention to break the gender bias habit for faculty at one institution: a cluster randomized, controlled trial. Acad Med. 2015;90(2):221–30.

Sexual Harassment

6

Christina Girgis

Subtitles

- Frequency of occurrence.
- Breakdown by perpetrator.
- Trainee issues.
- Common responses.
- Effects.
- Suggested responses.

Introduction

I was eager, young and inexperienced as a new intern in August 2005. It was my second month of psychiatry residency training and the first time I recall a patient making a sexually inappropriate remark to me. I was rounding on one of the two locked inpatient psychiatry units at Rush University Medical Center, where patients with psychiatric issues and substance use disorders were admitted for a few days to weeks at a time. As locked units, this

C. Girgis (✉)
Mental Health Service Line, Edward Hines Jr. VA Hospital,
Hines, IL, USA
e-mail: christina.girgis@va.gov

© Springer Nature Switzerland AG 2020
C. M. Stonnington, J. A. Files (eds.), *Burnout in Women Physicians*,
https://doi.org/10.1007/978-3-030-44459-4_6

meant that patients could not leave without a physician releasing them. It was a lot of power to hold as a newly graduated physician and 26-year-old woman. Each morning before we rounded with our attending psychiatrist, who supervised our cases, we would go in to see the patients on our own to check on how their night had gone. This patient, who I'll call Mr. J, was admitted for cocaine use and suicidal ideation, with severely depressed mood being a common symptom when withdrawing from cocaine. I knocked on the patient's room, said good morning, and asked him how his night was. Mr. J was lying in bed, sleeping, opened his eyes, looked at me, and said he was tired and didn't want to talk. I explained to him that I needed to see how he was doing so that we could plan his care for the day. Mr. J, becoming visibly irritated, said to me, "Baby girl, just come back later and we can talk then." Surprised, and not sure how to respond, I said, "Uh, okay, that's fine," and quickly left. I did not share the incident with my attending supervisor, though I did later tell my co-intern; we laughed about it and to this day she will still jokingly call me "baby girl."

A second incident occurred a few months later as I rotated through the emergency room, seeing patients with everything from heart attacks to broken bones to skin infections. One night, at maybe 2 or 3 in the morning, I was asked to see a man who was reporting abdominal pain. I announced myself and paused a moment before I walked into his room and found him lying in bed, openly masturbating. He looked up at me and, despite seeing me standing there, did not stop. I walked out and told my supervising physician. Her response? "You should be used to patients like this, you're going into psychiatry." The message was resoundingly clear: this was a normalcy in medicine, and I should stop complaining.

While these incidents may on the surface appear minor and seemingly insignificant, both stand out in my mind 14 years later, and I still regret not responding in some way to them. In retrospect, the first patient was likely trying to disturb the doctor-patient power dynamic (and he succeeded). The second patient may have been affected by psychosis, but his behavior was inappropriate and should still have been addressed and stopped, both for his sake and mine. At the time I also did not have a name for what had occurred: sexual harassment. This lack of recognition is not uncommon among women in academia, especially when the harassment is gender based [1]. What I have learned over the years is that these occurrences are highly familiar and to a great degree *expected* among women physicians. In this chapter, we will examine the following: the frequency at which sexual harassment toward women physicians occurs, what happens when the harasser is the patient, sexual harassment as it relates to trainees, how women physicians respond to and are affected by sexual harassment (including the effects on burnout), and, finally, what we can do as women physicians to address this ever-prevalent problem.

How Common Is Sexual Harassment Toward Women Physicians?

If you speak to any woman physician, ask her whether she has ever been sexually harassed at work. If you are expecting to hear a "no," then think again. This is unfortunately, and sadly, all too common-place. In one survey that was sent out in 2013 to medical students and residents at an academic institution in the Midwest, 81% of the women respondents had experienced at least one incident of sexual harassment by a patient in the past year [2]. This is consistent with other research findings and notably the 2018 National Academies of Sciences, Engineering and Medicine (NASEM) study that found rates of sexual harassment in science, technology, engineering, and medicine (STEM) fields are high, but the highest rates prevail in medicine. Nearly half (49.6%) of women medical students have experienced sexual harassment (especially gender harassment) versus only 40.8% of other women graduate students and 30.6% of women undergraduate students [3]. One landmark study performed in 1993 found that 77% of the 422 women physician respondents had been sexually harassed at least once in their career [4]. Perpetrators of the harassment included patients and colleagues and were primarily men. Since then, circumstances have not improved: a more recent 2018 study indicated that 76% of women physicians have experienced sexual harassment at work [5], with the perpetrators most commonly being colleagues and supervisors, the vast majority of whom were men.

One attending physician shares (All quotes in this chapter were obtained from women physicians in closed online groups and are published with permission.):

> I had the medical director ask me what I was doing in the hospital at 10:00 PM and why I wasn't home getting pregnant…And frankly, it was embarrassing to have the medical director alluding to my sex life, no matter how well intentioned his remarks were. I imagined he was trying to tell me I should go home and meant to be kind.

Interestingly, while the incident was clearly inappropriate, she rationalizes her medical director's behavior as simply misguided. Another physician tells her story:

> A former ICU director (now fired because of sexual harassment) once made a completely inappropriate joke in front of a patient and male resident. I was seeing a patient on the floor (the director was not at all a part of the patient's care). He was walking by the room and heard me speaking. He came in the room with the male resident who was following him. He tapped my shoulder and said "Excuse me nurse, nurse. I need some help," then chuckled to himself. He then followed this up while patting me on the back by saying to the patient "just kidding, she's a good doctor." He then walked out. Kindly enough the patient followed up with "Who was that jerk?"

So, do we need more research to validate that sexual harassment in medicine exists? Though it may be helpful to further study specific populations such as patients harassing women physicians [6], according to a recent perspective in the *New England Journal of Medicine*, the resounding answer is "No!" The data now speaks for itself and has spawned movements such as #TimesUp Healthcare," whose leaders state "We must hold professional organizations, research entities and academic institutions accountable for implementing systemic changes that support women and combat harassment [6]."

When Patients Sexually Harass Their Physician

One unique circumstance for women who work as physicians is that not only are they susceptible to sexual harassment from their supervisors and peers, but they are also subject to harassment from patients and their families. The data on this topic is limited, but several studies validate that women physicians get sexually harassed by their patients. One of the first, and largest, studies to find data supporting this notion dates back over 25 years and demonstrated that over 75% of women physicians had experienced sexual harassment by their patients sometime during their career [4]. While the most common location this occurred in was a private office, in other settings such as emergency rooms and clinics, unknown patients presented a proportionately higher risk. The most frequently reported behaviors included sexual remarks (59%), suggestive looks (53%), and suggestive exposure of body parts (31%) [4]. Despite the doctor-patient power differential for women physicians, this aspect of the relationship seems to be less of a factor than the gender differences. Gender appears to be a stronger contributory factor: one study found that 81% of women medical students versus 37% of male medical students reported at least one incident of inappropriate sexual behavior committed by a patient [2]. Other studies have shown that women students experience sexual harassment by patients at rates three to four times higher than that of male medical students [8, 9]. After training, women physicians continue to experience higher rates of sexual harassment by patients than male physicians; one study found that 33% of women physicians reported sexual harassment from patients versus 25% of men [5]. The higher than usual rate of sexual harassment in this study toward men may be accounted for by cultural differences (the study was conducted in Europe) and the way the question was worded [6].

Most recommendations in the medical literature, when addressing the doctor-patient relationship (even placing the term "doctor" before "patient") and the power dynamics, are patient-centric and focus on the power that the physician holds, encouraging patients to take charge of their healthcare [9]. However the fact that there is an additional population of potential harassers may be one of the reasons why rates of sexual harassment are higher in the field of medicine than they are in science, engineering, and technology. Women physicians are no different from other victims and are prone to blame themselves for sexual harassment and abuse [10]. Furthermore, it may be difficult to place blame on an ill patient who needs care. According to an attending physician:

> An elderly patient actually grabbed my breast one day while I was examining him at the VA but I think he was delirious and actually he died the next day.

Another story from a woman physician:

> A patient who was post-stroke and aphasic I was following for aspiration pneumonia issues. He seemed harmless and always wanted a hug after visits. I thought it was fine, until one day when the hug lasted too long, and he pulled me in and licked my ear. I ran out of the room and had one of my partner's take over his care. It really affected how I am with my patients from then on...I'm Med/Peds trained so hugging is normal for me in patient encounters, but this man ruined that for me.

These anecdotes highlight both the difficulty in identifying a patient as a sexual harasser and the effects that this harassment can have on a physician. While both of the examples above note that the patients have neurologic conditions that may have affected their behavior, it is notable that being harassed by an unwell patient still had a negative impact on the physicians. Sexual harassment from patients can lead to significant consequences that impact not only the person receiving the harassment but can also negatively influence patient care. One survey found that of medical students and residents who reported sexual harassment by a patient, 15% felt this negatively affected their ability to perform their duties, and 14% felt this negatively affected their attitude toward patients [2].

Further, there are numerous stories of patients *without* psychiatric or neurologic disorders who have sexually harassed their physician: either by asking them out on dates, commenting on their appearance, calling them pet names or other inappropriate behavior:

- "I was examining patient; patient tried touching my breasts. Patient had history of altered mental status, but I believe he was faking it. Since then I keep my distance and I am more careful with patients while examining."
- "A patient in a crowded elevator was groaning and rubbing his inner thigh while facing me and standing very close."
- "Patient looking at my chest throughout much of the session."
- "Patient made multiple uninvited attempts at requesting my telephone number and complimenting my appearance in an uncomfortable manner."
- "Patient came to appointment wearing white shorts, no underwear with testicles showing for part of the appointment. Behavior changed after I confronted him about this. He found my house on google maps. Never stalked me, but it made me uncomfortable."
- "Someone tried to kiss me (in front of his wife)."
- "I have been asked out by patients and other comments."

Regardless of whether patients carry a diagnosis that in part explains their behavior, sexual harassment can still have a negative impact: in one survey, increased experiences of harassment were independently associated with lower mental health, job satisfaction and sense of safety at work, as well as increased turnover intentions [11]. More research is needed to understand both the prevalence of sexual harassment by patients and the most effective solutions.

Sexual Harassment as It Relates to Trainees

In writing about this topic, I have come across many stories of women physicians who have experienced sexual harassment while working as a doctor. Above all, the most difficult stories to hear are the ones that occur to training residents and medical students, who particularly feel worried and uncomfortable speaking up from the bottom of the medical hierarchy. This bears out in the literature, with one study finding that only 15% of women residents who experienced harassment including sexual harassment reported the incident, most commonly (42%) giving the reason that they felt reporting would not be worthwhile [12]. One qualitative study looking at sexual harassment experienced by medical students found that they often stayed silent due to fear of retaliation, negative evaluations, feeling powerless and helpless, experiencing embarrassment and confusion, not wanting to offend patients and hearing their preceptors laugh along with the patient [13]. Another study found that 69% of women medical students experienced sexual harassment, with 40% experiencing this as distressing [14].

One resident physician tells her story:

> I think I have suppressed a lot of the memories because thinking about it too much makes me very angry. I was an intern on a consult rotation in another specialty and was the only woman on a team of men. One day my senior resident told me Indian girls are sluts because his girlfriend used to "do everything" to him and began to laugh. Later he asked me if I named my "beaver" and if I pet it. This occurred in front of a group of male residents. Another day, our conversation turned to sexual harassment (an attending had gotten fired or reprimanded because of it) and he laughed and looked at me and said, "I sexually harass you every day." At this point in the rotation, I had stopped talking to or reacting to him, especially when he would ask, "Hey, when this is over, are we hanging out?" as I had never given any indication we would. The comment about how he sexually harassed me happened on the last day of my rotation and I remember this rage going through me. He apologized but to this day, I think I should have gone further and reported him. I sometimes fantasize about finding and telling his ex-girlfriend just how racist he was (and probably still is).

There are multiple layers in this story that have a bearing on the situation, including both her race and that she was a resident physician rotating in a different specialty. But ultimately this woman physician, an intern, felt unable to speak up due to the hierarchy that exists in medicine and felt powerless as the only woman on the team. Medical students have similarly reported feeling unable to speak up due to multiple barriers including a lack of trust of those in positions of authority, the risk of poor evaluations, and being labeled weak [13]. This resident also felt a lack of support from her team members when they stood by and said nothing to assist her, which is an example of the well-known bystander response that has been documented in the medical literature [10].

The effects of sexual harassment on medical students and trainees can be significant and can have harmful consequences. One study showed that women who experienced sexual harassment prior to entering medical school were more vulnerable than other women or men to subsequent sexual harassment in medical school, leading to revictimization [9]. Another showed a different effect of sexual harassment in medical school—almost a quarter of the women who had been exposed to gender bias or sexual harassment reported this to be an influential factor in their choice of specialty [15]. Another large survey of medical students showed that when asked about sexual harassment, particularly discrimination, several themes emerged, including a fear of discrimination during medical school and in the future in residency, particularly in some specialties [16].

While all specialties in medicine are affected by sexual harassment and gender discrimination, some specialties are disproportionately affected and have historically reported higher rates. One study in cardiothoracic surgery revealed that 90% of women trainees had experienced sexual harassment [17]. Of women in general surgery training programs, 71% reported experiencing sexual harassment [18]. Another study in vascular surgery showed that 52% of women trainees had experienced sexual harassment, with the surgeon in the operating room most commonly being the perpetrator [12]. Notably this study also reported that 14% of respondents had witnessed sexual harassment (ambient sexual harassment), but did not separate this out by gender or classify this as sexual harassment (see next section for definition of "ambient sexual harassment"). In addition to surgery and surgical subspecialties, there has also been recent recognition of the problem of sexual harassment in other specialties, including otolaryngology [19], radiology [20], emergency medicine [21], dermatology [22] and obstetrics and gynecology [23].

Notably, perception of harassment (including sexual harassment and gender discrimination) has been found to decrease over time with training, as medical students have a higher perception than residents and fellows of the same behaviors [24]. This indicates that either trainees learn to normalize harassment as part of the culture of medicine, or they develop a sense of learned helplessness in order to make it through the grueling years of residency. We explore this further in the next section.

How Do Women Physicians Respond to Sexual Harassment?

After repeatedly experiencing sexual harassment in the workplace, to the point that it creates a hostile working environment, physicians—women in particular—most often do nothing. Previous data has shown that women physicians and medical students are typically very tolerant of sexualized comments and behaviors from male patients, often minimizing or denying any subsequent emotional impact [25]. Of surgery trainees that experienced sexual harassment, 93% did not report it, with 62% rationalizing that the harassment was harmless, 48% noting that reporting would be a waste of time, 38% being too busy and 32% feeling uncertain whether the behavior "counted."

One woman, a medical student, notes:

> I blew it off because of people joking about patients doing this kind of thing. I didn't really think of it as inappropriate or abnormal at the time.

Women physicians may also confide in colleagues who urge them not to say anything. As previously noted, sexual harassment by patients may be excused by attributing the behavior to a neurologic or psychiatric diagnosis. Furthermore, there may be a lack of awareness of ambient sexual harassment, most commonly defined as "the general or ambient level of sexual harassment in a work group as measured by the frequency of sexually harassing behaviors experienced by others in a woman's work group." [26] Women physicians may not know that, while not necessarily directed at them per se, this type of sexual harassment is in fact still illegal and harmful [3] and therefore important to consider. Other reasons for doing nothing can be fear of retribution for reporting behavior that has historically been accepted within the culture of many institutions, feeling embarrassed or fear of being labeled as too sensitive or a troublemaker [13]. This is particularly an issue in medicine when supervisors and program directors are responsible for writing recommendation letters for future jobs. Unfortunately, the concern about reporting due to the power differential is valid. While one physician eventually won a lawsuit, she never returned to a career in medicine after being dismissed from her residency program in 2009 in Indiana for reporting sexual harassment by her program director [27]. This can be just as difficult for bystanders; in 2011 a male emergency medicine physician in Illinois was fired after he reported a colleague for sexually harassing residents and medical students. He was eventually awarded $1 million as compensation [28].

Another reason for not reporting is that victims may lack confidence that they would receive help [8] or believe the claims will not be taken seriously or even worse will be viewed as the cause of the problem. I have seen this time and time again in medicine. To illustrate the point of victim blaming, a physician states:

> I reported it to my male supervisor and he just gave me advice to stop wearing skirts on days I was working with this person.

Such comments reinforce the message that it is not the harasser's responsibility to deal with his own inappropriate behavior. Women physicians and medical students also report concerns about "covert retaliation," particularly for those that wish to pursue careers in academia. Covert retaliation is defined as vindictive comments made by a person accused of sexual harassment about his or her accuser in a confidential setting, such as a grant review, award selection or search committee [29]. More subtle than overt retaliation, covert retaliation is understated and therefore more difficult to identify, however, can be equally damaging to one's reputation or career.

In those instances where sexual harassment is reported, the response can be inadequate. One study of medical students showed that those who reported sexual harassment to their preceptors felt that they ignored, condoned or dismissed their complaint; as a result, the students suffered feelings of shame, self-blame, confusion, humiliation, disrespect, fear or self-doubt [13]. Resident physicians who have experienced sexual harassment have also reported higher rates of ethical or moral distress, and lower levels of vitality, or being energized by work [30]. A different study surveying academic medical faculty showed that of women who reported severe forms of sexual harassment, 59% perceived a negative effect on confidence in themselves as professionals [31].

How Does Sexual Harassment Affect Women Physicians?

In considering how sexual harassment affects women physicians we must consider both the psychological impact and how it influences their future behavior:

> When I think about it, if I had been around that forever I would have lost my way in medicine. As trainees, we are lucky rotations come to an end. As an attending working in a rural region and now having experiences with racism and occasional sexism, I am already planning to leave as soon as my student loans are paid off which is a persistent thought that gets me through difficult days.

One study surveying medical students and residents showed that those who experienced sexual harassment also reported negative effects on feelings of safety and comfort at work, attitudes toward patients, ability to perform duties and general mental health [2]. As recently as 2019, another study showed that in response to sexual harassment, medical students described feeling vulnerable as learners, being concerned about receiving poor evaluations and generally feeling powerless [13].

Another physician notes her feelings of bewilderment and humiliation, as well as the disappointment in not having anyone stand up for her:

> I was at work today in the physician work room when a random doctor made a reference to me being an expert on human sex trafficking because I must have been a sex trafficking victim myself. I was in a room filled with other physicians and in the middle of staffing a patient. I was mortified and had no idea why he said this. I barely know him.

There have been multiple studies showing associations of sexual harassment with burnout. A study which surveyed surgeons showed that those experiencing sexual harassment had higher rates of burnout, as well as increased likelihood of declining or leaving a job [17]. Another study found an association between women physicians experiencing sexual harassment and lower job satisfaction [32]. Similarly there has been an association linking burnout to a decrease in job satisfaction and reduction in professional effort and the number of hours worked [32]. As early as medical school, mistreatment including sexual harassment of students has been linked to higher rates of burnout, particularly when the mistreatment is recurrent [33]. Furthermore, another study showed that while medical students are able to cope with trauma related to patients, when it comes to their own mistreatment they have higher rates of depression and stress and lower rates of resilience [34]. Recently new data has emerged showing that indirect harassment experiences increase burnout in women faculty and that social support does not mitigate burnout in women the way it does with men [35]. In one survey of women radiation oncology residents from 2019, 27% reported experiencing some type of sexual harassment, and 95% of the residents reported experiencing varying degrees of burnout [36]. Even more concerning is data showing that work stresses including harassment may increase the risk for suicide in women physicians, [37] particularly when we know that physicians are already at higher risk for suicide than the general population and that they are less likely to seek care for mental health issues [38]. It is clear that the issue of burnout in women physicians is complex and that we need thoughtful and effective strategies to address it.

In one survey looking at discrimination perceived by physician mothers, maternal discrimination (specific to pregnancy, maternity leave and breastfeeding) was associated with higher self-reported burnout (45.9% burnout in those with maternal discrimination vs 33.9% burnout in those without) [39]. Additionally the prevalence of attrition has been noted to be higher among women resident physicians than men in some specialties; in general surgery programs, for example, 25% of women compared to 15% of men leave residency, most commonly due to uncontrollable lifestyle changes [40]. Other factors accounting for this difference include lack of role models for women residents, perceptions of sex discrimination, negative attitudes toward women in surgery and sexual harassment; residents most often switch to specialties that are characterized as offering a better lifestyle [40].

While there have been studies looking at physical health outcomes of women in the general population who experience sexual harassment, comparable research looking at women physicians is limited. Although not specific to physicians, recent data has shown that a history of sexual harassment in women is associated with worse health outcomes later in life, including higher rates of depression, anxiety, insomnia, and hypertension [41]. Some of this also holds true for physicians. Internal medicine residents who have experienced all types of bullying, including sexual harassment, have reported feeling burned out (57%), worsened performance as a resident (39%), depression (27%), change in weight (15%) and coping with illicit drugs or alcohol (7%) [42].

We must also consider groups within medicine that face additional disparities, including those who identify as transgender and nonbinary (TGNB) or lesbian, gay, bisexual, transgender, and queer (LGBTQ). In one small study (the first of its kind), 69% of TGNB medical students and physicians reported experiencing sexual harassment, specifically gender discrimination [43]. Another study showed that women residents who identified as LGBTQ reported rates of sexual harassment at three times higher rates than those who did not (19% versus 6%) [44]. While there is limited data focusing specifically on sexual harassment of women physicians of color and physicians in the TGNB and LBGT communities, we would expect that any disparities and negative consequences would be amplified in these more vulnerable populations. Further research in these areas is needed.

Legal Aspects of Sexual Harassment in Medicine

Taking legal action is generally considered to be the last resort for addressing sexual harassment in the workplace and is typically pursued only if other measures, such as speaking to the perpetrator or internally reporting the situation, have failed. In 1964, the United States passed Title VII of the Civil Rights Act which makes it illegal to discriminate based on race, color, religion, sex, and national origin in the workplace, and later passed Title IX of the Education Amendments of 1972 in reference to institutions of higher learning [45]. Because there are two laws that may apply to trainees and physicians at academic institutions, there has been a lack of clarity as to which law takes precedence [46]. According to the U.S. Equal Employment Opportunity Commission, sexual harassment is illegal and can take place in two forms: "quid pro quo" (requiring a sexual favor in exchange for a work condition) or creating a hostile work environment [45]. While individual comments or isolated incidents in the workplace may not qualify as harassment, they can when they are frequent or severe enough to lead to a hostile working environment [45]. Retaliation against a person bringing to light such behavior is also illegal [45]. Despite these laws having been in existence now for decades, discrimination based on sex as well as sexual harassment continues to persist in medicine. Further, the NASEM study notes that academic institutions have focused on creating policies that comply with these regulations in order to primarily avoid liability, rather than prevent sexual harassment [3]. The study concludes that institutions must take greater responsibility and become proactive in addressing reports of sexual harassment [3]. The culture in medicine as it relates to women physicians must also be transformed, with efforts required from academic institutions including medical schools, as well as professional societies and organizational bodies [47, 48].

Solutions to Sexual Harassment in Medicine

In order to prevent and address sexual harassment of women physicians, and potentially drive lower burnout rates, I propose a multipronged approach. Strategies should be directed at individuals, academic institutions and healthcare organizations, professional societies and accrediting bodies, and, lastly, society. At the individual level, prevention strategies must be communicated to both men and women physicians and trainees. Information regarding reporting channels must be readily available [48]. Education strategies should include awareness of sexual harassment, whether for oneself or ambient sexual harassment (when witnessing the sexual harassment of another person) [36, 48]. It is also imperative that the topic of sexual harassment, including by patients, be given more attention in training [2, 4, 6, 8]. There have been some recommendations in the literature as to how physicians should respond to sexual harassment perpetrated by patients, including ensuring the safety of physicians and trainees, addressing the behavior or if feeling unsafe then leaving quickly [49]. To date, these have not yet been widely implemented in training. Were it to become a requirement for accreditation, this type of education would become commonplace in medical training. I propose the training and implementation of a memorable pneumonic and have developed the following illustrated below:

*N*otice if a patient is sexually harassing you or someone else.
*I*dentify any possible safety concerns in the room.
*C*ompose yourself in order to determine next steps.
*E*xit when feeling unsafe; **e**xpress yourself if feeling comfortable.
*T*alk about the behavior and not the person.
*R*epeat and redirect as needed during the discussion.
*Y*ou have a right to a safe and comfortable work environment.

Secondly, academic institutions and other healthcare organizations must contribute to preventing and addressing sexual harassment. Support must be offered to women to navigate their careers successfully, given that women are highly underrepresented in leadership positions [47, 48]. Conversely, support must be provided to women physicians, including physician mothers, in all aspects of their work and lives, in order to target burnout [39]. At most, institutions tend to address the individual but rarely the hierarchal system that contributed to the harassment [13]. Education for employees must include specific examples of what constitutes harassment, including ambient sexual harassment. In addition to educating physicians and other staff, academic institutions and other healthcare organizations must also foster a culture that allows for reporting without fear of retaliation, including anonymously, and their policies should reflect this [7, 48]. While all hospitals have a sexual harassment policy for employees, there are no guarantees that reporting will be effective or result in a positive outcome. Legally, all academic institutions must investigate formal complaints of sexual harassment, but they can additionally develop procedures to assist those who may be afraid to file a complaint, including interim measures such as separating the parties [48]. Institutions should also address recurrent patterns of behavior by specific individuals over time even without formal complaints [48]. Other strategies to prevent harassment and retaliation include medical schools and healthcare organizations declaring that there is zero tolerance for harassment and to require sexual harassment training.

Thirdly, professional societies and accrediting bodies have a duty to set standards tackling the issues around sexual harassment. While some professional societies have begun to address harassment within their own councils and annual meetings, many others have not yet followed suit [48]. The culture in medicine as it relates to women physicians must also be transformed, with efforts required from these same institutions. For example, the National Institutes of Health recently updated its sexual harassment policies, which is a step in the right direction [50].

Although there have been calls for action in the way that sexual harassment is reported in the medical setting [2, 3, 7], little policy or guidelines have been implemented by governing bodies for our most vulnerable population, resident physicians and medical students, despite that much attention has been paid to other issues impacting their well-being. One stark example is that the accrediting body for residency programs, the Accreditation Council for Graduate Medical Education (ACGME), has extensive and specific guidelines for sponsoring institutions for fatigue management for resident physicians [51]. These requirements include complying with duty hour limitations, monitoring duty hours closely, adjusting work schedules for fatigued residents, maintaining a working environment that facilitates fatigue mitigation providing adequate sleep facilities and safe transportation options for fatigued residents. There is a requirement that faculty and residents both demonstrate an understanding of their role in the recognition of impairment including from fatigue. ACGME has a provision stating that residents may be excused from their duties due to fatigue "without fear of negative consequences for the resident who is unable to provide the clinical work." Programs are required to educate both faculty and residents about recognition and mitigation of fatigue, and this education must come in the form of an annual educational program [51]. In addition to these specific and detailed policies, the Clinical Learning Environment Review (CLER, which is a part of ACGME) has published a 12-page issue brief in 2017 on the topic of fatigue management, mitigation and duty hours [52].

In contrast, the ACGME has one simple requirement about sexual harassment during residency training: that sponsoring institutions must have a policy, not necessarily GME-specific, that applies to all types of harassment and allows trainees to raise and resolve complaints as per applicable laws [51]. Similarly, the Liaison Committee on Medical Education (LCME), which accredits medical education programs leading to the M.D. degree, maintains within its standards a general antidiscrimination policy and a requirement that medical schools have policies against student mistreatment; however LCME standards do not contain any language specific to sexual harassment [53].

Likewise, the Joint Commission on Accreditation of Healthcare Organizations (JCAHO), the accrediting body for healthcare organizations, has extensive regulations for sexual abuse and harassment of *patients*, but does not have a specific workplace violence policy for healthcare workers [54].

Finally, change must occur at a societal level. The recent #MeTooMedicine and #TimesUpHealthCare social media campaigns have brought attention to the ever-prevalent issue of sexual harassment that women physician and trainee experience, as well as efforts at organized change [55]. This has included raising money for a legal fund to assist with costs for specific cases of sexual harassment or related retaliation in the healthcare workplace [56]. While nearly 50 healthcare organizations and academic institutions have signed on as allies to the movement, it is unclear as of now what this will tangibly translate to in the future [57]. States can and should also require training; for example, as of January 1, 2020, all professionals including physicians who wish to renew their license in Illinois will be required to complete sexual harassment training first [58]. Other states should do the same.

In 2019 the NIH director himself publicly called for an end to "manels," otherwise known as all-male panels [59]. Women in medicine need more men in leadership positions to take similar positive stances and set an example for others.

Men also need to be educated and supported. An unintended consequence of the #MeToo movement has been that some men now have a fear of being falsely accused and therefore have backed away from mentoring women [60]. It is important, however, to note that relatively few claims of sexual assault are found to be false and ranges from 2% to 10% of all claims [61]. One academic center that summarized its own responses to sexual harassment complaints discovered only one unfounded claim in 10 years [62]. Men must also be trained in management of sexual harassment, including the bystander effect, in which if they see something, they say something. They must be made to feel empowered and obligated to intervene without a fear of punishment when they inevitably witness sexual harassment.

Sexual harassment has significantly negative effects on women medical trainees and physicians, as well as the system around them. There has been a recent upsurge in the literature examining sexual harassment in medicine and offering solutions. What is clear is that no one is exempt from responsibility in confronting this pervasive problem, and we will all lose if we allow it to continue.

References

1. Lindquist C, McKay T. Sexual harassment experiences and consequences for women faculty in science, engineering, and medicine. Research Triangle Park, NC: RTI Press; 2018. RTI Press Publication No. PB-0018-1806.
2. Sanders K, Khatkhate G, Girgis C. Don't call me baby: unwanted sexual attention towards medical students and residents by patients. Unpublished manuscript, Loyola University Medical Center, Maywood; 2018.
3. National Academies of Sciences, Engineering, and Medicine. Sexual harassment of women: climate, culture, and consequences in Academic Sciences, Engineering, and Medicine. Washington, D.C.: The National Academies Press; 2018.
4. Phillips SP, Schneider MS. Sexual harassment of female doctors by patients. N Engl J Med. 1993;329(26):1936–9.
5. Jenner S. Djermester P, Prugl J, Kurmeyer C, Oert-Prigione S. Prevalence of sexual harassment in academic medicine. JAMA Intern Med. 2019;179(1):108–11.
6. Girgis C. Khatkhate G, Mangurian C. Patients as perpetrators of physician sexual harassment. JAMA Intern Med. 2019;179(2):279.
7. Choo EK, van Dis J, Kass D. Time's up for medicine? Only time will tell. N Engl J Med. 2018;379:1592–3.
8. Fnais N, et al. Harassment and discrimination in medical training: a systematic review and meta-analysis. Acad Med. 2014;(89)5:817–27.
9. Banerjee A, et al. Dynamics of doctor patient relationship: a cross-sectional study on concordance, trust, and patient enablement. J Fam Community Med. 2014;19(1):12–9.
10. Stone L, et al. Sexual assault and harassment of doctors, by doctors: a qualitative study. Med Educ. 2019;53(8):833–43.
11. EA Vargas, ST Brassel, LM Cortina, IH Settles, TRB Johnson, and R Jagsi. #MedToo: a large-scale examination of the incidence and impact of sexual harassment of physicians and other faculty at an Academic Medical Center. J Women's Health. Published Online: 12 Sep 2019 https://doi.org/10.1089/jwh.2019.7766Med Educ. 2009;43(7):628–36. https://doi.org/10.1111/j.1365-2923.2009.03388.x. Universal problems during residency: abuse and harassment. Nagata-Kobayashi S, Maeno T, Yoshizu M, Shimbo T.
12. Nukala M, Freedman-Weiss M, Yoo P, Smeds MR. Sexual harassment in vascular surgery training programs. Ann Vasc Surg. 2019. pii: S0890–5096(19)30414–5. https://doi.org/10.1016/j.avsg.2019.05.011. [Epub ahead of print].
13. Susan P. Phillips et al. Sexual harassment of Canadian medical students: a national survey. EClinical Medicine Published by the Lancet. 2019;7:15–20. Open Access Published:February 07, 2019.

14. Siller H, Tauber G, Komlenac N, Hochleitner M. Gender differences and similarities in medical students' experiences of mistreatment by various groups of perpetrators. BMC Med Educ. 2017;17(1):134. https://doi.org/10.1186/s12909-017-0974-4.

15. Stratton TD, et al. Does students' exposure to gender discrimination and sexual harassment in medical school affect specialty choice and residency program selection? Acad Med. 2005;80(4):400–9.

16. Mansh M, White W, Gee-Tong L, Lunn MR, Obedin-Maliver J, Stewart L, Goldsmith E, Brenman S, Tran E, Wells M, Fetterman D, Garcia G. Sexual and gender minority identity disclosure during undergraduate medical. Education: "In the Closet" in medical school. Acad Med. 2015;90:634–44. First published online February 16, 2015.

17. Ceppa DP, Dolejs SC, Boden N, Phelan S, Yost KJ, Donington J, Naunheim KS, Blackmon S. Sexual harassment & cardiothoracic surgery – #UsToo? Ann Thorac Surg. 2020;109:1283.

18. Freedman-Weiss MR, Chiu AS, Heller DR, Cutler AS, Longo WE, Ahuja N, Yoo PS. Understanding the barriers to reporting sexual harassment in surgical training. Ann Surg. 2019;271:608. https://doi.org/10.1097/SLA.0000000000003295.

19. Tang AL, Seiden AM. Sexism and sexual harassment: considering the impact on medical students, residents, and junior faculty. Laryngoscope. 2018;128(9):1985–6.

20. Camargo A, Liu L, Yousem DM. Sexual harassment in radiology. J Am Coll Radiol. 2017;14(8):1094–9. https://doi.org/10.1016/j.jacr.2017.02.054. Epub 2017 Apr 29.

21. Marco CA, Geiderman JM, Schears RM, Derse AR. Emergency medicine in the #MeToo era. Acad Emerg Med. 2019;26(11):1245–54. https://doi.org/10.1111/acem.13814. [Epub ahead of print].

22. DeWane ME, Mattessich S, Wu R, Whitaker-Worth D. A survey study of resident experiences of sexual harassment during dermatology training. J Am Acad Dermatol. 2019. pii: S0190–9622(19)32381–3. https://doi.org/10.1016/j.jaad.2019.07.023.

23. Nuthalapaty FS. Sexual harassment in academic medicine: it is time to break the silence. Obstet Gynecol. 2018;131(3):415–7. https://doi.org/10.1097/AOG.0000000000002473.

24. Kulaylat AN, Qin D, Sun SX, Hollenbeak CS, Schubart JR, Aboud AJ, Flemming DJ, Dillon PW, Bollard ER, Han DC. Perceptions of mistreatment among trainees vary at different stages of clinical training. BMC Med Educ. 2017;17:14. https://doi.org/10.1186/s12909-016-0853-4. Published online 2017 Jan 14. PMCID: PMC5237524 PMID: 28088241.

25. Babaria P, et al. "I'm too used to it": a longitudinal qualitative study of third year female medical students' experiences of gendered encounters in medical education. Soc Sci Med. 2012;74:1013–20.

26. Glomb TM, Richman WL, Hulin CL, Dragow F, Schneider KT, Fitzgerald LF. Ambient sexual harassment: an integrated model of ante-

cedents and consequences. Org Behav Human Decision Proc. 1997;71(3):309–28.

27. https://www.indystar.com/story/money/2015/06/05/st-vincent-hospital-settles-sexual-harassment-case/28574997/. 6/5/2015. Accessed 3/26/19.

28. https://www.chicagotribune.com/business/ct-advocate-doctor-1-million-judgment-1005-biz-20161004-story.html, October 5, 2016. Accessed 3/26/19.

29. Binder R, Garcia P, Johnson B, Fuentes-Afflick E. Sexual harassment in medical schools: the challenge of covert retaliation as a barrier to reporting. Acad Med. 2018;93(12):1770.

30. Pololi LH, Brennan RT, Civian JT, Shea S, Brennan-Wydra E, Evans AT. Us, Too. Sexual harassment within academic medicine in the United States. Am J Med. 2020;133(2):245.

31. Jagsi R, Griffith KA, Jones R, Perumalswami CR, Ubel P, Stewart A. Sexual harassment and discrimination experiences of academic medical faculty. JAMA. 2016;315(19):2120–1. https://doi.org/10.1001/jama.2016.2188.

32. West CP. et al. Physician burnout: contributors, consequences and solutions. J Intern Med. 2018;283(6):516–29.

33. Cook AF, et al. The prevalence of medical student mistreatment and its association with burnout. Acad Med. 2014;89(5):749–54.

34. Haglund ME, et al. Resilience in the third year of medical school: a prospective study of the associations between stressful events occurring during clinical rotations and student well-being. Acad Med. 2009;(84)2:258–68.

35. Takeuchi M, Nomura K, Horie S, Okinaga H, Perumalswami CR, Jagsi R. Direct and indirect harassment experiences and burnout among Academic Faculty in Japan. Tohoku J Exp Med. 2018;245(1):37–44. https://doi.org/10.1620/tjem.245.37.

36. Osborn VW, Doke K, Griffith KA, Jones R, Lee A, Maquilan G, Masters AH, Albert AA, Dover LL, Puckett LL, Hentz C, Kahn JM, Colbert LE, Barry PN, Jagsi R. A survey study of female radiation oncology residents' experiences to inform change. Int J Radiat Oncol Biol Phys. 2019. pii: S0360–3016(19)30726–6. https://doi.org/10.1016/j.ijrobp.2019.05.013. [Epub ahead of print].

37. Fridner A, Belkic K, Marini M, Minucci D, Pavan L, Schenck-Gustafsson K. Survey on recent suicidal ideation among female university hospital physicians in Sweden and Italy (the HOUPE study): cross-sectional associations with work stressors. Gend Med. 2009;6(1):314–28. https://doi.org/10.1016/j.genm.2009.04.006.

38. Gold KJ, Sen A, Schwenk TL. Details on suicide among US physicians: data from the National Violent Death Reporting System. Gen Hosp Psychiatry. 2013;35(1):45–9. https://doi.org/10.1016/j.genhosppsych.2012.08.005. Epub 2012 Nov 2.

39. Adesoye T, Mangurian C, Choo EK, Girgis C, Sabry-Elnaggar H, Linos E. for the Physician Moms Group Study Group. Perceived discrimination experienced by physician mothers and desired workplace changes a cross-sectional survey. JAMA Intern Med. 2017;177(7):1033–6. https://doi.org/10.1001/jamainternmed.2017.1394.
40. Khoushhal Z, Hussain MA, Greco E, Mamdani M, Verma S, Rotstein O, Tricco AC, Al-Omran M. Prevalence and causes of attrition among surgical residents a systematic review and meta-analysis. JAMA Surg. 2017;152(3):265–72. https://doi.org/10.1001/jamasurg.2016.4086.
41. Abbasi J. Sexual harassment and assault associated with poorer midlife health in women. JAMA. 2019;321(3):234–6.
42. Ayyala MS, Rios R, Wright SM. Perceived bullying among internal medicine residents. JAMA. 2019;322(6):576.
43. Dimant OE, Cook TE, Greene RE, Radix AE. Experiences of transgender and gender nonbinary medical students and physicians. Transgend Health. 2019;4(1):209–16. https://doi.org/10.1089/trgh.2019.0021. Published online 2019 Sep 23. PMCID: PMC6757240.
44. Pololi LH, Brennan RT, Civian JT, Shea S, Brennan-Wydra E, Evans AT. Us, Too. Sexual harassment within academic medicine in the United States. Am J Med. 2020;133(2):245.
45. https://www.eeoc.gov/laws/statutes/index.cfm
46. Silver J, et al. Sexual harassment in medicine: toward legal clarity and institutional accountability. EClinicalMedicine. 2019;7:3–4.
47. Morgan AU, Chaiyachati KH, Weissman GE, Liao JM. Eliminating gender-based bias in academic medicine: more than naming the "Elephant in the Room". J Gen Inter Med. 2018;33(6):966–8.
48. Bates CK, Jagsi R, Gordon LK, Travis E, Chatterjee A, Gillis M, Means O, Chaudron L, Ganetzky R, Gulati M, Fivush B, Sharma P, Grover A, Lautenberger D, Flotte TR. It is time for zero tolerance for sexual harassment. Acad Med. 2018;93(2):163–5.
49. Viglianti EM, Oliverio AL, Meeks LM. Sexual harassment and abuse: when the patient is the perpetrator. Lancet. 2018;392(10145):368–70. https://doi.org/10.1016/S0140-6736(18)31502-2.
50. Update on NIH Policies/Approaches to Prevent and Address Sexual Harassment, National Institutes of Health (December 13, 2018) Available at: https://acd.od.nih.gov/documents/presentations/12132018Harassment Policy.pdf.
51. https://www.acgme.org/Portals/0/PFAssets/ProgramRequirements/CPRs_2017-07-01.pdf.
52. https://www.acgme.org/Portals/0/PDFs/CLER/CLER_Issue_Brief_FATIGUE_FINAL.pdf.
53. https://lcme.org/publications/#Standards.
54. https://www.jointcommission.org/questions_answers_hospital_accreditation_standards_workplace_violence/.
55. https://twitter.com/TIMESUPHC.

56. https://www.timesupnow.com/times_up_legal_defense_fund.
57. https://www.timesuphealthcare.org/signatories?fbclid=IwAR3WBkYKk
H1nsr6qdraj5WkHEYcFnXRl_1vXyaPeiUjiD3rhMW9JDk24XF8.
58. https://www.isms.org/News_and_Publications/Publications/Physician_
Advocate/2019/0329/ISMS_Offers_Free_Courses_Designed_to_Fulfill_
Your_Licensure_Requirement_for_Sexual_Harassment_Prevention_
Training/.
59. https://www.nih.gov/about-nih/who-we-are/nih-director/statements/
time-end-manel-tradition.
60. Byerley JS. Mentoring in the era of #MeToo. JAMA. 2018;319(12):1199–
200.
61. Lisak D, et al. False allegations of sexual assault: an analysis of ten years
of reported cases. Violence Against Women. 2010;16:1318.
62. Best CL, Smith DW, Raymond JR Sr, Greenberg RS, Crouch
RK. Preventing and responding to complaints of sexual harassment in an
academic health center: a 10-year review from the Medical University of
South Carolina. Acad Med. 2010;85(4):721–7. https://doi.org/10.1097/
ACM.0b013e3181d27fd0.

Work-Life Conflicts

7

Eva Elisabeth Weinlander

Introduction

> Your father is on the other end of the speaker phone, from a
> 1000 miles away, raising his voice in poorly disguised panic: "your
> mom is not doing well". Your teenager's car, which you are driving
> (as yours is in the shop), smells like weed, or is that sweaty cleats?
> Your middle schooler had just texted you (and you peeked): "Mom
> I really really want you to drive me and my friend for the arbore-
> tum class trip- you never do". Your cell phone is simultaneously
> getting other texts, one from the lab "orders were accidentally
> released, pls reorder, patient is waiting," and the caretaker of an
> elderly patient (you only give your cell phone out to a select few
> over 85 ...) writes in all caps: "THE ITCHING IS GETTING
> WORSE AND NOTHING IS HELPING!"

As the number of women physicians grows, so does the imperative to improve work-life integration within the practice of medicine. Since 2017 the number of women entering US medical
schools has exceeded the number of men, most recently 52.4%,
and 2019 marks the first year that the majority of all US medical
students are women, at 50.5%. More than ever, these young

E. E. Weinlander (✉)
Department of Medicine, Division of Primary Care and Population
Health, Stanford University School of Medicine, Palo Alto, CA, USA
e-mail: evaew@stanford.edu

© Springer Nature Switzerland AG 2020   129
C. M. Stonnington, J. A. Files (eds.), *Burnout in Women Physicians*,
https://doi.org/10.1007/978-3-030-44459-4_7

women have indicated that having a work-life balance, rather than a "stable, secure future" or the "ability to pay off debt," was an "essential consideration" in their career path considerations after medical school [1]. "Work-life balance" refers to the balance that an individual needs between time allocated for work and other aspects of life, for example, personal interests, family, and social or leisure activities. However, creating hard boundaries between work and the rest of life is nearly impossible and injecting a bit of life into work and vice versa can increase overall fulfillment. For example, although the mobility of the electronic health record (EHR) has its down sides by encroaching on homelife, it also allows parents to get home for dinner and bedtime and resume work thereafter, rather than having to stay or return to clinic or hospital. Similarly, other technologies allow us to address home issues during downtime with a quick text or FaceTime break. Therefore, for the purpose of this chapter, I will instead use the terms "work-life integration" to refer to a synergy and satisfaction with both work and life and "work-life conflict" to refer to the barriers of achieving that synergy and satisfaction, that is, simultaneous expectations from work and home life that cannot both be accommodated in a manner considered to be satisfactory to both. Professional fulfillment throughout one's career requires recognition of work-life conflicts, strategies to navigate the conflicts (both individually and organizationally), and a supportive culture. While a concern for both men and women physicians, work-life conflicts remain a larger source of distress among women physicians than their male counterparts [31, 112]. Thus, with women on the verge of representing half the physician workforce, it is critical we find solutions to these conflicts and make work-life integration easier to attain.

Work-life integration and conflict will vary and evolve over the life span of the physician and will depend on specialty choice, type of practice (academic/private/government/safety net, etc.), setting (urban/rural), responsibilities (clinical/education/research), full-time vs part-time status, personal characteristics, family unit composition and support, country of residence, and many other factors. For example, for US surgeons, number of hours worked weekly, having children, being female, and practice setting (Veterans Administration and academic center) were independently associated with an increased risk for conflict between work and home life responsibilities [28]. Work-life integration, that is, balancing and harmonizing a meaningful medical career with a joyful and thriving home life, means integrating responsibilities across multiple domains, and many of these are unique to women physicians [31, 75, 109, 112]. It is imperative that work-life conflicts are addressed as they are an especially important driver of burnout as women face the monumental challenge of responding to the often-competing demands of work and home.

Work-home conflicts are strongly associated with higher burnout, lower mental and physical (e.g., fatigue) quality of life, symptoms of depression with positive depression screens, and difficulties in relationships (lower satisfaction with their partner and more likelihood to be contemplating separation or divorce) [31]. In fact, physicians, both women and men, with a recent work-life conflict, if able to revisit their decision, reported they would be less likely to choose to become a physician again (63.0 vs 77.2%) and were less likely to choose the same specialty (65.7 vs 76.0) [30].

Specialty Characteristics/Hours and Income

Specialty Choice/Income

> I loved all my rotations, and what I loved best was how the family medicine docs had such meaningful long-term relationships with their patients. Some of them had 4 generations in their practice! So cool! But they were so busy, and some of them look a bit burned out. The hours were crazy and that was just at work: I know they were spending hours in the evenings and on weekends in front of the computer, because that's when they would send me their feedback. And they don't make a lot of money; a lot of them have partners who bring in the real dough. I don't think I want to live that life, but I am so torn. I love that continuity of care...

The characteristics of work-home conflicts differ among the specialties. Specialty choices influence income and hours worked and all three have an important effect on work-life integration. Women have historically been attracted to *specialties that involve longitudinal care.* The draw to deliver continuity of care starts early, with female medical students gravitating toward residencies and specialties that involve long-term patient relationships. In the USA, in 2018, 65% of all applicants to Pediatrics were women, in Family Medicine they made up 50.5%, and in OB/Gyn 77% [3]. Women in these fields have reported greater satisfaction with their choice of specialty and relationships with patient and colleagues than their male counterparts [82]. Wages vary substantially across physician specialties, however, and are lowest for primary care specialties [67]. Shanafelt and colleagues found significant variation in burn-out among specialties and highest among those at the front line of access, that is, primary care (Family Medicine and General Internal Medicine) and Emergency Medicine [104]. In older studies, specialties such as Pediatrics, Child and Adolescent Psychiatry, Obstetrics and Gynecology, and Internal Medicine tended to have a relatively lower physician job satisfaction [82] and also tended to have *longer hours.* Women in these fields reported they were less likely to be satisfied with salary and resources, workplace control, and relationships with the community.

While women physicians tend to see the same number of complex patients as their male counterparts, they additionally care for proportionally *more female patients with multifaceted psychosocial problems* who on average seek help more often than male patients. They are rarely compensated for the extra time they take to care for this complicated patient population. In fact, women physicians express the need for 36% more time allotted, compared to men at 21% [82]. Not only do they tend to take *more time with patients* during in-person visits, the advent of the EHR patient portal has further increased time spent with work tasks, especially in ambulatory care [102], and thus disproportionally for women. Women tend to respond back to EHR notes with lengthier messages. The EHR, in its current state, has increased time away from home and even enters and directly competes for time within the home, with "pajama time" and "date night" hours [102]. Many women physicians still believe that significantly more time is needed than allotted for these activities and they often use their own time to complete their work [25], adding to work-life conflicts and contributing to burnout [105].

Shanafelt and colleagues found that satisfaction with work-life balance was not always correlated with burnout, however. Physicians in the specialties of Dermatology, Physical and Rehab Medicine, and Emergency Medicine, while expressing higher work-life satisfaction, also had higher burnout. Neurosurgeons, General Surgeons, and Pediatric subspecialists registered lower on both work-life satisfaction and burnout [104]; however, a follow-up, 2017 survey of US physicians found that Emergency Medicine, general surgery subspecialties, neurosurgery, and pediatric subspecialties were independently associated with higher rates of burnout [106]. Emergency Medicine has also been associated with a high burnout rate compared to many other specialties elsewhere. In a study of Emergency Medicine residents in Qatar citing "stressful work," social reasons, and a desire for "better work and life balance in primary health care," graduating female residents reported significantly higher burnout compared to their male counterpart (22.6% vs 2.3%) although the same proportion of women vs men left the specialty [7].

Work Hours/Income

"Something has to give. I haven't had a break for months. I get home at 6:30, cranky, starving and angry. And after a quick microwave dinner I am back at my charts. Weekends aren't much better lately, and I haven't exercised for weeks. But we really need the money. Amari's private school costs as much as college and I have to be fulltime to get that university tuition break for Arjana. I never thought it would be this hard! You look great; that part-time practice seems to be doing wonders for you–I am so tempted!"

Satisfaction in work-life integration for both men and women physicians decreased significantly between 2011 and 2017 (42.7% vs 48.5%) despite a stable median number of hours worked per week [106]. As noted above, women have tended to gravitate toward specialties involving longitudinal care. Because of the workload involved in maintaining continuity of care, however, many of these specialties also impose long work hours. Longer work hours have been shown to be a driver of burnout and especially in specialties focused on longitudinal care [104].

In a study of US physicians in primary and specialty nonsurgical care, women had 1.6 times the odds of reporting burnout compared to men and this increased by 12–50% for every additional 5 hours worked over the 40-hour work week. Importantly, this could be mitigated, and burnout decreased by 40%, when supportive colleagues and partners helped integrate home and work life [82].

The choice of specialties that involve long hours among female trainees is not unique to the USA. In the United Kingdom, female medical students choose General Practice almost twice as often as men (32% vs 18%). This is despite the fact that three quarters of these women weighed hours and working condition as well as domestic circumstance as being crucial to honor work-life integration and did significantly more so than their male counterparts. Thirty-two percent of women who chose Psychiatry also did so for "domestic circumstances" [45]. Among a small group of English residents ($n = 96$) across six specialties (General Practice, Medicine, Ob/Gyn, Psychiatry, Radiology, and Surgery), focus groups and interviews revealed that existing work-life conflicts significantly challenged learning and training. Many traveled great distances, separating them from their support groups, leading to low morale and harm to well-being, which made coping with personal pressure even more challenging. Many reported feeling dehumanized. Work-life conflict especially affected women with children, those working full-time, and those exposed to gender discriminatory attitudes. While women residents more often felt compelled to choose a specialty such as General Practice in an attempt to mitigate these conflicts [100], they may have been surprised that this did not materialize as they hoped. For example, over three quarters of female physicians who chose General Practice were compelled to do so for "hours/working conditions," and over half rated "domestic circumstances" as paramount to their choice, compared to 34% and 19%, respectively, of those intending to be hospital doctors [65]. Similarly, in Belgium, primary care specialties (Family Medicine and General Internal Medicine) were also more likely to be sought out by women compared to men. And again, there was a notably higher rate of dissatisfaction with work-life conflicts attributed to a lack of adequate time for family and private life compared to other specialties [23]. In Scandinavia, where proportionally more women practice medicine than in the United States (47% of physicians are women, compared to the US's 35%) [101], trends in specialty choice were similar. Despite enviable work-life policies, such as Norway's sponsored day care centers, paid parental, and sick child leave, there were fewer women in the field such as Surgery and Internal Medicine, and in fact both men and women increasingly engaged in part-time work. For women, persistent challenges combining family responsibility with specialties involving night duties and heavier workloads, inflexible work hours, gender discrimination, and a lack of female role models partially explained these trends [44].

It may be that an increasing awareness of these challenges is behind the more recent shift in women not pursuing specialties offering continuity of care with long hours as often as they traditionally have (AAMC 3- Table C-1 [2]/Excel link; [66]). Whereas previously, among American women residents, work-life integration has been cited as the single most common reason for not choosing specialties such as Emergency Medicine, Hospitalist, Pediatrics, OB/Gyn, and Surgery (e.g., choosing the latter 12% of the time compared to men at 32%) [65], the ability to work fixed shifts and work fewer hours overall specific to specialties such as Emergency Medicine and Hospitalist Medicine [68] is increasingly considered by women, for example [1].

According to a 2005 national survey of physicians, well over double the number of female physicians in academic medicine worked *part-time* compared to their male counterparts (20% vs 7%). These part-time physicians had higher job satisfaction, higher productivity, and equal performance [82]. When part-time tenure track faculty at the University of Illinois College of Medicine were queried, women and men had different underlying reasons for choosing to work part-time: women did so to allow for family responsibilities whereas male physicians did so because of competing demands from another job [41]. In addition to many Emergency Medicine and Hospitalist practices,

Family Practice provides some choice in number of hours worked. It is near the middle of the hours ranking but unfortunately is associated with some of the lowest wages [67]. Many female physicians feel compelled or choose to work fewer hours to maintain a positive home environment and have lower incomes for this reason. In a survey of academic family physicians, Shrager and colleagues found that half of the women worked full-time compared to 87% of their male colleagues [107]. In her essay, a response and rebuttal to a provocative exhortation in *The New York Times* Op Ed that physicians not be allowed to work part-time because of the resources invested in them, Dr. Shrager concludes: "Working part time will enable me to continue working happily for many years to come" [108].

Surgical and procedural specialties, those that involve crisis management and caring for patients under extreme circumstances and more often chosen by men, are paid significantly more than cognitive specialties. Neurosurgery, for example, receives the highest wage although it was not among the highest in total hours worked. Dermatology is the only specialty in the top 10 most highly paid specialties where women outnumber men at 64.4%. It also ranks among specialties with the lowest hours worked [68]. It is important to keep in mind, however, that hours worked and career satisfaction are not always inversely related: neonatologists and perinatologists, for example, despite having high average hours, also had high career satisfaction [104].

Choices and factors that affect work hours have significant downstream implications for women physicians well into their career. Although women physicians in the middle stages of their careers work fewer hours overall, they were more likely to experience a work-life conflict that was resolved in favor of work. Resolving a work-life conflict in favor of work leads to high levels of emotional exhaustion and professional and career choice dissatisfaction and occurred more frequently than for male mid-career physicians. These mid-career women physicians are more likely to be burned out than their early or late career colleagues. Although they are at a phase in their career when physicians are the most productive clinically, middle career physicians are more likely to plan on leaving their current practice to pursue a career that did not include seeing patients or to leave medicine altogether [30].

Given that higher incomes might mitigate some of a woman physician's work-life conflicts, it is important to understand the additional reasons that women may not choose some of those higher-paid specialties. In Denmark, for example, *lack of self-confidence and competitive work environments* were cited for why women tended to shy away from the more lucrative technical specialties versus person-oriented specialties [92]. In an older study among Swedish medical students, more women than men reported *degrading experiences and harassment* in the surgical fields, fewer opportunities to perform minor surgery and examine patients, and mistreatment by nurses and staff, leading them to shy away from some of these more highly paid specialties [101].

And just as it is important to note that hours worked and career satisfaction are not always inversely related [104], for women physicians, hours worked are not necessarily correlated with income levels, for example, in Dermatology. Several recent reports revealed that women received considerably *lower incomes after accounting for hours worked* ([68, 91]; Doximity Physician Compensation Report). In a study of internists and family physicians, part-time physicians were more satisfied, with less burnout and more work control than full-time physicians [83]. The gender wage discrepancies among female and male physicians that persist even after accounting for age, experience, specialty, faculty rank, and clinical and research productivity are explored further in Chap. 11 (Mind the Gap: Career and Financial Success for Women in Medicine).

Home and Childcare Responsibilities

In our current medical work environments, having children and raising them may limit opportunities and advancement for women physicians and introduce significant work-life conflicts, particularly during training and early and middle career.

Childcare Planning and Paternal Leave Among Trainees

> Jack just had his second kid, and his wife never bothers him about anything. They even come by the hospital and bring Jack warm lunches. She's at home doing crafts with the kids and making cupcakes for the resident room! Chris and I wanted kids by now but there is no way; I would be training forever, and it would take years to get to sit my boards.

Trainees have indicated that having work-life balance was more important to them than a "stable, secure future" or the "ability to pay off debt" [1]. Women in general tend to value "life goals" and find power "less desirable" than family and lifestyle [43, 120].

Women who choose to start a family may very well be pregnant or raising children during the lengthy medical training, placing an additional responsibility on them. Medical school, residency, and fellowship training, especially in some subspecialties, can span some of the most fertile years of a woman's life; delaying childbirth to minimize the disruption of advancement and promotion or to spare colleagues because of lack of support for those left covering, increases the risk of fertility problems for women; their male counterparts often do not have to grapple with this scenario [8, 113].

Attitudes among administrators and *policies surrounding parental leave and accommodations around childbirth and child-rearing vary significantly* among residency training programs. When surveyed, residents have found these policies range from supportive to hostile. Many have shared direct negative career consequences, loss or delay of fellowship positions, and even adverse pregnancy outcomes because of inadequate understanding of maternal health needs. Even after finishing residencies and fellowships, practicing physicians continue to experience work-life conflicts and inadequate support, citing lack of access to paid leave, physical difficulties with pregnancy and breastfeeding (many organizations have no policies reducing workload for lactation and have no specific place to privately and hygienically pump), career opportunity loss, and workplace discrimination [47].

The head of the American Academy of Pediatrics has publicly endorsed a minimum of six months of paid family leave (a recommendation based on the child's medical and developmental needs). The mean length of paid leave offered at the top US medical schools however is only about 8 weeks.

Two research letters published late in 2018 examined childbearing and family leave policies at 15 programs associated with the 12 top US graduate medical education sponsoring institutions. Although all 12 schools provided paid childbearing or family leave for faculty physicians, only 8 of the 15 programs did so for residents. Among those that did provide benefits to trainees, residents received on average 6.6 weeks paid leave compared to the 8.6 weeks provided to faculty [77, 115]. More recently however 12 weeks of paid parental leave has been offered to both residents and faculty in at least one institution known to this author (Christiana Care Health System).

The Family and Medical Leave Act, last updated in 1993, requires that employees be allowed 12 weeks of unpaid leave per year. Despite the benefits of paid childbearing leave for parents and infants, no federal law requires US employers to provide paid childbearing leave and it is up to the discretion of the employer. Medical students are not in control of exactly where they match for residency and may end up in spots with very little family or community support, often in urban areas with high cost of living. This is a significant impediment to many female residents in terms of setting up their families and possibly also affecting which programs they choose to apply to and rank highly. Although it is important that medical students make themselves aware of family leave benefits at the institutions they apply to for their residencies, they would often be doing so at a time when they may likely feel vulnerable bringing these issues up during the competitive interview season.

Of course, residents must comply with their certifying board on the amount of time off allowed per year and thus may not even be able to take advantage of generous policies. Each board has their own rules and training time may additionally need to be extended to sit for board exam and certification.

The marital and family profile of female and male residents differs and the specialty they train in also affects that profile. Among *surgical residents*, in a pattern similar to those in later career stages, female surgical residents are just as likely as their male counterparts to be married (68% vs 64%); however, they were twice as likely to be married to a professional (82% vs 41%), twice as likely to be married to a physician (43% vs 18%), and more likely to have a spouse employed full-time (93 vs 54%) [8]. There are implications this profile has on division of household and parenting duties, especially if children are part of that union. Women in surgical residencies were thus more likely to have delayed the birth of their first child until after medical school (100% vs 46%), and many delayed having children until they were through their surgical residency (77% vs 19%). In fact, female trainees were more likely to not have children at all compared to male residents (82% vs 33%). Those that did have children were more likely to be responsible for childcare planning. They nonetheless reported similar satisfaction regarding personal life and in overall work-life integration. However, they reported lower satisfaction with their working life, which has implications for burnout and professional fulfillment and for programs that aim to entice, support, and promote women surgeons [8].

Home Care Responsibilities Among Trainees

Among American general surgery residents who had at least one child during their residency, professional dissatisfaction, thoughts about changing career trajectories, and/or recommendation to medical students to avoid a surgical specialty was associated with three work-life conflicts: having to alter fellowship training plans because of difficulty balancing childbearing with the original choice of subspecialty, lack of formal maternity leave policies, and perception of stigma associated with pregnancy [98]. These findings represent an obvious opportunity for organizations and institutions to step up to the plate and put in place policies and resources to promote diversity by helping woman remain in their chosen field.

In a study of 190 Radiation Oncology residents, half were parents and 44.2% reported a pregnancy during residency. Compared to their female counterpart, males had more children, were in a higher level of training, were older (median age of 32 vs age 30), had more PhDs, were more often married (99% vs 43%), and significantly more often had a partner who did not work outside the home (24.7% vs 1.9%). Although childcare was considered a shared duty, female residents were frequently responsible for more childcare duties than males. Despite this they had similar career aspirations and research productivity. Of those with children, the number of manuscripts published was similar between women and men, as was the number of residents who stated their intention to pursue an academic career [54]. The determination and stamina that women physicians often possess means they are frequently juggling significantly more tasks than their male counterparts.

Among female Dermatology residents in the USA, *the need to extend their training if they had a child* during training was the most concerning impediment to childbearing. This work-life conflict makes them significantly less likely to have a child during residency than their male counterparts. About a third made a deliberate choice of career success over starting a family, although about a third were committed to having children later in life. As they moved on from training, having children also played into job choice. While 10% of women without children felt they sacrificed an ideal job because of their spouse's career choices, twice that many who did have children reported doing so. Of those without children, over a third responded positively to the question "Did you choose success in your career rather than a family?" [80]. Of those women with children, 40% responded yes to the question "Did you feel you missed out on your child(ren)'s milestones?". Again, the determination and stamina of women physicians, coupled with societal norms, can undermine successful work-life integration.

Beyond Training

Early investigations reported that women physicians placed a higher value on the quality of their personal and work lives than their male counterparts and ranked these higher than institutional stature and or earning potential [16]. Many women who left careers in academic medicine did so because they felt that their *expectations and their personal views of success were at odds with their institution* or that they would not be able to achieve the success they desired without compromising their own values and priorities [69]. Although many organizations and institutions have worked hard to develop policies to promote flexibility in academic medicine, these are often stereotypically stigmatized and are not used to their full advantage [109]. This is important for institutions to recognize and work against when attempting to hire and maintain a diverse faculty.

Given the challenges inherent in trying to juggle a medical career and personal life, women physicians will often choose to *delay entering into committed relationships*, and a lack of a supportive relationship at home may further fuel work-life conflicts. In a study of deferred personal life decisions, which was reported by 64% of the female physician respondents, 22% reported waiting to get married and 86% reported waiting to have children. Interestingly, while 71% of those who deferred either decision indicated that they would choose medicine again as a career, more women who did not defer (85%) would choose medicine again, highlighting that perhaps deferring marriage and children may have in fact decreased professional fulfillment [11]. In her exploration of the meaning of success and creating a life of well-being, Arianna Huffington reflects that having children was the best possible antidote for her workaholic "always on" tendencies, providing her with perspective, an effective detachment from the stressors of work, and helping her prioritize in a healthier manner [55]. This may explain the greater professional fulfillment in those women physicians who did not defer entering committed relationships or starting families.

> I could tell my chief was holding his breath, and he certainly looked at me sideways and turned a deeper shade of purple when I said I wanted to take the 12 weeks maternity leave. I already felt so bad thinking about my colleagues being stuck with all my patients and in-basket; I don't understand why they won't cover me with a locum! And my poor husband, he only gets two weeks and with our last one that was spent in the NICU- he barely knows his son.

As noted previously, the latest Family and Medical Leave Act (1993) provides certain employees up to 12 weeks of unpaid job-protected leave and requires that group health benefits be maintained during the leave. A few states require employers to offer family leave with partial pay, for example, New York, and some teaching hospitals provide paid leave to care for a child. The Family Act (S 337), introduced in Feb 2017 [38], recommends 60 days of paid family leave. Leave allowances are available to compare online, and among 12 of the top medical schools, leave and salary support varies significantly between institutions. Average leave with full salary support during childbearing leave was 8.6 weeks but ranged from 6 through 16 [56]. Of concern was that many had policies that included the constricting verbiage "at the discretion of the department" or "practice leadership." This may allow supervisors to "encourage" women to cut short their leave or lead them to do so their own to appear as better workers, both equally harmful to work-life integration [78]. *Some policies did not include partners*, which further disadvantages the primary caregiver, usually women, by not allowing for shared responsibility at home and parenting in a cooperative manner [56]. This can be most challenging for women given that almost half the time they are in *dual-physician partnerships*, and their partner may often be at the same institution [78].

Family composition notably affects work-life integration. Dyrbye and her colleagues found that even though male and female physicians in the *early stages of their career* worked comparably fewer hours and took less call duty than those in later stages, they were more likely to experience significant work-home conflicts. This could well be because they, and their children, were likely to be younger and hence the added challenge of equitably navigating both home and work. Unfortunately, these early career physicians were the least likely to report being able to resolve the conflict in a manner that allowed both home and work responsibilities to be met to some satisfactory degree [30]. Whether this was due to personal characteristics, a lack of experience, or lack of autonomy or flexibility remained unclear to the authors. In the UK, early career female physicians with children felt less supported and mentored than their male counterparts. Although they were more satisfied with their income and leisure activities/friendships than their male counterparts, they were plagued with greater work-life conflicts and were significantly more likely to curtail work hours, avoid academia or larger hospitals, less likely fill senior positions, and avoid what might be considered prestigious surgical fields [19]. Given that work-home conflicts and how they are ultimately resolved are known to affect career satisfaction, burnout, and impactful career decisions, this finding is of great importance and may represent a true opportunity.

Among early career physicians in Ontario, Canada, many women having children felt guilty taking the fully legislated pregnancy leave allowed and often curtailed that leave [88]. Similarly, in a large American medical school, although most felt that their family leave policies were fairly implemented, almost half the women faculty were *concerned about the reaction of their colleagues* if they took time to attend their family [10]. In addition to other lifestyle considerations, this worry may impact the decision to have children: in one-physician couples, the average number of children was higher when the male was a physician (1.86) versus when the female was a physician (1.40) [75]. Thus, in addition to their stamina, resilience, poor self-care skills, a tendency to self-sacrifice, and persistent societal norms, underdeveloped and/or underutilized institutional policies can interfere with successful work-life integration.

In her essay "Promoting Sensible Parenting Policies: Leading by Example" [27], Diamond references a report evaluating parental leave policies of 141 countries, which demonstrated that increasing maternity leave by 10 weeks was associated not only with a 10% reduction in neonatal infant mortality but also a decreased mortality of children younger than 5 years (by 9%) [51]. Furthermore, access to paid family leave correlated with decreased parental stress and a longer interval of breastfeeding. A retrospective study of 14,000 families demonstrated that less than 12 weeks of maternity leave or 8 weeks of paid leave was associated with an increase in postpartum depression in mothers; fewer than 8 weeks of paid leave was also associated with a reduction in overall maternal health [26].

Increasing paternity leave, modeled after Swedish policy, significantly reduces the risk of postpartum mothers experiencing adverse physical health complications and improves her mental health. A study from Stanford's Institute for Economic Policy Research [94] suggests career costs of family formation secondary to lack of workplace flexibility are exacerbated by a father's inability to respond to domestic and newborn needs, further exacerbating the maternal health costs of childbearing.

> "I walk in the door and start picking up toys so I don't kill myself. I am always putting everybody's things away. You all leave the dishes in the sink; don't you know what this dishwasher is for? I have cooked dinner 5 days this week and while I appreciate you grilling the burgers, it would really help if you helped out with a few more chores."

Results from the American Time Use Survey between 2003 and 2016 confirmed that among physicians who were married, sex differences exist in *time spent on household activities* (e.g., cleaning and cooking) and childcare (e.g., bathing and homework). Female physicians, even after adjusting for work hours out of the home, spent significantly more time per day on household activities and childcare than their male counterparts, specifically 100.2 minutes more [75]. Across most western countries where the proportion of women physicians is reaching 40%, women remained responsible for most domestic tasks and responsibilities and thus over 90% of US women physicians reported poor work-life integration [112]. Similarly, among physicians in Newfoundland and Labrador, female physicians reported spending significantly more time on childcare activities and domestic activities than their male counterparts. They bore most of the responsibility for day-to-day functioning of the family unit, whereas male physicians were more readily able to rely on their female partner to carry out these responsibilities. Women physicians faced with these work-life conflicts additionally reported feeling more guilt over their performance as mothers [91]. A 2016 survey of French women physicians revealed similar work-life conflicts, with 41% reporting their careers significantly impacting their child-rearing plans [37].

For those choosing an *academic* medical career, long hours are the norm, compounding work-life conflicts. Patient care, call, high expectations for research with increasing competition for funding, teaching assignments, committee work, as well as professional society and organizational commitments to demonstrate local regional and national recognition are all required for academic advancement. Female doctors entering academia, in comparison to their male counterparts, additionally spent *more hours on childcare and domestic chores* and reported higher level of conflict between their work obligations and family life [59]. Academic productivity of early career faculty was adversely and differentially affected by child-rearing responsibilities. In Jolly and colleague's exploration, these faculty members overwhelmingly believed that their career progress productivity was slowed by having children. Some career development grants are limited to physicians who finished training within the last 10 years, limiting women physician's flexibility to take time off to raise their children or to work part-time [78]. It is not surprising then that academic women physician-researchers do not achieve career success at the same rate as their male counterparts. Jolly and colleagues suggest differences in nonprofessional responsibilities may partially explain this gap. In their study of gender differences in time spent on parenting and domestic responsibilities of nearly 1500 high-achieving academic physicians with K grants between 2006 and 2009, women physicians were more likely than their male counterparts to have partners who worked full-time themselves (86% versus 49%) and they spent an average of 8.5 more hours per week working around the home. Among those who had children, women worked more hours in total, but 7 fewer (paid) hours than men, particularly research hours, and spent 12 hours more on parenting or domestic tasks per week. These married or partnered women researchers with children did 43.8% (vs men at 25.2%) of the total parenting or domestic tasks time themselves. Spouses or partners of male physicians dedicated a greater number of hours on these tasks than spouses of women physicians (60.2% vs 32.4%). In the physician faculty with children and with spouses employed full-time, women spent 46.3% of the total time on parenting or domestic tasks themselves, whereas men only spent 31.1%. Women were significantly more likely to report using day care (38.8% vs 30.6%), nanny, or babysitter services (44.3% vs 32.3%) and were less likely to rely on their spouses or domestic partners (29.5% vs 54.9%). Men and women who were married/partnered but did not have children spent similar hours at work and home, which suggests that gender issues surrounding childcare were the major differentiator: women with children were spending substantially more time on parenting or domestic activities than their male peers. Time spent on home responsibilities was found to compete primarily with flexible research hours [59].

Similarly, in narratives of *physician-researchers* and their mentors, significantly more women than men physicians identified the burden of work-life conflicts they face as factors in being less likely to pursue the academic milestones needed for promotion. Although both male and female academic physicians prioritize personal and home life, gendered societal expectations of the woman's role were still considered to significantly and negatively impact female physicians' academic achievements. Women's narratives additionally exposed the guilt surrounding having to compromise time spent with family while at the same time feeling they were neglecting their research careers. Deeply rooted challenges to work-life integration exist within the professional culture of academic medicine, including the stigma attached to taking advantage of, in some cases generous, work flexibility policies [109]. Strong and colleagues cite research in management and psychology that confirms that both women and men are perceived as less committed to their career if they become a parent or use the existing leave policies; thus their fear is not unfounded [109]. Actively promoting and *destigmatizing use of these policies is essential* to attracting and retaining a diverse faculty.

There has been a slow but steady rise in the number of women entering the *surgical* fields. This parallels a rise in dual-physician partnerships, which introduces its own set of work-life challenges (and not just among surgeons). In an exploration by Baptiste and colleagues of *early career surgeons*, the home life profile of men and women differed significantly but was not all that different from surgical trainees. Women were more likely than men to be married and married to a professional (90% vs 37%), and that partner was more often working full-time (74% vs 18% of men's partners). Women were more likely than men to report having delayed childbearing until after medical school (100% vs 60%) or residency (81% vs 50%), and overall, they had fewer children and their children tended to be younger. Similar to the trainees, early career women surgeons were more likely to be primarily responsible for childcare planning, meal planning, grocery shopping, and vacation planning. The policy of clock stopping was implemented to support women faculty; delaying promotion following an already long and arduous training, however, was seen by some as being punitive. Nevertheless, women faculty had significantly lower satisfaction in personal life but, surprisingly, in their study there was no difference in overall work-life balance satisfaction between genders or among the different career stages [8].

Satisfaction with one's career plays into how one shows up at work. Engagement and "citizenship" can affect one's ability to effectively contribute to a supportive and productive work environment for the whole team, significantly impacting workplace culture [57, 76]. Given that a workplace culture of wellness (along with personal resilience and efficiency of practice) is one of the three reciprocal domains fundamental to improving and sustaining professional fulfillment [14], the importance of supporting all physicians with household responsibilities is an additional opportunity to enhance overall wellness and work performance and reduce burnout. Many day care facilities often have year-long wait periods (my own had the option of entering "estimated date of confinement," expecting couples to sign up even before the child was born!), which needs to be addressed.

Maternal Discrimination and Microaggression

"I am not sure about your order Marcie (AKA Dr. Marcia Rise). Dr. Yung (AKA known as Dr. Mark Yung) mentioned this morning that we should stop the heparin, not continue it. You look so tired, poor thing. That little bun in the oven is sure taking a toll on you; my memory went to pieces too when I was pregnant!"

In addition to work-life conflict, microaggressions and workplace hostility contribute to work stress and have also been shown to play a role in the struggle of women to attain the rank of full professor [13]. Women physicians are more often targeted with microaggressions, such as having their medical orders questioned and challenged more frequently and being addressed more casually and less respectfully than male peers [40].

Interested in exploring perceived discrimination regarding motherhood, an online survey of the Physician Moms Group was launched. Of 5782 respondents, over a third reported gender and maternal discrimination, most commonly disrespectful treatment by nurses or support staff (based on pregnancy or maternity leave (89%) and breastfeeding (48%)), being excluded from administrative decision-making, as well as receiving lower pay and benefits than their male counterparts. Importantly, burnout was reported in 45.9% in those women physicians who experienced maternal discrimination vs 33% of those who did not [6]. Addressing microaggression and maternal discrimination begins with recognizing that it exists. Advocating for education and policies to eradicate microaggressions and implicit bias should considerably improve the experience of women in medicine.

Domestic Responsibilities and Work-Life Conflict Among Middle Career Physicians

It is established that women physicians are at high risk of work-family conflict just from the dual role of being a physician and a mother. In the same 60,000 participants of the online Physician Moms Group referenced previously, in addition to frequently bearing the greater load of domestic duties and child-rearing, physician mothers' roles as caretakers often means they are additionally caring for spouses, parents, friends, and others with a serious health problem, long-term illness, or disability. Not surprisingly this subset of physician mothers (16.4%) with additional work-life conflict had higher self-reported mood and anxiety disorders (aRR 1.21) as well as burnout (aRR, 1.25) [122].

In a study of *middle career women surgeons,* personal life satisfaction was on par with trainees and early-stage surgeons, but less than late-stage surgeons. Additionally, these mid-career women surgeons reported lower satisfaction scores in work-life than surgeons in all stages, that is, residents and early and late career surgeons. Within these practices, women surgeons were more likely to be on the clinical track. They tended to have younger children and were more likely to have experienced a recent work-home conflict, the latter known to factor into burnout and depression [8].

In contrast to other physicians, work hours among male and female surgeons are relatively similar. In a study of almost 8000 American surgeons by Dyrbye and colleagues, men and women both worked about 60 hours a week and had similar numbers of nights per week taking call (2–3) [28]. Women, however, spent less time in the operating room per week and held lower academic rankings. Far fewer women surgeons compared to men felt their work schedules allowed them time enough for personal and family life (29.8% versus 37.4% of men). Most of the male surgeons had a life partner (90%), and half of those did not work outside the home. These surgeons were much more satisfied with their career than those with spouses who did work outside the home. Women were twice as likely to have a working spouse (83.1% vs 47.8%). Sixteen percent of surgeons overall were married to other physicians. Similar to surgical residents and early career surgeons, a much greater percentage of women surgeons were married to physicians (43%); and in 27% of cases they were married to other surgeons. In comparison, male surgeons were married to physicians only 28% of the time and in only 5% of these cases these were surgeons. Career conflicts between spouses of dual-physician household were more commonly reported in women. *The conflict was resolved in favor of the surgeon if he were male 87% of the time but only 59% of the time if the surgeon was a woman.* Surgeons married to physicians tended to *delay having children.* There was a significant difference in the perceived effect having children had on career advancement, with more than half (57.3%) of the women surgeons reporting that raising children slowed the advancement of their career compared to 20.2% of men. Compared to their male counterparts, they were less likely to rely on their partner to take care of a sick child or a child out of school. They were five times more likely to use a nanny. Thus, it is understandable that women surgeons were significantly more likely than their male counterparts to have had a recent work-life conflict (62 vs 48%). These conflicts were rarely resolved in favor of personal responsibilities; rather, overwhelmingly they resolved either in favor of work or in a manner that met both responsibilities, although perhaps suboptimally. Women surgeons endorsed slightly more depressive symptoms, were more likely to feel burned out (43 vs 39%), and had a lower mental quality of life, but these differences disappeared when controlling for age, having children, and hours worked. Similar to Internal Medicine physicians [29], after controlling for personal and professional characteristics among surgeons, three themes emerged that were all independently associated with burnout: each additional hour worked per week, a work-home conflict within the last 3 weeks, and resolving that conflict in favor of work [28].

The work-life conflicts described above were even more exaggerated in women surgeons married to other surgeons. Households where both partners were surgeons tended to be younger and newer to their practice. Latent gender discrimination was endorsed by 41% of women surgeons in a dual surgeon US cohort, who felt that the most recent career conflict was resolved in favor of their spouse/partner—more than three times that reported when querying males [28]. These findings suggest that traditionally held societal beliefs about women's role in the home and workforce remain true today for a large segment of the US women surgeon population. In an older study, and in stark contrast, among practicing women surgeons in Canada, a much lower percentage, 10%, thought that their spouse/partner expected his career advancement to take priority over their own career [86].

Among gynecology subspecialists, once again more woman than men felt that their careers more significantly impacted decisions made on parenting: they often felt that their academic and clinical work was negatively impacted by having children [52].

In a sample of almost 50,000 American physicians, not differentiated by specialty (31,000 men and 18,000 women) surveyed 2000–2015, significant differences between female and male doctors were noted in levels of home support. Only 8.8% of women physicians had partners who did not work outside the home, compared to 46% of male physicians. Whereas 31% of the women physicians were married to other physicians, only 17% of the male physicians were, meaning significantly less support at home for female physicians [74]. As the number of paid work hours of spouses of female physicians increased, professional adjustments were made, with more hours spent taking care of household responsibilities and fewer paid hours. In an older study, 82% of the male physicians' spouses performed most or all of the duties at home compared with 5% of the female physicians' spouses [118]. In dual-physician families there can be significantly more challenge integrating work and home life for women physicians than for the male physicians, and in general women physicians in dual-physician marriages end up working fewer paid hours than their male counterparts because of greater pressure to allocate more time to household and childcare responsibilities [74].

There are more similarities than differences in the work-life conflicts felt by women physicians in other countries across the globe. An extensive 2014 examination of women physicians' experiences in Japan, Scandinavia, Russia and Eastern Europe highlighted significant gender-based concerns that contributed to work-life conflicts [80, 97]. In Russia, where medicine had become one of the lowest paid professional careers under Soviet rule, women have comprised about 70% of that work force since the 1950s [50, 80, 101]. Wages are poor to begin with, and medical careers likened to blue-collar jobs. Differences in primary household and childcare responsibilities for women resulted in a 10-hour difference in hours worked per week and women physicians' salaries were found to be 65% of male physicians, who were often found in academic and tertiary care careers [101]. In Hungary, 52% of physicians in 2012 were female and were expected to prioritize family life. At the same time, they reported lack of social support and female mentorship, lower job satisfaction, and higher levels of work-family conflict resulting in lower incomes and higher levels of burnout than their male counterparts [4, 5]. Similarly, in Serbia, where women comprise 64% of the physician workforce, and only 1% of the workforce works part-time, childcare is primarily the responsibility of women, and work-family conflict and burnout are thus significantly higher in women physicians (OECD 2012 Health Data/[95]).

In Japan, where only 20% of physicians are women, they reported discrimination regarding choice of career, discrimination and sexual harassment in the workplace, a paucity of both spousal and institutional support surrounding pregnancy and childcare, and high levels of work-family conflict [121]. Japanese female surgeons noted a lack of family support as their most significant challenge [63]. Only half of Japanese women OB/GYNs were able to secure any maternity leave [110] and only half of hospitals had on-site childcare centers [121]. Thus, Japanese female OB/GYNs frequently gave up surgery and deliveries, worked significantly fewer hours and fewer nights, and made significantly less money [110]. Female physician employment at 9 years after graduation decreased by 75%, [121] with a marked decline in their late 20s and 30s; workforce participation of male physicians, in contrast, remained high until the age of 65 [60]. Cultural expectations and the challenges of meaningful work-life integration result in the workforce participation of Japanese female physicians resembling the M-shaped curve: "starting low but rapidly increasing as women first enter the workforce; declining as women temporarily withdraw from the labor market to have and raise children; increasing again when those children grow a little older and women reenter the workforce; and then declining again as all workers, men and women, reach retirement age" [60]. Finnish women were less likely to need to sacrifice their work-life for childcare responsibilities because of their country's robust social resources [101].

Work-life conflicts are more burdensome for female physicians for many of the reasons elucidated above. Although, in general, physician marriages tend to be longer lasting and the overall divorce rate lower than nonphysician marriages, it may not be surprising then that *female physicians are significantly more likely to be divorced than male physicians*. Lack of shared responsibility and cooperative parenting further impedes harmonious work-life integration. The divorce rate in female physicians is positively correlated with the number of hours worked per week, suggesting that there is a *differential response to working longer hours*, both paid and unpaid, and which may have a significant impact on the primary relationship [73].

Late Career

> "I miss the kids like crazy, but I have to say, I am loving having the time to do some writing, and you know, I really like it! And "call" used to throw me for a loop, but it doesn't seem to bother me now. I have finally come to a place where I don't feel I need to play to the crowd; I am comfortable with my values and priorities and that feels wonderful!"

Late career physicians of both genders appear to be doing much better. They report greater professional fulfillment and are more satisfied with their career choices. Although they hold fewer leadership positions than men overall, women physician's publication rates increase and actually exceed those of men in the latter stages of careers [99]. They worked fewer hours, took less night call, and had fewer instances of work-life conflict. Their most recent conflict was considerably more likely to have been resolved in favor of both work and personal life (e.g., utilizing the workplace benefit of in-home or center-based replacement care for one's child or elderly parent: https://stanford.app.box.com/s/0a16dfy52pu3s8wtf0sexdiaw2heb4u5). They exhibit less emotional exhaustion and depersonalization than their younger colleagues and are overall less burned out [30]. While demands at home may be less, given children who are more independent or out of the house, perhaps the years of experience additionally allows them to more successfully navigate work and home life conflicts and develop the ability to resolve issues more equitably.

Intermittent focus on career advancement because of childcare and responsibility to the family is a thread oft woven throughout a woman's medical career. As emphasized by Huffington, home life can also be an effective antidote to the stressors of a career, providing healthy perspective and clearer means to prioritize. Austrian women physician leaders recognized and appreciated the power of positive effects and energy that is derived from a rich family life. Harmony, happiness, well-being, and health had a constructive spillover into work and helped enhance the work-life relationship (which they termed "work-family enrichment") [103]. Along a similar vein, in an opinion piece by pediatrician Dr. Mayte Figueroa, she celebrates the changing work-life integration that occurs through various career stages as contributing to the daily and overall sense of achievement and enjoyment [39]. The Austrian cohort also felt however that early recognition and management of stress, boredom, personal overload, and family-work conflict was important for continued engagement and fulfillment [103].

"To achieve a measure of inner peace with our roles, sacrifices, and decisions, women should realize that our bodies are different from those of men physically, hormonally, and mentally; learn to embrace these differences; cherish our roles; set realistic expectations; and take pride in our individuality. It eventually comes together in unexpected ways, with unforeseen twists and turns. That's the beauty of life. Motherhood is an important role for those who take that road, but it's best savored in stages" [85].

Academic Advancement and Mentorship

Challenges to successfully integrate work and home life for women in academic medicine appear to be deeply embedded in today's professional culture and include the stigma attached to taking advantage of work flexibility (timing and work location) that has been made available and the lack of adequate mentorship [109].
My husband is in the academic tenure track line, with all its research and publication timeline requirements, but I couldn't imagine I was going to be happy there. First of all, there were no women in the tenure track in my division, so it must be impossible. And so here I am, 10 years later, and still an assistant professor in the clinical educator line. I am so busy in clinic and teaching, I don't have any time to even think about writing up my research, and they sure aren't giving me anyone to help. I feel so guilty about having to ration my time between work and the kids. I feel I have been left behind! No one is really looking out for me. I think I am

going to leave academia and go into private practice; for all the
time I am putting in I would certainly make more money...

Many medical schools offer work flexibility and for a variety of
reasons, women often end up in tracks that may make academic
advancement more challenging. Of 83 medical schools that offer
a clinician educator track (CET), which includes primarily inpatient and outpatient care and medical education rather than the
expectation of publishing high-quality data in peer-reviewed
medical and scientific journals, 77% of them reported that significantly more women than men pursued this option. Of the 102
medical schools offering the traditional tenure track, 80% have a
higher proportion of males engaged. Although many institutions
claim to value their CET faculty, tenure track professors are twice
as likely to be promoted. Not surprisingly, faculty in the CET,
mostly women, were more likely to leave academia and seek
employment elsewhere [119].

A survey to explore *barriers to advancement*, sent to 1456
clinical and research faculty at or above the rank of assistant professor faculty at a large Midwestern academic Institution, identified work overload and lack of self-advocacy skills as significant
challenges. Forty-two percent responded to the survey and women
faculty, especially clinicians, reported that the demands of their
current positions prevented them from adopting additional roles,
despite how desirable they might be or important they were to
advancement. These women also reported that acknowledgment
of their work and support from leadership required considerable
efforts in self-promotion [35], a skill that may remain societally
underdeveloped in woman in general and female faculty specifically. A lack of leaning into promotions and leadership roles
because of work-life concerns, work roles, work overload, and
organizational factors appears to be more of a factor for female
clinical faculty rather than female research faculty [34].

The additional time spent by academic women physicians on
household duties and childcare was found to compete primarily
with flexible research hours [59]. Given that research, grant acqui-

sition, and publications are so critical to advancement in the academic arena, this may significantly curtail the academic success of talented, competent, and motivated women. Furthermore, due to the poor appreciation of work-home conflicts by their male colleagues and superiors, policy changes that would allow women to integrate and thrive in both realms are often not even considered at some institutions [59]. A decrease in faculty applying for academic promotion overall, and the underrepresentation of women compared to men in senior leadership, independent of policy awareness, may challenge that assumption and underscore that these supposed family-friendly policies are simply not meeting the needs of women physicians. There is, however, evidence of a shift toward recognizing the importance of work-life flexibility and increasing awareness of the need to address gender differences in life-work conflict. For example, attempts to identify and remedy *gender-biased descriptors* in letter of recommendation have resulted in a noted equalization of hiring at the assistant professor level at some institutions [116].

While many academic medical schools have valuable stop-the-clock programs and other supports in place to help support woman in their academic goals and improve work-home integration, women are often reluctant to utilize them for fear of perpetuating stereotypes that unfairly stigmatize women. There is a perception, for example, that men who leave work to attend a soccer game are viewed differently from women who do the same [109]. In a study of faculty at a large American medical school by Becket and colleagues, balancing career and family obligations posed significant challenges for both women and men. Interestingly, in their study, they found no differences in satisfaction across gender or faculty rank in clinical and non-clinical faculty [10]. Nevertheless, women physicians were more likely to report that conflicts between work and family might contribute to a decision to leave academic medicine than men (32% versus 18%). It is important to note that for women, reaching the associate professor rank was associated with greater career satisfaction than it was for men. But despite women entering careers in academic medicine in greater numbers than men, they are more likely to leave academic medicine before achieving the rank of associate or full professor [90]. Likewise, a study of biomedical PhDs highlighted that women who had a child within 5 years of taking a tenure track faculty position were significantly less likely to make tenure than their male counterparts [79]. More than 10 years later, a recent study showed that women in medicine are still more likely to leave academic medicine before achieving the rank of associate full professor than men [56]. Over the years, many medical schools developed *flexible policies attempting to reducework-life conflicts*. As of 10 years ago almost half of schools offered probationary periods beyond 8 years for clinical or basic science faculty as well as the ability to stop the tenure clock for childcare, medical disability, or care of an ill or elderly family member. However, part-time employment options are offered less frequently to tenure tract faculty, with only a third offering this opportunity [20]. Recently even more flexible career policies have been offered by several top medical schools; however, *low utilization of these policies* has been noted, indicating they do not meet the true needs of faculty. Reasons for not taking advantage of these options include *financial barriers, perceptions regarding commitment, and concerns about colleagues left with a greater burden*. At UC Davis, for example, despite the school's efforts to broadly communicate the many family-friendly policies that exist, there is still considerable underuse. Although the number of women in the biomedical sciences taking the maximum 12-week maternity leave tripled, the percentage of women who took less than 4 weeks remained the same, again raising concern that awareness may not be widespread or women are concerned they may be stigmatized and face repercussions [116]. Increased support, encouragement, and normalization of using flexible policies may be essential to support the academic advancement of women physicians.

In an older study, less than 20% of highly productive academic pediatricians were women. Among over 4000 pediatric faculty at 126 academic pediatric departments, women reported having *less protected time* and working fewer hours (60 vs 64 hours) weekly than males. Among instructors and assistant professors, women spent significantly more time teaching and in direct patient care (40 hours vs 35 hours weekly) and less time in research (15 hours vs 20 hours per week). This was perceived to be a consequence of receiving less protected time and decreased access to research space provided by their leaders [61]. A more recently published study of over 1200 faculty at 24 US medical schools over 17 years attempted to identify factors predicting academic promotion, retention, and attainment of senior leadership positions. Gender differences still remain with women less likely to reach senior levels compared to men, even adjusting for numbers of publications [24]. Examining overall career productivity in academic physicians, women publish about a third fewer articles than men and their h-index remains lower throughout their work-life. In their later years however, their productivity increased and was equal or greater than their male counterparts. It appears that whereas women may have been deterred from academic advancement because of *greater family responsibilities* and additional factors explored previously, they were often able to make up for that later in their careers if they remained in academia [36, 99].

In their study of Viennese women physicians, the dearth of *women in senior leadership positions* led to significant underrepresentation of their individual and collective voices and opinions in policy and decision-making. The lack of networking or encouraging role models and same-sex mentoring for younger women may decrease their motivation to aim for top careers in medicine. Conversely, implementation of these opportunities was considered crucial to academic advancement. Effective faculty mentoring and fellowship activities promoting networks of similarly academically productive colleagues having frequent discussions about projects and grants were considered essential for academic achievement. For women, more so than men, this was challenging to develop and engage in and took time from their highly valued family life; thus, their networking was less efficient. An early anticipation and planning for academic advancement and consideration of flexible timelines was also deemed important for the advancement of women [103]. Given that gender preferences and practices regarding work-life integration affect time dedicated to clinical, educational, and research efforts, and very likely contribute to the variances in retention and academic advancement, it is important to be aware of family leave policies where one works. This was previously explored in the section on family responsibilities.

> "Tricia, (AKA Dr. Patricia Rose) would you like to be a mentor for Dr. Kirby?" "Who me? I never had a mentor; can't I have one??"

In the latest data currently tabulated by the AAMC, 2015, only 15.9% of department chairs in academic medicine were women [2]. As such there are few *effective role models* for women physicians who may enter medicine aspiring to advanced leadership roles but who also place value on creating and participating in a fulfilling family life. It is not surprising then that although women may enter medicine with goals of academic advancement, they are not as successful as their male colleagues and there is significant attrition along the way. In addition to fewer female role models and mentors, the generational values and the quality of mentorship from male role models and mentors are important. Several years ago, women at one academic institution cited a lack of role modeling on how to combine career and home life and deal with the research frustrations and an institutional culture that appeared to favor men [69]. Although currently there is an appreciation of the emotional and psychological support women often receive from male mentors, in Strong's 2013 examination of narratives of physician-researchers and mentors, the lack of real life strategies and advice about how "to do it," that is, specifically and successfully manage to integrate work and home life, was notable lacking "as they never had to deal with it" [109].

Valentine and Sandborg from Stanford highlighted early on that the lack of women physician role models in leadership positions relays a clear message that women must choose between academic advancement and their personal life. "Even more pernicious is that this message creates a vicious cycle of inequity and transforms our robust pipeline into a funnel" [114].

Seventy-five percent of medical schools offer mentoring for their female students, but even at this level of training the quality of mentoring has been highlighted as a concern, with women medical students reporting less satisfaction (42% vs 53%) than their male counterparts. This dichotomy represents a significant challenge as both job satisfaction and career advancement rely heavily on effective mentorship; in fact, the presence of a good mentor has been shown to double a physician's chance of promotion [9]. In general, mentors who are cognizant and skilled in adapting to the gender-related needs of mentees will contribute to the retention and development of women in academic medicine, expanding leadership diversity and capacity [12].

Given these findings, a *mentoring program*, which began with a robust Mentee Needs Assessment Form, was created specifically for junior women faculty at Wake Forest School of Medicine. Mentorship included discussion on career development, research, promotion seeking, available administrative resources/services, and well-being. Not surprisingly, significant benefits included promotions, grant applications/awards, articles, presentations, and professional memberships [117].

At the Mayo Clinic, where there were not enough senior women physicians to mentor junior women, a facilitated peer mentorship pilot was developed. Senior women physicians with significant experience acted as facilitators for a group of junior women, who then served as their own peer mentors. Participants in the pilot program benefited from more published papers, skills acquisition, and promotion in academic rank [81].

Role modeling and exposure are critical to academic advancement. Departmental and divisional leaders, mentors, and sponsors are increasingly trying to combat a much tweeted about occurrence, conference "manels," or *male-dominated panels*. Not unique to medicine, this refers to the persistent and pervasive gender bias in those invited to present or sit on expert panels at conferences and other events. For example, between 2010 and 2015 every annual critical care conference was male dominated, and other specialties report a similar pattern [84]. Women, especially those in early training, need to see other women in these positions in order to envision themselves in similar situations. Many conference organizers are making efforts to invite and include women to take part and increasingly male academicians are refusing to participate unless women are present. Although some may consider it patronizing being the token women given these efforts, the effect on members of the female audience is nonetheless important and essential in normalizing the diversity and eliminating bias.

> "Hey Maria, you going to cocktail hour?" "No, Mario, my daughter has afterschool ballet and my son has soccer, so I am going to pick them up, and get dinner going, but say hi to the chief for me."

Social capital is an important factor in professional advancement in many realms. Women physicians in particular, because of the already long hours, tend to engage less in the informal networking that frequently takes place in after-hours meetings and gatherings as it often interferes with homelife and childcare [103]. This is where garnering important relationships and sponsorships takes place, however. Strong and supportive mentorship relationships with well-placed individuals, as well as connections with powerful networks, help propel women by allowing her efforts to build social capital to proceed far more efficiently [33]. Informal networks often connect physicians with legitimate sponsors in positions of power who are able to advocate for one's career advancement and promotion in various ways, including provision of protected time and workload [53]. In the corporate world, having sponsors significantly increased advancement of women into upper levels of leadership [111]. In medicine, it appears that men are more likely to have these resources than women. Social capital is important for professional advancement and promotion, and men are more likely than women to invest in and use these informal but powerful networks.

Self-Advocacy, Setting Limits, and Self-Care

"I don't understand why I didn't get asked to apply for that position. I didn't even know they were looking for someone. Here I am killing myself at work. I am on two committees, I'm precepting (now I have PA students in addition to the med student), I am teaching a class (with no support I might add), I just finished up a chapter, and a journal article, and presented at a national conference. I just don't get it." "Ya, but did they know all that??"

Women are socialized to introduce their suggestions as questions, in an effort to promote consensus and avoid appearing forward or abrasive [58]. Whereas exercising power and volubility in meetings can be very effective for men, studies show that women can be penalized for such behaviors [15]. As such, *self-perpetuating cycles* ultimately develop as these socialized behaviors are adopted: as women physicians soften their edges, they may appear less competent and promotable. This can lead to women doubting their own capabilities and contributing or deepening their sense of *imposter syndrome*. Imposter syndrome is characterized by self-doubt and fear of being found out as an intellectual fraud. Women in medicine are plagued by imposter syndrome more often than their male counterparts [89]. It can lead to hypervigilance and overwork and decreased time for self-care, and understandably it is highly associated with psychological stress and burnout. Ariana Huffington, in her book, *Thrive*, describes how imposter syndrome can drive women to overcompensate by working harder and longer. Woman too often feel they do not "belong" in what traditionally has been a boys' club atmosphere and their overwork may help them feel that they fit in and allow them to gain a measure of security. This may be tantamount to a Pyrrhic victory, however, as overextending themselves at work negatively impacts their health (e.g., through lack of sleep), which then negatively affects their performance [55].

Although women who become physicians are often highly driven, ambitious, and resilient, characteristics that align with success in their profession, they may also be less skilled at and *less likely to self-advocate*. The "unnaturalness" and effort required to self-promote often leads to lack of notice or acknowledgment of their work [35]. Putting oneself up for opportunities, having established name recognition, and knowing people can lead to collaboration and career advancement opportunities are often lacking in women. In mixed gender environments, in order to maintain or promote relationship prospects, women tend to minimize ambitions and salary expectations [21]. Viennese academic women leaders, in an attempt to understand the general lack of women in leadership, additionally described a tendency to poor self-assessment and understatement, with inadequate presentation of skills, personality, and successes, as potential barriers to medical career advancement. Women physicians tended to underplay the softer "female" skills of empathy, grit, and resilience, as well as their ability to function well within teams, and encouraged a greater appreciation and valuing of these skills, which are increasingly recognized as valuable leadership qualities [103].

> Lucky for us...(unspoken)... "you don't have kids, is it ok if I put you on call over the holidays? Jack and Tom were planning on taking their families skiing."

Women physicians often *struggle with setting limits*. For example, despite committing more time to domestic and child-rearing duties, a Swedish study of female physicians reported that women were more likely to show up to work despite being unwell (sickness presenteeism) than their male colleagues. The inability to effectively set limits becomes apparent when examining their reasons for doing so, that is, "concern for others and workload," cited significantly more often by women than men [48].

> "Sandy, you need to get help!" "There is no way I am going to do that. As soon as I admit I am depressed my licensing fiasco starts. And I think it might give my chief more ammunition to further ostracize me. I can do this but I admit, I'm scared, I can barely get up in the morning these days."

Mood disorders and **mental health concerns** can both contribute to and be exacerbated by work-life conflicts. Although matriculating medical students have fewer depressive symptoms than comparable undergraduates, by their second year this pattern is reversed [32]. There is a significant increase in depressive symptoms for both women and men during the internship year, though statistically significantly greater for women versus men (PHQ–9 increase of 3.2 vs 2.5). *Accounting for work-family conflict decreased this difference by a third.* Support at home has been shown to significantly reduce work-life conflicts [82], and when fathers are provided with, and take, paternity leave, maternal post-partum physical health complications and mental health status are significantly improved [94].

Female physicians are 2.2 times more likely to die by suicide than female nonphysicians. Promoting self-care, addressing work-life integration, and providing mental health support are essential, not only to support women in medicine but to allow them to thrive. Overt efforts to address and decrease both work-life conflict and depression may also promote retention and advancement of women in academic medicine [49] and contribute to the diversity of successful role models for subsequent generations.

> "So how is your NEST? (Nutrition, Exercise, Sleep, Time to be/ Time management). You know how important it is to get your rainbow-colored fruits and vegetables daily; how about your aerobic exercise and stretching? Yoga is good for that. And don't forget strengthening, so important. And Sleep- you need 8 hours a night, time to clear out all that metabolic waste among other things (cancer risk, memory issues, infections). And no iPhone or computer for an hour before, right? Do you have the CBTi app? And you know, there is so much known now about the need to just "be". Meditation is so good for you; do you have that Headspace or Calm app?" "Hmm, I don't know doc, do you do all that yourself?"

The pressures and expectations of the medical profession may lead women to unwittingly sacrifice their own well-being and that of their family in order to meet the needs of their patients and the often-unarticulated expectations of the profession. Self-care, including getting adequate sleep, exercise, good nutrition, and time for reflection, can often be seen as selfish but is in fact essential to providing the kind of patient care that women physicians aspire to provide. For example, in a New Zealand study of trainees, women residents were more likely than their male counterparts to report never/rarely waking refreshed and suffering from excessive sleepiness [42]. Acute sleep deprivation creates challenges in committing to regular activities outside of work, being too fatigued to maintain these activities; disruptive night and weekend shift work and having to study while working were additional work patterns that negatively affected life away from work and contributed to a lack of time for partners, children, and families [42].

Whereas residents and early career faculty may be sleep deprived from overnight shifts and youngsters at home, women in the later stages of their career who may be traversing perimenopause may be sleep deprived due to a number of other factors. The emotional dysregulation resulting from *poor sleep* can make the challenge of work-life integration even harder, as is dealing with potentially hormonal and dysregulated teenagers. Add a threatened marital relationship and work-life integration is further jeopardized. Women physicians in *late career stages* are often at a crossroads. They have accumulated a vast experience and wisdom in their clinical/research/educational endeavors, potentially reached positions of leadership, and may be in supportive primary relationships or past the turmoil of ending them. However, they may also be both caring for their parents and caring for or launching their older children, in the midst of experiencing unexpected perimenopausal hormonal changes and symptoms. Ageism is a known entity in America, and not much is written or shared about these particular struggles, which often remain a personal journey due to lack of time for social connection, embarrassment, or shame. At the same time, women physician at this stage are also looking ahead and deciding how to reconcile the challenges of their medical careers with the desires for a healthy, fulfilling, and meaningful future (see Chap. 17 on late career solutions).

Solutions and Resources

Organizational and Practice-Based Solutions: Flexible Hours, Workflow, Extended Tracks, etc.

- Offer residency couple match for medical students in relationships.
- Offer shift work and job sharing for residents and faculty with small children. For example, the American Board of Family Medicine has clear guidelines for shared or part-time residency training.

- Focus early on gender bias and confidence building within the medical school curriculum such that certain specialties are not considered by women to be out of reach [92].
- In recruitment of dual-physician couples offer tandem recruiting for faculty such that both hiring units or departments synchronously engage in the recruiting process so that both partners feel equally valued. Fund spouses using a combination of funds from both departments with additional support from the deans and/or provost office [96].
- Offer high-quality mentorship; for example, the Doris Duke charitable fund has provided support to medical schools to make mentorship more available and increase career development opportunities for physicians in the early stage of their career.
- Prioritize educating senior faculty on the unique challenges facing women physicians in integrating career and home life while navigating their institution's advancement and promotions pathway [9]. Facilitate discussion groups and have women from this cohort on the A&P committee, with protected time.
- Use a Mentee Needs Assessment Form to individualize the mentoring relationship [117].
- Offer generous parental leave for residents. Some progress: The Board of Plastic Surgery has proposed modifying their requirement of 48 weeks of training per year to 94 weeks in the final 2 years, thus providing for two additional weeks off.
- Destigmatize parental leave policies for both parents—make utilization the expected norm. Offer guaranteed temporary replacement for physicians on leave [88].
- Provide adequate (sufficient, nearby, hygienic) lactation facilities at all clinical sites [63]. No more pumping in dirty bathrooms! Or provide the time to walk to another building. Provide the amenities required for efficient, clean, private pumping including on-site pumps.
- Make efforts to reduce maternal discrimination, through raising awareness, education, and bias training as well as deliberate appreciation and support of women physicians who are also mothers, with explicit workplace changes including longer paid maternity leave, backup childcare, and support for breastfeeding [6].

- Offer high-quality affordable on-site childcare as well as on-site backup sick childcare facilities, with extended hours for night shifts and conferences.
- Eliminate compensation practices that dis-incentivize practitioners from using vacation time [105].
- Offer financial advising resources regarding school debt, mortgages, etc. [87].
- Offer (but don't insist) *flexible and extended clinic hours*, which also maximizes use of space.
- Create programs to retrain women and men who wish to return to medicine after taking time off to care for children [62].
- Address gendered stereotypes, for example, by recognizing when it happens and raising awareness [121] and advocating for education that address socially constructed gender-based assumptions that negatively influence the medical careers of female physicians [22].
- Offer transparent and equitable compensation and bonus plans.
- Offer concierge health services for faculty.
- Fund (FTE and Budget) departmental or divisional wellness directors, who work to improve the work-life experience of their faculty and can also work to make changes that appeal to diverse faculty.
- Offer videoconferencing and telemedicine for improved work-life integration.
- Offer EMR Concierge training to all physicians, often!
- Provide high-quality transcription services (e.g., Dragon DMO) which allows you to dictate into/through your own phone, at work, at home, on the road.
- Provide reliable, well-trained, and experienced scribes.
- Expand AI to perform mundane tasks and free up time for physicians to work at the top of their licensure [70].
- Cover the costs of clinical licensing, board (re)certification, DEA, conferences required to maintain licensure, and conferences at which physicians are presenting.
- "Clock stopping" for their tenure track faculty, for example, the NIH has recognized this priority and automatically extends "early investigator status" allowing women researchers to

apply for additional support without penalties if they give birth during their grant period.

- Include a diversity and inclusion review of institutional educational programs, panels, and hiring practices to ensure women and minorities are adequately recruited and represented.
- Proactively identify qualified women, for example, looking at lists like those of fellows and editors, so that all those in positions to provide sponsorship can easily identify women who might otherwise not immediately come to mind; apply a "Rooney Rule" equivalent, already adopted by the National Football League, requiring that minority candidates at least be included among those considered for a senior position [64].
- Offer leadership programs to faculty; we are all leaders and benefit from the multitude of skills offered starting with self-awareness, values clarification, etc.
- Discourage "sickness presenteeism" by providing adequate coverage that would mitigate concerns of overtaxing colleagues, as well as schedule templates that allow for timely rescheduling of patients.
- Given that women tend to devote a good portion of their "extra time" to family care, rather than reserving it for grant writing, provide a grant office and admin staff that can better cater to their needs/time schedules [9].
- Promote men and women faculty equitably, timely, efficiently, and transparently.
- Sponsor/pay for high-quality childcare at faculty and professional meetings/conferences [59, 71].
- Schedule meetings and committee work during work hours, not before or after the day, or during lunch.
- In addition to mentors, offer sponsors who are in positions of power to advocate publicly for the advancement of women in academia [111].
- Leaders should take advantage of practice improvement processes that have been successfully implemented in other organizations. The AMA STEPS Forward website highlights many resources and modules for physicians in general with a host of

topics/real-life examples, such as addressing the EHR and in-basket restructuring and how to efficiently manage the in-basket, engaging and empowering the entire team, improving work culture and workflow, the use of huddles, strengthening working relationships to improve practice efficiency, appreciative inquiry around fostering positive culture, protecting against burnout, and fostering self-care: https://edhub.ama-assn.org/steps-forward/pages/professional-well-being.

- Organizations should recognize the subtle ways in which women are socialized to behave in public spaces that can prevent them from being recognized for their contributions and be proactive about setting rules and norms that seeks to recognize women physicians for excellent work. Offer education to bring awareness and counter such behavior and allocate resources toward leadership training on these issues to both genders.

- Work closely with local, state, and federal agencies and legislatures to develop policies that support institutional, cultural, and individual efforts, for example, shifting from volume-based to value-based care reimbursement models, eliminating questions about mental health diagnoses from medical license renewal, financial credits to organizations that provide paid parental care and on-site day care, eliminating barriers to telehealth models, etc.

Examples of Practice-Based Programs Offered at Various Institutions

- The New York-Presbyterian Hospital, in addition to medically necessary time off for a woman giving birth, employees, including residents, can take 6 weeks of paid parental leave for the primary care-giving parent and 2 weeks for the secondary parent. This is available to all parents, women and men, whether for birth, adoption, or surrogacy.

- Stanford University offers Child Care Subsidies and Assistance, based on income. It offers Junior Faculty up to $1000 as a Dependent Care Grant for expenses incurred when travelling to professional meetings/conferences. They offer an emergency and backup dependent care for kids and for elderly both in home and in center with copay: https://stanford.app.box.com/s/0a16dfy52pu3s8wtf0sexdiaw2heb4u5. They maintain a comprehensive database for self-pay services such as nannies, babysitters for evenings and weekends, discounts and preferential enrollment in certain day cares, Test prep, tutoring, pet sitters, house keepers, Elder Care resources/referrals, and free social worker consultation.

- Christiana Health offers 12 weeks of paid paternity leave for all faculty and residents.
- Stanford's "time bank" program (initially a department-wide pilot, currently only continued by the Stanford Emergency Medicine program) provides options to participate in service work (filling in last minute, taking an extra shift, mentoring, serving on committees, or deploying in emergencies) to collect time bank credits. Credits can be used to free up time to spend with family and get help with grant writing, free meals, house cleaning, and eldercare. (Credits cost "far less" than 1% of the budget.) The department also pays for medical scribes.
- Stanford's Emergency Medicine residency program has a transparent return to work policy for new parents—no overnight shifts, no sick call, and no more than three shifts in a row while fully staffing clinical sites [46].
- University of California,Davis, created a Women in Medicine and Health Science Advisory Board, which develops programs to retain women in the early career stages as well as attract more mid-career and senior women faculty members. They have an annual leadership with the intent of investing in and cultivating women's careers in academia and growing them into leaders [116].
- The AAMC's Group of Women in Medicine and Science (GWIMS) offers a 2-volume toolkit with a variety of excellent presentations that speak to "Leveraging your Career" (Vol 1) and "Institutional Strategies for Advancing Women in Medicine" (Vol 2) https://www.aamc.org/members/gwims/toolkit/343518/toolkithometsr.html.

- Stanford Family Medicine extended its hours, now open 7 am to 7 pm, providing flexibility for both patients (more afterhours availability for the employed and students), physicians (increased flexibility to get kids to school in the morning by shifting clinics later or be there to pick them up after school by shifting clinics earlier), and staff (who often commute very long distances and now had the option of working fewer longer shifts, cutting down on commute hours, and helping with retention).
- In June 2018, the American Society for Radiation Oncology (ASTRO) adopted a new policy to provide on-site childcare at its annual meeting.
- The Stanford Division of Primary Care and Population Health provides funding for a Director of Faculty Wellness as well as a budget for activities that increase wellness and professional fulfillment. Clinic-based wellness champions help decide what works for them, for example, funds for wellness-based conferences, physician health coaching, leadership coaching, babysitting dollars for date night, healthy snacks, exercise equipment, "commensality" dinners, and Physicians and Literature groups/Narrative Medicine/Balint meeting. A divisional website lists resources and events and highlights wellness activities of its faculty.

Cultural (Supportive Networks, Mother's Groups, Reducing Stigma Regarding Help Seeking, Sharing Stories)

- Provide divisional or clinic-based funding for activities that increase wellness, decided upon by faculty or wellness directors/champions, for example, additional funds for wellness-based conferences, physician health coaching, leadership coaching, babysitting for date night, healthy snacks, exercise equipment, Physicians and Literature groups/Narrative Medicine/Balint group).
- Support each other in taking a stance against microaggression.
- Support each other with interventions to foster resilience among women physicians, for example, SPACE.

- Training to recognize early sign of depression, normalization of mental health counselling, supportive debriefs and check-ins after near miss events of patient deaths, disaster efforts, etc.
- Offer social gatherings for faculty that include activities for young families/children.
- Provide funding and time for faculty-invested and faculty-led practice improvement projects.
- Consider joining a Physician Mothers social media group.

Examples of Programs that Promote a Culture of Wellness Offered by Some Institutions

- Departmental, divisional, or clinic-based funding for wellness directors and funds for activities that promote a culture of wellness (not specific to women) (e.g., in the Stanford Division of Primary Care, bringing together young families, "Spring Fling"; in Primary Care and the associated University Health Alliance "Commensality"/"Comraderie" gatherings, monthly small group paid dinner gatherings of 6–8 faculty, loosely facilitated, with the first 20 minutes dedicated to a topic of physician-hood with each member given time to share; Physicians and Literature groups/Narrative Medicine gatherings/Balint groups).
- Authentic connections: https://authenticconnectionsgroups. org, facilitated colleague support groups for women fostering collegiality, which significantly lowered depression and global symptoms, with notable improvement in self-compassion, feeling loved, physical affection received, and parenting stress [72]. It was first tested at the Mayo Clinic in Arizona as a means of reducing burnout among physicians, physician assistants, and nurse practitioners, all of whom are mothers.
- Mayo Clinic in Arizona offers facilitated support groups for women (six women per group) that occur during working hours (e.g., 8–9 am), offer CME credit, and are supported by use of a single trip day for the 8 weekly sessions.
- Christiana Care Health System in Delaware offers small group coaching cohorts for women physician leaders. Additionally, although not aimed specifically to women they host COMPASS

(Clinician-Organized Meetings to Promote and Sustain Satisfaction), the goal of which is to encourage physician collegiality, shared experience, mutual support, and meaning in work to decrease burnout and promote well-being. Each COMPASS group consists of 6–8 physicians who meet over a 6-month period to share a meal while a facilitator leads discussion on topics such as medical mistakes and the wounded healer, personal and professional balance, and finding sources of meaning.

- Although not aimed only at women, but heavily women subscribed, Stanford University School of Medicine's Department of Medicine offers facilitated faculty groups that promote a culture of wellness and collegiality called SPACE ("Tending your Nest" and "Making SPACE for What Matters Most) with a goal of enabling physician participants to develop *skills, behaviors, and attitudes* that promote *physical, emotional, and professional well-being* and contribute to their *resilience and leadership potential*: http://medicine.stanford.edu/faculty/professionalDevelopment.html.
- UCSF is starting facilitated learning/support groups for women physicians aimed at creating community/support and well-being at work and developing skills in self-advocacy. The book *How Women Rise* (Sally Helgesen and Marshal Goldsmith), about women in the workplace, is a focal point.

Individual-Personal Wellness: Self-Care, Self-Advocacy, and Limit Setting

- Know (and celebrate) that you are worth it!
- Acknowledge that times have changed, and your life and job depend on taking care of and standing up for your most valuable asset—*You*!
- Build and prioritize your NEST (nutrition, exercise, sleep, and time management) to make SPACE for What Matters Most to you (∗Stanford SPACE © program). Keep a calendar and schedule in sleep, movement, and exercise, in addition to your meetings, conferences, call schedule, vacations, and the birthdays of those you love!

- Seek out effective mentors (and more than one!).
- Premeds—If you have decided early to pursue medicine, do your research—don't be surprised when you get to the application phase, or medical school, by those who have been planning for years. If it is important to you or you have a specific specialty in mind, optimize your resume/CV with competitive standardized test scores (i.e., take the time out to dedicate to preparation time if you can, others do!), pursue leadership experiences that you enjoy (beyond just showing up: lead but develop new ideas/directions; can you leave a legacy?), pursue shadowing experiences, and find or create opportunities to be involved with publications.
- Medical students—if your well-being includes entry into a certain specialty, ensure the appropriate rotations early enough and aggressively seek out effective role models and sponsors. If you anticipate your career path may include an academic focus, identify and speak to mentors you hope to emulate early on and make a plan for academic advancement that includes planning for relationships and family building. Seek out opportunities/information/seminars on career planning, exploring flex time, and flexible career structures [18].
- Medical students—Consider the couple match if you are in a strong relationship.
- Residents—The American Medical Association (AMA) divides resident well-being into six, evidenced-based categories: nutrition, fitness, emotional health, financial health, preventative care, and mindset and behavioral adaptability. Devote time to seek out classes, conferences, and programs that teach and promote these. Practice them! Partner with others for support and hold one another accountable.

- Take advantage of programs to help manage the stress of medicine including:
    - Learning and practicing interpersonal skills that increase the availability of social support
  - Appropriate prioritization of personal, work, and educational demands

- Techniques to increase stamina and attend to self-care needs
- Recognition and avoidance of maladaptive responses
  - Positive outlook skills/focus on values, meaning.

- The AMA has amalgamated resources in their STEPS Forward program: https://edhub.ama-assn.org/steps-forward.
- Read the chapter Self-Care, Resilience, and Work-Life Balance by Worley and Stonnington in Physician Mental Health and Well-Being- Research and Practice. Kirk J. Brower, Michelle B. Riba Editors Page 238–258- many excellent resources!
- Take pride in the softer "female" skills including the ability to function well within team, grit, resilience, and empathy (Schueller- Weidekamm el al. 2012). The Mayo Clinic has a yearly GRIT Conference. Get a group together and go!
- If you marry, choose a supportive spouse! One who is knowledgeable and understanding of your commitments and shares your values. Engage early and frequently with your partner regarding your career goals, family plans, daily grrs, and victories. One who will help with household duties and childcare. Have discussions early regarding shared decision-making, role clarity, reasonable expectations, and acknowledging the benefits that living with a doctor, or both being doctors, brings to the marriage [93].
- If you have a partner, schedule date night/time alone—just do it! Take advantage of institutional support for personal time; for example, the Stanford Primary Care Director of Wellness has a budget that among other things financially supports date night.
- Take advantage of parental leave (for both partners). Educate yourself about your organization's policies and negotiate (and advocate) for paid and even unpaid time off—10 years from now you will rarely regret taking time off, but you may regret leaving time on the table.
- Encourage your partner to take advantage of parental leave.
- Engage with your peers for support and resources regarding childbirth, childcare, domestic help, and fun things to do outside of work.
- Seek help from extended family but educate yourself and take advantage of employer-based benefits.

- Consider extending the roles of your home help—shopping, meal prep, cooking, cleaning, personal assistance.
- Meal prep services—there are many, with a variety of options (daily, 3 times a week, weekly, some prep, full prep, vegan, vegetarian, etc.).
- Consider shared jobs with other residents or physicians in a similar situation.
- Engage with mentors and leaders to consider and strategically plan temporary career breaks to prioritize child-rearing in a manner that will minimize academic disruption to academic promotion and career development. Make efforts to normalize this.
- Consider and negotiate flexible hours. Extending the use of office space to earlier or later hours, if that suits you, may also be a smart use of already existing space. Flexible hours for an MA or an extra MA costs little compared to losing or significantly curtailing the hours of a physician.
- Advocate for increased physician control in the workplace; participate in process improvement projects that support work-life integration and wellness (we just did one called Wanted: Healthy and Delicious Lunches for Faculty and Staff Meetings—wow what a success—problem now is that we are overeating because the food is so delicious!!).
- Say yes to breaking up manels (male-dominated panels).
- Engage with your institution and colleagues to recognize, call out, and take a stance against implicit bias and microaggression toward yourself and others. Offer implicit bias training.
- Live close to work to minimize commute and stress from traffic.
- Ask for and take part in a physician leadership program, early.

Examples of Wellness Programs Offered by Some US Institutions

- Johns Hopkins Medical School has instituted physical and emotional wellness programs for medical students, residents, and fellows to prevent burnout. Their website is replete with resources: http://wellness.som.jhu.edu/.
- Stanford has a general trainee website with wellness information and resources: http://med.stanford.edu/gme/housestaff/all-topics/wellness.html.

- Stanford's Surgery and Anesthesia department has also aimed efforts at preventing and addressing resident burnout. The Surgery department created Balance in Life (BIL), a holistic, multifaceted program with the primary aim of educating about and facilitating physical and mental health among resident trainees. They link residents to mentorship and social events, provide access to healthy food, and have mandatory time-protected meetings with a psychologist exploring difficult conversations and situations, as well as access to individual sessions.
- The Stanford Medicine Residency Program has faculty encouraging and modeling exercise and socializing with residents in their REACH program (Resiliency, Education, Advocacy, Community, Health) (medicine: http://medicine.stanford.edu/2019-report/residency-training-with-a-side-of-wellness.html).
- Stanford's Emergency Medicine residency program offers their trainees customizable 12 hours of well-being credit that can take the place of their usual Wednesday conference. Some go for a hike; some try their hand at teaching. All residents are offered 12 free counselling sessions.
- The Stanford O'Conner Family Medicine residency has "Wellness Wednesdays" with a featured wellness topic during noon conference series. Additionally, they have a monthly evening Wellness Group meeting, protected time for first and second years and optional for final year residents, which includes dinner/debrief (45 mins) and a wellness topic/activity (45 mins). Residents also complete the MDI twice per year and receive 1:1 feedback session with their advisor, along with quarterly check-ins.
- Stanford/Lucille Packard Children's Hospital residents have a Wellness Curriculum which includes a humanism program http://med.stanford.edu/peds/prospective-applicants/resident-life/wellness.html. Additionally, weekly email announcements promote various events/activities. Social chairs and well-being chairs on their residency council take the lead on planning/advertising these events as well.
- Mayo Clinic Rochester, Arizona, and Florida campuses all support the "fellow and residents health and wellness initiative" FERSHAWI, with the aim of engaging trainees and

improving self-care, and to combat fatigue, stress, and low motivation among graduate medical trainees. The program includes art projects (watercolor painting, screen printing, and origami) as well as discussions of artwork and guided visual imagery. They have a monthly noontime conference reserved for "Humanities" Thursdays. The Florida Campus supports a quarterly wellness fair at the Florida campus where residents and fellows may participate in arts, chair massage, yoga, and Pilates, visit vendors to gather information such as healthy eating, etc., for a 3-hour period. The program won awards from the accreditation council for graduate medical education ACGME and shared their story in an online module within AMA's STEPS Forward™ collection of practice improvement strategies: https://edhub.ama-assn.org/steps-forward/module/2702541.

- Other residency wellness program successes are also highlighted on the AMA website: https://edhub.ama-assn.org/steps-forward/module/2702511.
- AMA STEPS Forward website has many resources and modules for physicians in general with a host of topics/real-life examples, such as how to efficiently manage your in-basket, engaging and empowering the entire team and improving work culture and workflow, huddles, strengthening working relationships and improving practice efficiency, appreciative inquiry around fostering positive culture, protecting against burnout and fostering self-care, addressing the EHR and in-basket restructuring, etc.: https://edhub.ama-assn.org/steps-forward/pages/professional-well-being.
- Although not gender specific, a one-time 8-hour training session "Relationship: Establishment, Development and Engagement" is offered by the Cleveland Clinic and shown to reduce physician burnout [17].
- The Cleveland Clinic offers peer coaching which aims to increase job satisfaction, engagement, resilience, and professional goal attainment.
- The Stanford University Department of Medicine "SPACE" program focuses on self-care professional fulfillment and leadership while promoting physician collegiality across divisions

(building your NEST: nutrition, exercise, sleep optimization, and time management so that you can make SPACE—through serenity, presence, appreciation, compassion, equanimity—for What Matters Most): http://medicine.stanford.edu/faculty/professionalDevelopment.html.

- Stanford has a website exploring microaggression and micro−/ cross-cultural communication: https://respect.stanford.edu/.
- There are many organizations and conferences that support women. For example, TOOER (Through Our Own Eyes Retreat) is a network of women physicians "dedicated to empowering ourselves to enact positive change in our personal lives, workplaces and communities; through continuing education activities with focus on incorporating self-care and well-being practices into all aspects of our careers in medicine." Their mission is to provide regular educational meetings with the following purposes: to develop, promote, and sustain a community of women physicians, dedicated to development of self-care and healing practices that support our work as healers, to provide a safe, nurturing space for women physicians to define their values and goals and to formulate a plan to live those values and attain those goals in their personal and professional lives, and to incorporate teachings that enhance our leadership and mentoring skills and enhance patient care: https://www.tooer.org/.
- Mayo Annual Conference: GRIT for Women in Medicine: Growth, Resilience, Inspiration, and Tenacity. Goal is to empower women in medicine (men invited too) with the skills and resources to remove barriers and bias of women in leadership positions specific to the challenges in healthcare. Leaders in business and healthcare present evidence-based strategies to promote professional development and enhance personal well-being. Addresses the growing need for improved clinician wellness and development for a gender-balanced leadership healthcare team. Participants learn to enhance communication with colleagues and team members to improve team-based care and to better manage conflict, identify symptoms of burnout in themselves and will be able to describe strategies to manage these symptoms, and formulate action plans to create and support a diverse healthcare team: https://gimeducation.

mayo.edu/store/GRIT-for-women-in-medicine-promote-
professional%20development-remove-bias-of-women-in-
leadership-in-healthcare.

Work-life conflict in medicine abounds, for both men and
women. Acknowledging and addressing these challenges from
various angles, personally, culturally, and institutionally (including government, licensing, and healthcare policies that are in synergy with organizational efforts) is essential. Taking personal
responsibility to care for oneself, although often monumentally
challenging, is paramount and of course more likely if there is
institutional support. Remaining open to opportunities to weave
together work and life, that is, using technology to accomplish
some work tasks while at home, and some home/life duties and
responsibilities while at work, that is, work-life integration, will
"allow us to come to work whole" (Logghe 2018) and help mitigate some of the challenges faced. While many institutions have
made significant commitment and inroads to lessoning work-life
conflict, some, for various reasons, have not. Heightening awareness and sharing of best practices is a first step to addressing some
of the inequities. Aligning institutional values with the personal
values that initially calls most individuals into medicine is imperative. Given the increased burden on women physicians over their
training and careers it is in fact a huge testament to their courage
and resilience that they have accomplished so much in medicine.
The goal now is to make this challenging and meaningful journey
one filled with significantly more resources and support such that
joy and celebration prevail every step of the way.

Bibliography

1. AAMC-1.   https://www.aamc.org/system/files/2019-11/2019_FACTS_
   Table_A-1.pdf.
2. AAMC-3.   https://www.aamc.org/download/481198/data/2015table9a.
   pdf.
3. AAMC-4.   https://www.aamc.org/download/321558/data/factstablec1.
   pdf.

4. Adám S, Györffy Z, Susánszky E. Physician burnout in Hungary: a potential role for work-family conflict. J Health Psychol. 2008;13(7):847–56. https://doi.org/10.1177/1359105308095055.

5. Adám S. High prevalence of work-family conflict among female physicians: lack of social support as a potential antecedent. Orv Hetil. 2009;150(50):2274–81. https://doi.org/10.1556/OH.2009.28583.Hungarian.

6. Adesoye T, Mangurian C, Choo EK, et al. Perceived discrimination experienced by physician mothers and desired workplace changes: a cross-sectional survey. JAMA Intern Med. 2017;177(7):1033–6. https://doi.org/10.1001/jamainternmed.2017.1394.

7. Aziz AA, Kahlout BH, Bashir K. Female physicians suffer a higher burnout rate: a 10-year experience of the Qatar EM Residency Training Programme. J Coll Physicians Surg Pak. 2018;28(8):651–2. https://doi.org/10.29271/jcpsp.2018.08.651. PMID: 30060800.

8. Baptiste D, Fecher A, Dolejs S, Yoder J, Schmidt M, Couch ME, Ceppa D. Gender differences in academic surgery, work-life balance, and satisfaction. J Surg Res. 2017;218:99–107. PMID: 28985884.

9. Beasley BW, Simon SD, Wright SM. A time to be promoted. The prospective study of promotion in academia (prospective study of promotion in academia). J Gen Intern Med. 2006;21(2):123–9. Epub 2005 Dec 7. PubMed PMID: 16336619; PubMed Central PMCID: PMC1484667.

10. Beckett L, Nettiksimmons J, Howell L, Villablanca AC. Do family responsibilities and a clinical versus research faculty position affect satisfaction with career and work–life balance for medical school faculty? J Women's Health. 2015;24(6):471.

11. Bering J, Pflibsen L, Eno C, Radhakrishnan P. Deferred personal life decisions of women physicians. J Womens Health (Larchmt). 2018;27(5):584–9. https://doi.org/10.1089/jwh.2016.6315. Epub 2018 Mar 12.

12. Bickel J. How men can excel as mentors of women. Acad Med. 2014;89(8):1100–2. https://doi.org/10.1097/ACM.0000000000000313.

13. Blithe SJ. Gender inequality in the academy: microaggressions, work-life conflict, and academic rank. J Gend Stud. https://doi.org/10.1080/09589236.2019.1657004.

14. Bohman B, Dyrbye L Sinsky D, Linzer M, Olson K, Babbott S, Murphy M, PP de Vries, Hamidi MS, Trockel M. Physician well-being: the reciprocity of practice efficiency, culture of wellness, and personal resilience. NEJM Catalyst April 2017.

15. Brescoll V. Who takes the floor and why: gender, power, and volubility in organizations. Adm Sci Q. 2011;56:622–41. https://doi.org/10.1177/0001839212439994GoogleScholar.

16. Brown AJ, Swinyard W, Ogle J. Women in academic medicine: a report of focus groups and questionnaires, with conjoint analysis. J Womens Health (Larchmt). 2003;12:999–1008.

17. Boissy A, Windover A, Bokar D, Karafa M, Neurendorf K, Frankel R, Merlino J, Rothberg M. Communication skills training for physicians improves patient satisfaction. J Gen Intern Med. 2016;31(7):755–61.
18. Buddeberg-Fischer B, Herta KD. Formal mentoring programmes for medical students and doctors–a review of the Medline literature. Med Teach. 2006;28(3):248–57. Review.
19. Buddeberg-Fischer B, Stamm M, et al. The impact of gender and parent-hood on physicians' careers – professional and personal situation seven years after graduation. BMC Health Serv Res. 2010;10:40. PubMed PMID: 20167075; PubMed Central PMCID: PMC2851709.
20. Bunton SA, Corrice AM. Evolving workplace flexibility for U.S. medical school tenure-track faculty. Acad Med. 2011;86(4):481–5. https://doi.org/10.1097/ACM.0b013e31820ce51d.
21. Bursztyn L, Fujiwara T, Pallais A. "Acting wife": marriage market incen-tives and labor market investments. Am Econ Rev. 2017;107:3288–319. https://doi.org/10.1257/aer.20170029GoogleScholar.
22. Carnes M. Commentary: deconstructing gender difference. Acad Med. 2010;85:575–7. [PubMed]. https://doi.org/10.1097/ACM.0b013e3181d983de.
23. Deliege D. The opinions of Belgian physicians about their practice. Cah Sociol Demogr Med. 2004;44:443–506.
24. Carr PL, Raj A, Kaplan SE, Terrin N, Breeze JL, Freund KM. Gender differences in academic medicine: retention, rank, and leadership com-parisons from the National Faculty Survey. Acad Med. 2018;93(11):1694–9.
25. Cassidy-Vu L, Beck K, Moore JB. Burnout in female faculty members. J Prim Care Community Health. 2017;8(2):97–9. https://doi.org/10.1177/2150131916669191. Epub 2016 Sep 21. PubMed PMID: 27650035; PubMed Central PMCID: PMC5932657.
26. Chatterji P, Markowitz S. Family leave after childbirth and the mental health of new mothers. J Ment Health Policy Econ. 2012;15(2):61–76.
27. Diamond R. Promoting sensible parenting policies: leading by example. JAMA. 2019;321(7):645–6. https://doi.org/10.1001/jama.2019.0460.
28. Dyrbye LN, Shanafelt TD, Balch CM, Satele D, Sloan J, Freischlag J. Relationship between work-home conflicts and burnout among Ameri-can surgeons: a comparison by sex. Arch Surg. 2011;146(2):211–7. https://doi.org/10.1001/archsurg.2010.310.
29. Dyrbye LN, West CP, Satele D, Sloan JA, Shanafelt TD. Work/home con-flict and burnout among academic internal medicine physicians. Arch Intern Med. 2011;171(13):1207–9. https://doi.org/10.1001/archin-ternmed.2011.289. PubMed PMID: 21747018.
30. Dyrbye LN, Varkey P, Boone SL, Satele DV, Sloan JA, Shanafelt TD. Phy-sician satisfaction and burnout at different career stages. Mayo Clin Proc. 2013;88(12):1358–67. https://doi.org/10.1016/j.mayocp.2013.07.016.

31. Dyrbye LN, Sotile W, Boone S, West CP, Tan L, Satele D, Sloan J, Ores-kovich M, Shanafelt T. A survey of U.S. physicians and their partners regarding the impact of work-home conflict. J Gen Intern Med. 2014;29(1):155–61. https://doi.org/10.1007/s11606-013-2581-3. Epub 2013 Sep 17. PubMed PMID: 24043567; PubMed Central PMCID: PMC3889954.

32. Dyrbye LN, West CP, Satele D, Boone S, Tan L, Sloan J, Shanafelt TD. Burnout among U.S. medical students, residents, and early career physicians relative to the general U.S. population. Acad Med. 2014;89(3):443–51. https://doi.org/10.1097/ACM.0000000000000134.

33. Eagly AH, Carli LL. Women and the labyrinth of leadership. Harv Bus Rev. 2007;85:62–71, 146

34. Ellinas EH, Fouad N, Byars-Winston A. Women and the decision to leave, linger, or lean in: predictors of intent to leave and aspirations to leadership and advancement in academic medicine. J Womens Health (Larchmt). 2018;27(3):324–32. https://doi.org/10.1089/jwh.2017.6457. Epub 2017 Oct 19.

35. Ellinas EH, Kaljo K, Patitucci TN, Novalija J, Byars-Winston A, Fouad NA. No room to "lean in": a qualitative study on gendered barriers to promotion and leadership. J Womens Health (Larchmt). 2019;28(3):393–402. https://doi.org/10.1089/jwh.2018.7252. Epub 2018 Nov 27.

36. Eloy JA, Svider PF, Cherla DV, Diaz L, Kovalerchik O, Mauro KM, Bare-des S, Chandrasekhar SS. Gender disparities in research productivity among 9952 academic physicians. Laryngoscope. 2013;123(8):1865–75. https://doi.org/10.1002/lary.24039. Epub 2013 Apr 8.

37. Estryn-Behar M, Fry C, Guetarni K, Aune I, Machet G, Doppia MA, Lassaunière JM, Muster D, Pelloux P, Prudhomme C. Work week duration, work-family balance and difficulties encountered by female and male physicians: results from the French SESMAT study. Work. 2011;40(Suppl 1):S83–100. https://doi.org/10.3233/WOR-2011-1270.

38. FAMILY Act, S 337, 115th Cong (2017–2018). https://www.congress.gov/bill/115th-congress/senate-bill/337. Accessed 22 Jan 2019.

39. Figueroa M. Work-life balance does not mean an equal balance. Front Pediatr. 2016;4:18. https://doi.org/10.3389/fped.2016.00018.eCollection 2016. Review. PubMed PMID: 27014668; PubMed Central PMCID: PMC4789363.

40. Files JA, Mayer AP, Ko MG, Friedrich P, Jenkins M, Bryan MJ, Vegunta S, Wittich CM, Lyle MA, Melikian R, Duston T, Chang YH, Hayes SN. Speaker introductions at internal medicine grand rounds: forms of address reveal gender bias. J Womens Health (Larchmt). 2017;26(5):413–9. https://doi.org/10.1089/jwh.2016.6044. Epub 2017 Feb 16.

41. Fox G, Schwarz A, Hart KM. Work-family balance and academic advancement in medical schools. Acad Psychiatry. 2006;30(3):227–34.

42. Gander P, Briar C, Garden A, Purnell H, Woodward A. A gender-based analysis of work patterns, fatigue, and work/life balance among physicians in postgraduate training. Acad Med. 2010;85(9):1526–36. https://doi.org/10.1097/ACM.0b013e3181eabd06.
43. Gino F, Wilmuth CA, Brooks AW. Compared to men, women view professional advancement as equally attainable, but less desirable. Proc Natl Acad Sci U S A. 2015;112(40):12354–9. https://doi.org/10.1073/pnas.1502567112. Epub 2015 Sep 21. PubMed PMID: 26392533; PubMed Central PMCID: PMC4603465.
44. Gjerberg E. Gender Similarities in Doctors' Preferences- and gender differences in final specialization. Soc Sci Med. 2002;54:591–605. Edit Citation.
45. Goldacre MJ, Fazel S, Smith F, Lambert T. Choice and rejection of psychiatry as a career: surveys of UK medical graduates from 1974 to 2009. Br J Psychiatry. 2013;202(3):228–34. https://doi.org/10.1192/bjp.bp.112.111153. Epub 2012 Oct 25. PubMed PMID: 23099446; PubMed Central PMCID: PMC3585421.
46. Gordon AJ, Sebok-Syer SS, Dohn AM, Smith-Coggins R, Ewen Wang N, Williams SR, Gisondi MA. The birth of a return to work policy for new resident parents in emergency medicine. Acad Emerg Med. 2019;26(3):317–26. https://doi.org/10.1111/acem.13684. Epub 2019 Feb 5.
47. Gottenborg E, Maw A, Ngov LK, Burden M, Ponomaryova A, Jones CD. You can't have it all: the experience of academic hospitalists during pregnancy, parental leave, and return to work. J Hosp Med. 2018;13(12):836–9. https://doi.org/10.12788/jhm.3076.
48. Gustafsson Sendén M, Schenck-Gustafsson K, Fridner A. Gender differences in Reasons for Sickness Presenteeism - a study among GPs in a Swedish health care organization. Ann Occup Environ Med. 2016;28:50. https://doi.org/10.1186/s40557-016-0136-x. Published 2016 Sep 20.
49. Guille C, Frank E, Zhao Z, Kalmbach DA, Nietert PJ, Mata DA, Sen S. Work-family conflict and the sex difference in depression among training physicians. JAMA Intern Med. 2017;177(12):1766–72. https://doi.org/10.1001/jamainternmed.2017.5138. PubMed PMID: 29084311; PubMed Central PMCID: PMC5820732.
50. Harden J. 'Mother Russia' at work: gender divisions in the medical profession. Eur J Womens Stud. 2001;8:181–99.
51. Heymann J, Raub A, Earle A. Creating and using new data sources to analyze the relationship between social policy and global health: the case of maternal leave. Public Health Rep. 2011;126(Suppl 3):127–34. https://doi.org/10.1177/00333549111260S317.
52. Hill EK, Stuckey A, Fiascone S, Raker C, Robison K. Gender and the balance of parenting and professional life among gynecology subspecialists. J Minim Invas Gynecol. 2018;26(6):1088.

53. Hitchcock MA, Bland CJ, Hekelman FP, Blumenthal MG. Professional networks: the influence of colleagues on the academic success of faculty. Acad Med. 1995;70:1108–16.

54. Holliday EB, Ahmed AA, Jagsi R, Stentz NC, Woodward WA, Fuller CD, Thomas CR Jr. Pregnancy and Parenthood in Radiation Oncology, Views and Experiences Survey (PROVES): results of a blinded prospective trainee parenting and career development assessment. Int J Radiat Oncol Biol Phys. 2015;92(3):516–24. https://doi.org/10.1016/j.ijrobp.2015.02.024. Epub 2015 Apr 16.

55. Huffington A. Thrive the third metric to redefining success and creating a life of well-being, wisdom, and wonder. New York: Harmony Books; 2014.

56. Jena AB, Khullar D, Ho O, Olenski AR, Blumenthal DM. Sex differences in academic rank in US medical schools in 2014. JAMA. 2015;314(11):1149–58.

57. Johnson CA, Johnson BE, Liese BS. Dual-doctor marriages: career development. Fam Med. 1992;24(3):205–8.

58. Johnson SK. What the science actually says about gender gaps in the workplace. Harvard Business Review blog. https://hbr.org/2017/08/what-the-science-actually-says-about-gender-gaps-in-the-workplace. Posted August 17, 2017. Accessed 8 July 2019.

59. Jolly S, Griffith KA, DeCastro R, Stewart A, Ubel P, Jagsi R. Gender differences in time spent on parenting and domestic responsibilities by high-achieving young physician-researchers. Ann Intern Med. 2014;160(5):344–53. https://doi.org/10.7326/M13-0974. PubMed PMID: 24737273; PubMed Central PMCID: PMC4131769.

60. Kaneto C, Toyokawa S, Inoue K, Kobayashi Y. Gender difference in physician workforce participation in Japan. Health Policy. 2009;89(1):115–23. https://doi.org/10.1016/j.healthpol.2008.05.010. Epub 2008 Jun 30.

61. Kaplan SH, Sullivan LM, Dukes KA, Phillips CF, Kelch RP, Schaller JG. Sex differences in academic advancement. Results of a national study of pediatricians. N Engl J Med. 1996;335(17):1282–9.

62. Kawakami K. Support systems for women doctors. JMAJ. 2011;54(2):136–8.

63. Kawase K, Kwong A, Yorozuya K, Tomizawa Y, Numann PJ, Sanfey H. The attitude and perceptions of work-life balance: a comparison among women surgeons in Japan, USA, and Hong Kong China. World J Surg. 2013;37(1):2–11. https://doi.org/10.1007/s00268-012-1784-9.

64. Knoll MA, Glucksman E, Tarbell N, Jagsi R. Putting women on the escalator: how to address the ongoing leadership disparity in radiation oncology. Int J Radiat Oncol Biol Phys. 2019;103(1):5–7. https://doi.org/10.1016/j.ijrobp.2018.08.011.

65. Lambert T, Goldacre R, Smith F, Goldacre MJ. Reasons why doctors choose or reject careers in general practice: national surveys. Br J Gen Pract. 2012;62(605):e851–8. https://doi.org/10.3399/bjgp12X659330.

66. Leigh JP, Tancredi DJ, Kravitz RL. Physician career satisfaction within specialties. BMC Health Serv Res. 2009;9:166. https://doi.org/10.1186/1472-6963-9-166. PubMed PMID: 19758454; PubMed Central PMCID: PMC2754441.

67. Leigh JP, Tancredi D, Jerant A, Kravitz RL. Physician wages across specialties: informing the physician reimbursement debate. Arch Intern Med. 2010;170(19):1728–34.

68. Leigh JP, Tancredi D, Jerant A, Kravitz RL. Annual work hours across physician specialties. Arch Intern Med. 2011;171(13):1211–3. https://doi.org/10.1001/archinternmed.2011.294.

69. Levine RB, Lin F, Kern DE, Wright SM, Carrese J. Stories from early-career women physicians who have left academic medicine: a qualitative study at a single institution. Acad Med. 2011;86(6):752–8. https://doi.org/10.1097/ACM.0b013e318217e83b.

70. Lin SY, Mahoney MR, Sinsky CA. Ten ways artificial intelligence will transform primary care. J Gen Intern Med. 2019;34(8):1626–30. https://doi.org/10.1007/s11606-019-05035-1.

71. Logghe HJ, Scarlet S, Jones CD, Aggarwal R. Work-life integration: being whole at work and at home. American College of Surgeons, Division of Education: RISE article https://www.facs.org/education/division-of-education/publications/rise/articles/work-life. Posted June 2018.

72. Luthar SS, Curlee A, Tye SJ, Engelman JC, Stonnington CM. Fostering resilience among mothers under stress: "Authentic Connections Groups" for medical professionals. Womens Health Issues. 2017;27(3):382–90. https://doi.org/10.1016/j.whi.2017.02.007. Epub 2017 Apr 14. PubMed PMID: 28410972.

73. Ly DP, Seabury SA, Jena AB. Divorce among physicians and other healthcare professionals in the United States: analysis of census survey data. BMJ. 2015;350:h706. https://doi.org/10.1136/bmj.h706. PubMed PMID: 256e94110; PubMed Central PMCID: PMC4353313.

74. Ly DP, Seabury SA, Jena AB. Hours worked among US dual physician couples with children, 2000 to 2015. JAMA Intern Med. 2017;177(10):1524–5. https://doi.org/10.1001/jamainternmed.2017.3437. PubMed PMID: 28828476; PubMed Central PMCID: PMC5820690.

75. Ly DP, Seabury SA, Jena AB. Characteristics of U.S. physician marriages, 2000-2015: an analysis of data from a U.S. Census Survey. Ann Intern Med. 2018;168(5):375–6. https://doi.org/10.7326/M17-1758. Epub 2017 Nov 21.

76. Lyu HG, Davids JS, Scully RE, Melnitchouk N. Association of domestic responsibilities with career satisfaction for physician mothers in procedural vs nonprocedural fields. JAMA Surg Published online April 10, 2019. https://doi.org/10.1001/jamasurg.2019.0529.

77. Magudia K, Bick A, Cohen J, Ng TSC, Weinstein D, Mangurian C, Jagsi R. Childbearing and family leave policies for resident physicians at top

training institutions. JAMA. 2018;320(22):2372–4. https://doi.
org/10.1001/jama.2018.14414.

78. Mangurian C, Linos E, Sarkar U, Rodriguez C, Jagsi R. What's holding
women in medicine back from leadership. Harv Bus Rev. 2019 2018
UPDATED NOVEMBER 07, 2018. https://hbr.org/2018/06/whats-
holding-women-in-medicine-back-from-leadership.

79. Mason MA, Goulden M. Do babies matter (part II)? Closing the Baby
Gap Academe. 2004;90(6):10–15 Published by: American Association
of University Professors Stable URL: http://www.jstor.org/sta-
ble/40252699.

80. Mattessich S, Shea K, Whitaker-Worth D. Parenting and female derma-
tologists' perceptions of work-life balance. Int J Womens Dermatol.
2017;3(3):127–30. https://doi.org/10.1016/j.ijwd.2017.04.001. eCollection 2017 Sep. PubMed PMID: 28831421; PubMed Central PMCID:
PMC5555353.

81. Mayer AP, Blair JE, Files JA. Peer mentoring of women physicians. J
Gen Intern Med. 2006;21(9):1007. https://doi.
org/10.1111/j.1525-1497.2006.00577.x.

82. McMurray JE, Linzer M, Konrad TR, Douglas J, Shugerman R, Nelson
K. The work lives of women physicians results from the physician work
life study. The SGIM Career Satisfaction Study Group. J Gen Intern
Med. 2000;15(6):372–80. PubMed PMID: 10886471; PubMed Central
PMCID: PMC1495474.

83. Mechaber H, Levine R, Manwell LB, Mundt MP, Linzer M. Part-time
physicians… prevalent, connected, and satisfied. J Gen Intern Med.
2008;23(3):300–3. https://doi.org/10.1007/s11606-008-0514-3.

84. Mehta S, Rose L, Cook D, Herridge M, Owais S, Metaxa V. The speaker
gender gap at critical care conferences. Crit Care Med. 2018;46(6):991–
6. https://doi.org/10.1097/CCM.0000000000003114.

85. Mezu-Chukwu U. Balancing motherhood, career, and medicine. JAMA
Cardiol. 2017;2(7):715–6. https://doi.org/10.1001/jamacar-
dio.2017.0983.

86. Mizgala CL, Mackinnon SE, Walters BC, Ferris LE, McNeill IY,
Knighton T. Women surgeons: results of the Canadian Population Study.
Ann Surg. 1993;218(1):37–46.

87. McCue JD, Sachs CL. A stress management workshop improves residents' coping skills. Arch Intern Med. 1991;151(11):2273–7.

88. Mobilos S, Chan M, Brown JB. Women in medicine: the challenge of
finding balance. Can Fam Physician. 2008;54(9):1285–1286.e5.
PubMed PMID: 18791106; PubMed Central PMCID: PMC2553450.

89. Mullangi S, Jagsi R. Imposter syndrome: treat the cause, not the symptom. JAMA. 2019;322(5):403–4. https://doi.org/10.1001/jama.2019.9788.

90. Nonnemaker L. Women physicians in academic medicine — new
insights from cohort studies. N Engl J Med. 2000;342:399–405. https://
doi.org/10.1056/NEJM200002103420606OECD2012healthdata. www.
oecd.org/health/healthpoliciesanddata/oecdhealthdata2012.htm.

91. Parsons WL, Duke PS, Snow P, Edwards A. Physicians as parents: parenting experiences of physicians in Newfoundland and Labrador. Can Fam Physician. 2009;55(8):808–809.e4. PubMed PMID: 19675267; PubMed Central PMCID: PMC2726099.

92. Pedersen LT, Bak NH, Dissing AS, Petersson BH. Gender bias in specialty preferences among Danish medical students: a cross-sectional study. Dan Med Bull. 2011;58(9):A4304.

93. Perlman RL, Ross PT, Lypson ML. Understanding the medical marriage: physicians and their partners share strategies for success. Acad Med. 2015;90(1):63–8. https://doi.org/10.1097/ACM.0000000000000449.

94. Persson P, Rossin-Slater M. When dad can't stay home: fathers' workplace flexibility and maternal health. May 2019 Stanford Institute for Economic Policy Research. https://siepr.stanford.edu/research/publications/when-dad-can-stay-home-fathers-workplace-flexibility-and-maternal-health.

95. Putnik K, Houkes I. Work related characteristics, work-home and home-work interference and burnout among primary healthcare physicians: a gender perspective in a Serbian context. BMC Public Health. 2011;11:716–26. https://doi.org/10.1186/1471-2458-11-716. PubMed PMID: 21943328; PubMed Central PMCID: PMC3189139. [PMC free article] [PubMed].

96. Putnam CW, DiMarco J, Cairns CB. Recruitment of dual-career academic medicine couples. Acad Med. 2018;93(11):1604–6.

97. Ramakrishnan A, Sambuco D, Jagsi R. Women's participation in the medical profession: insights from experiences in Japan, Scandinavia, Russia, and Eastern Europe. J Womens Health (Larchmt). 2014;23(11):927–34. https://doi.org/10.1089/jwh.2014.4736. Epub 2014 Oct 16. Review. PubMed PMID: 25320867; PubMed Central PMCID: PMC4235590.

98. Rangel EL, Lyu H, Haider AH, Castillo-Angeles M, Doherty GM, Smink DS. Factors associated with residency and career dissatisfaction in childbearing surgical residents. JAMA Surg. 2018;153(11):1004–11. https://doi.org/10.1001/jamasurg.2018.2571.

99. Reed DA, Enders F, Lindor R, McClees M, Lindor KD. Gender differences in academic productivity and leadership appointments of physicians throughout academic careers. Acad Med. 2011;86(1):43–7. https://doi.org/10.1097/ACM.0b013e3181ff9ff2.

100. Rich A, Viney R, Needleman S, Griffin A, Woolf K. 'You can't be a person and a doctor': the work-life balance of doctors in training-a qualitative study. BMJ Open. 2016;6(12):e013897. https://doi.org/10.1136/bmjopen-2016-013897. PubMed PMID: 27913563; PubMed Central PMCID: PMC5168633.

101. Riska E. Medical careers and feminist agendas: American, Scandinavian, and Russian women physicians. New York: Aldine de Gruyter; 2001.

102. Saag HS, Shah K, Jones SA, et al. Pajama time: working after work in the electronic health record. J Gen Intern Med. 2019; https://doi.org/10.1007/s11606-019-05055-x.

103. Schueller-Weidekamm C, Kautzky-Willer A. Challenges of work-life balance for women physicians/mothers working in leadership positions. Gend Med. 2012;9(4):244–50. https://doi.org/10.1016/j.genm.2012.04.002. Epub 2012 May 23.

104. Shanafelt T, Hasan O, Dyrbye L, Sinsky C, Satele D, Sloan H, West C. Changes in burnout and satisfaction with work-life balance in physicians and the general US working population between 2011 and 2014. Mayo Clin Proc. 2015;90(12):1600–13.

105. Shanafelt TD, Dyrbye LN, Sinsky C, et al. Relationship between clerical burden and characteristics of the electronic environment with physician burnout and professional satisfaction. Mayo Clin Proc. 2016;91(7):836–48.

106. Shanafelt TD, West CP, Sinsky C, Trockel M, Tutty M, Satele DV, Lindsey E, Carlasare LE, Dyrbye LN. Changes in burnout and satisfaction with work-life integration in physicians and the general US working population between 2011 and 2017, MD, MHPE Mayo Clin Proc. September 2019;94(9):1681–94. https://doi.org/10.1016/j.mayocp.2018.10.023, www.mayoclinicproceedings.org.

107. Shrager S, Kolan A, Dottl SL. Is that your pager or mine: a survey of women academic family physicians in dual physician families. WMJ. 2007;106(5):251–5.

108. Shrager S. Working part time in academic family medicine -narrative essay 738. Fam Med. 2012;44(10):737–8.

109. Strong EA, De Castro R, Sambuco D, Stewart A, Ubel PA, Griffith KA, Jagsi R. Work-life balance in academic medicine: narratives of physician-researchers and their mentors. J Gen Intern Med. 2013;28(12):1596–603.

110. Sugiura-Ogasawara M. Reply to: an insight on career satisfaction level, mental distress and gender differences in working conditions among Japanese obstetricians and gynecologists. J Obstet Gynaecol Res. 2013;39(1):469. https://doi.org/10.1111/j.1447-0756.2012.01965.x. Epub 2012 Nov 14.

111. Travis EL, Doty L, Helitzer DL. Sponsorship: a path to the academic medicine C-suite for women faculty? Acad Med. 2013;88(10):1414–7.

112. Treister-Goltzman Y, Peleg R. Female physicians and the work-family conflict. Isr Med Assoc J. 2016;18(5):261–6.

113. Turner PL, Lumpkins K, Gabre J, Lin MJ, Liu X, Terrin M. Pregnancy among women surgeons: trends over time. Arch Surg. 2012;147(5):474–9.

114. Valantine H, Sandborg CI. Changing the culture of academic medicine to eliminate the gender leadership gap: 50/50 by 2020. Acad Med. 2013;88:1411–3. [PMC free article] [PubMed] [Google Scholar].

115. Varda BK, Glover M 4th. Specialty board leave policies for resident physicians requesting parental leave. JAMA. 2018;320(22):2374–7. https://doi.org/10.1001/jama.2018.15889.

116. Villablanca AC, Li Y, Beckett LA, Howell LP. Evaluating a medical School's climate for Women's success: outcomes for faculty recruitment, retention, and promotion. J Womens Health (Larchmt). 2017;26(5):530–9.
117. Voytko ML, Barrett N, Courtney-Smith D, Golden SL, Hsu FC, Knovich MA, Crandall S. Positive value of a women's junior faculty mentoring program: a mentor-mMentee analysis. J Womens Health (Larchmt). 2018;27(8):1045–53. https://doi.org/10.1089/jwh.2017.6661. Epub 2018 May 29.
118. Warde CM, Moonesinghe K, Allen W, Gelberg L. Marital and parental satisfaction of married physicians with children. J Gen Intern Med. 1999;14(3):157–65. PubMed PMID: 10203621; PubMed Central PMCID: PMC1496552.
119. Wietsma AC. Barriers to success for female physicians in academic medicine. J Community Hosp Intern Med Perspect. 2014;31:4. https://doi.org/10.3402/jchimp.v4.24665. eCollection 2014. PubMed PMID: 25147633; PubMed Central PMCID: PMC4120052.
120. Wilmuth CA. Gender Differences in Professional Advancement: The Role of Goals, Perceptions, and Behaviors. Doctoral dissertation, Harvard University, Graduate School of Arts & Sciences. 2016. https://dash.harvard.edu/handle/1/33493559.
121. Yamazaki Y, Kozono Y, Mori R, Marui E. Difficulties facing physician mothers in Japan. Tohoku J Exp Med. 2011;225:203–9. [PubMed] PubMed PMID: 22027270.
122. Yank V, Rennels C, Linos E, Choo EK, Jagsi R, Mangurian C. Behavioral health and burnout among physician mothers who care for a person with a serious health problem, long-term illness, or disability. JAMA Intern Med. 2019;179(4):571–4. https://doi.org/10.1001/jamainternmed.2018.6411.

Isolation, Lack of Mentorship, Sponsorship, and Role Models

8

Anita K. Blanchard and Janice C. Blanchard

Chapter Objectives
- Describe the gender inequity in career advancement for women in academic careers
- Emphasize the importance of gender climate as a modifier of professional isolation
- Identify factors that contribute to workplace isolation and proposed solutions

Vignette

An early career African American physician has a thriving clinical practice at an academic institution but has limited insight into promotion strategies. She is often asked to participate in hospital

A. K. Blanchard (✉)
Medical Education, University of Chicago, Chicago, IL, USA
e-mail: ablancha@bsd.uchicago.edu

J. C. Blanchard
Emergency Medicine, George Washington University,
Washington, DC, USA

© Springer Nature Switzerland AG 2020
C. M. Stonnington, J. A. Files (eds.), *Burnout in Women Physicians*,
https://doi.org/10.1007/978-3-030-44459-4_8

committees and recruit patients for studies but feels like a "token representative" in these activities. She is one of the few women in her department and the only underrepresented minority (UIM) faculty member. Her chairman is cordial and meets with her to review her relative value unit (RVU) success but dismisses requests to meet and discuss research ideas and pathways to promotion. He values her clinical contributions to the department and includes her in the photo opportunities to highlight diversity but never engages her in a plan for further career development.

She is so busy clinically and with committee work that she never has the opportunity to activate her ideas about institutional initiatives, develop new investigative strategies, or partner on publications. Junior-level male faculty are hired with similar credentials but are given protected time to pursue academic and professional interests. She discovers in casual conversation that they have higher salaries despite what she knows to be equal or less clinical productivity. The chairman meets regularly with male faculty to discuss career interests, possibly due to their common shared experiences. She was surprised to receive a smaller clinical bonus that academic year and wonders if this was related to her attempt to discuss the differences in faculty support between her and her male colleagues she observed with her chairman.

Introduction

Women have become increasingly prevalent in medicine. According to the American Association of Medical Colleges, the percentage of women medical school graduates has increased from 7% in 1967 to 46%.in 2016 [1]. In 2018, there were more women than men matriculating at United States medical schools [2]. Despite this trend, gender gaps in career choices still exist across many specialties. Women are most widely represented in the specialties of pediatrics, internal medicine, and family medicine and less likely represented in fields such as surgery [1]. Underrepresented minorities represent only a quarter of women medical school matriculants [3]. Defined by the AAMC in 2004, an *underrepresented minority in medicine (UIM) means those racial and ethnic populations that are underrepresented in the medical profession relative to their numbers in the general population* [4]. While the overall trends of women in medicine are improving, there are still significant differences in pay, academic rank, and leadership [5].

Despite the increase in the number of female medical graduates, few women choose academic medicine. Only 27% of medical school faculty are women with medical degrees (MDs) [1]. Among women who develop academic careers, few earn tenure and rise to the level of senior leadership. While women represent 51% of clinical instructors, they represent only 20% of all full professors with MDs [1]. Women represent only 15% of department chairs. In addition, women represent only 16% of all medical school deans; most instead hold midlevel or associate dean positions [6, 7].

This lack of parity in female advancement in academic medicine has been documented extensively in the literature [1, 8, 9]. While women may develop thriving clinical practices and excel at teaching, these attributes tend to be weighed less favorably toward promotion, as compared to more traditional scholarly activity, such as research publications. Historically, women have had lower numbers of peer-reviewed research publications, driven initially by the smaller number of women in medicine [10, 11]. As the number of women in academic medicine has risen, the proportion of women authors has also increased, including those with first authorship roles [12]. In some specialties, when adjusting for the number of years in practice and stratifying by rank, women publish at equal rates to men [13, 14]. Despite similar trends in productivity, the outcomes are not equal. Female faculty who publish at a similar rate to their male colleagues in the same specialties still have discordant career trajectories, with many women plateauing at the rank of associate professor [1, 8, 9, 14].

According to a survey performed by Carr et al., there are five overarching barriers women face in academic career advancement: (1) a perceived wide spectrum in gender climate, (2) lack of parity in rank and leadership by gender, (3) lack of retention of women in academic medicine (the "leaky pipeline"), (4) lack of gender equity in compensation, and (5) a disproportionate burden of family responsibilities and work-life balance on women's career progression. Survey respondents noted that the "gender climate" differed by academic rank for women, with lower ranks being perceived as more welcoming for women as compared to more isolating senior ranks [8, 15].

The remainder of the chapter will focus on the gender climate in academic medicine, with a specific focus on the impact of professional isolation on this climate. It will also explore ways to recognize the sequelae of isolation as well as steps needed to address it.

Isolation in Professional Careers

Isolation is defined as the state of being in a place or situation that is separate from others [16]. Isolation related to workplace interactions is most often described in the educational, sociological, and business literature. Isolation can interfere with collaboration and professional development. Inadequate support structures, including mentorship, may impede insight, feedback, and professional growth. According to a Harvard Business Review survey, solitude is associated with higher learning. Loneliness and less workplace support are more common in individuals who have advanced degrees than those who have only attained undergraduate or high school degrees. Respondents with professional degrees in law and medicine are the loneliest; according to the survey, they are 25% lonelier than respondents with bachelor's degrees and 20% lonelier than those with Doctor of Philosophy degrees [17].

Isolation has not been extensively addressed in the medical literature; most of the literature that does exist is primarily centered around rural medicine [18]. However, isolation occurs beyond the context of geography. Professional isolation refers to a lack of networks or a sense of isolation from professional peers, which may result in a sense of estrangement from work identity and practice currency. Individuals with professional isolation feel that they lack colleagues with whom to discuss work-related issues [19]. Components of professional isolation include making decisions alone, deficient collaboration, not being a part of the work community, and lack of mentorship [20]. Professional isolation can occur at any stage of career. It is not limited to specialty type, length of time in the profession, or gender.

Gender-based professional isolation is a generational construct of academic culture stemming from a historic paucity of women in academic medicine. Lack of a critical mass of women in general and women in leadership create this imbalance. Gender-based professional isolation may include a psychological, qualifiable component that affects self-confidence and motivation. Lack of women role models at the highest levels of leadership can limit the outlook of what is achievable for women at junior levels. Gender-based professional isolation is also a condition of physical quantifiable work-environment barriers that impede success. Studies show that resources for women including space, salary, and ability to participate in outside professional activities are inequitable [21–23]. Though these inequities have been identified for decades, they continue to exist. In a 17-year follow-up study of a survey initially conducted in 1995, Freund et al. found that a 10% lower salary persists for women compared to men [24]. Women in academic medicine may face inequities in assignment location and effort allocation that may contribute to professional isolation in the academic system. Women may be more likely to choose flexible schedules for work-life integration or may seek community-based practices with academic affiliation and instead may spend more time performing educational and clinical duties over research efforts [25]. Temporary leave from the workforce for childbearing, child care, and elder care may delay promotion, may interrupt research endeavors, and can derail tenure time- specific goals. Women with children also spend a disproportionate amount of time performing parental duties as compared to their male counterparts. In a study comparing obstacles in career success, both male and female surgeons reported social and family issues as major concerns. Men noted a higher tendency to miss family activities due to job demands. Women were significantly more likely to miss work activities due to family responsibilities [26]. Female physicians with children spend an average of 11 hours less time at work than male colleagues due to domestic duties, including child care and elder care [27]. Extrapolated over 1 year, this leads to a time difference of 572 hours that can contribute to lagging career success and isolation from colleagues. The differences in priorities of work and home are changing with more enlightened dual-career couples. Over time, the home responsibilities of women and men in medicine may reach better parity. However, even though there are fiscal and/or professional costs for time that women take off in their careers for home and child care responsibilities, the limits on academic progress may be persistent and out of proportion to the time lost [5].

Even women who remain full time in the academic setting with robust research careers may experience professional isolation due to lack of clear pathways to success. Gender may influence career goals of academicians. In a survey of motivations, goals, and aspirations of male and female faculty, both groups equally perceived the importance of career goals related to publication quality and quantity, clinical care, and teaching. Male faculty were more likely to consider earning a high salary, having national and international reputation as an expert, and achieving a leadership role as important career goals than female faculty [28, 29]. The paucity of female role models at the highest levels may not only influence top male leaders but may have a rate-limiting effect on career aspirations in other women. Without clear and abundant examples of female faculty succeeding in all aspects of academic medicine, there may be limited perspective of possibilities in career growth leaving women with lower sets of expectations.

Leadership may have gender bias in the recognition of accomplishments. Women may be overlooked for selection for new opportunities and promotion. When women have achieved success in research and have reached the full professor status, they are still overlooked for top leadership roles. They remain penalized by cultural stereotypes and are relegated to the "out group" when top positions are available [30]. For example, while men are stereotypically recognized as possessing the agentic traits of logic, independence, and leadership, women are thought to possess the more communal traits of kindness, dependency, and being group oriented, which may diminish consideration from traditionally male-dominated leadership roles. These character trait assumptions and associations may make women's accomplishments less recognized in departmental and institutional cultures. These disadvantages become more prominent with career stage advances [30–32].

In business literature, the majority of leaders advocate for protégés who remind them of themselves. Unconscious and affinity biases motivate leaders to seek the company of individuals who make them feel comfortable: those who share their race, gender, upbringing, culture, and religion. This advocacy for majority of men is a roadblock to widespread sponsorship for underrepresented groups. The majority of corporate America is led by white males, which may be self-perpetuating, keeping diverse talent outside of the C-suite ("chief" officer suite) [33].

The business literature further supports this concept of professional isolation experienced by women and minority leaders who do achieve senior-level positions. Women business leaders often find loneliness at the top and can experience peril if they advocate for other women, resulting in negative performance reviews. In a survey of 350 executives, Hekman and colleagues concluded that individuals engaging in diversity-valuing behavior were evaluated less favorably than those who did not actively promote balance [34]. In response to inequality of opportunities by gender and race, there is a tokenism that is also perpetuated that further marginalizes women who have ambition. Anne McNulty notes "some senior-level women distance themselves from junior woman, perhaps to be more accepted by their male peers…it's easy to believe that there's limited space for people who look like you at the top when you can see it with your own eyes." [35]

The professional isolation documented in the general education and business environments similarly affects both women and underrepresented minorities in medicine. Recognition of isolation may be subtle at first, but there may be social clues. The isolated physician may be more withdrawn and less likely to speak up in group professional settings. This is paralleled in UIM data on social isolation of medical students. Students, who are not welcomed in a social network, can be mistakenly perceived as less interested, unprofessional, or lacking knowledge [36]. Similarly, faculty who are isolated may not be perceived as professionally engaged in the culture of the organization. Women and UIM faculty who experience ongoing frustrations with the institutional framework may move from passive behavior eventually asserting themselves or issuing complaints. Unlike men in the academic majority who speak up and are favorably perceived as self-advocates, women and UIM faculty are perceived as unwelcomingly aggressive [36].

The long-term sequelae of professional isolation may be disengagement, career dissatisfaction, and attrition. The three most common reasons that women and minority faculty cite for leaving academic medicine include lack of career/professional advancement, salary inequity, and chairman/departmental leadership issues, including harassment and discrimination [37]. In a survey on workplace discrimination, women were more likely than men to file a complaint of discrimination (14.6% vs 8.1%) but were more likely to report a worsening situation following the complaint as compared to men (26.7% vs 5.3%) [38]. The discriminatory actions and the lack of response and resolution of the situations are equally damaging. If professional isolation is not addressed, it may lead to the three dimensions of burnout: emotional exhaustion, depersonalization, and personal accomplishment [39]. Effects of burnout are numerous and can affect patient care, health system outcomes, and physician health. These results of burnout can lead to lower quality of patient care, medical errors, lower patient satisfaction, reduced physician productivity, increased physician turnover, and increased health-care costs. Finally, isolation, loneliness, and burnout can lead to the adverse physician health effects of substance abuse, depression, suicidal ideation, poor self-care, and motor vehicle accidents [40–42].

As professional isolation is linked to deficiencies in promotion and career success, these determinants are multifactorial and include lack of mentorship, coaching, and sponsorship, unclear or circuitous pathways to success, limited feedback, and lack of a conducive organizational structure. In order to move forward to solutions, these factors must be addressed. Sustained transformation of the gender climate to reduce professional isolation and inequity requires change at individual, organizational, and national levels. The academic culture must shift to allow for this progress in four key areas (Fig. 8.1).

1. Mentorship, Coaching, and Sponsorship

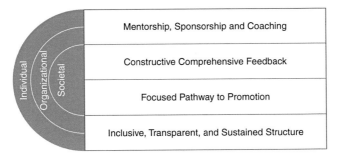

Fig. 8.1 Ending professional isolation by changing the culture of academic medicine

Mentorship, coaching, and sponsorship are all on the continuum of professional development and facilitate professional engagement on an individual level. Definitions and characteristics of these roles vary in career development literature. Some aspects of mentoring, coaching, and sponsorship are intertwined. All help move the protégé to a higher goal. Mentorship typically occurs in the same field of expertise. The mentorship relationship can either be a one-on-one relationship, a group relationship with one mentor and several mentees, or a peer-based relationship [43]. Mentors are role models at the same institution or at other academic organizations. Mentors provide feedback, encourage professional growth, foster networking, and can give insight into the culture of an organization.

Coaches may not have expertise in the same area but can still provide the protégé the ability to self-reflect on his/her actions and help develop a career advancement strategy. In the business setting, Cummings and Worley define coaching as working with organizational members, managers, or executives on a regular basis to help them clarify their goals, deal with potential stumbling blocks, and improve their performance. It is typically a personal one-on-one interaction and helps the targeted individual gain perspective about career goals. Unlike coaching, mentoring is often more directive with the mentor intentionally transferring specific knowledge and skill and guiding the client's activities [44].

Sponsors differ from mentors in that they are always in positions of leadership. Sponsors go beyond giving feedback and advice for an individual; a sponsor actively advocates to help an individual gain visibility. In the business literature, sponsorship is defined as active support by someone appropriately placed in the organization who has significant influence on decision-making processes and who is advocating, protecting, and fighting for the career advancement of an individual [6, 45, 46]. A sponsor has the capacity to appoint or elevate his/her protégé into a role that will lead to career advancement. In medicine, sponsors open doors to opportunities for scholarship, funding, or the establishment of a regional/national reputation for his/her protégé that are otherwise unattainable [6]. The roles of mentor and sponsor are not necessarily mutually exclusive and can have overlapping traits. One person may serve in both of these capacities for a protégé. Distinguishing these roles as separate but related activities may help female faculty develop appropriate relationships. Women are half as likely to have sponsorship than men, yet the significance of mentorship and sponsorship has been demonstrated in all professional fields including business, law, and health care [47].

Mentorship, both alone and in the context of sponsorship, improves professional productivity, career development, job satisfaction, perceived institutional support, and faculty retention [48–50]. Women tend to have difficulty finding mentors, and when they are mentored, they have less successful outcomes [45]. Mentorship is gender neutral; male and female faculty are equally capable of providing mentorship. Familiarity drives aspects of mentorship for both the mentor and protégé. Leaders prefer to mentor individuals who have shared qualities and traits. The protégé may feel uncomfortable approaching someone with a different background in anticipation of a greater likelihood of rejection. The benefits of gender-matched mentorship include shared experiences and roadblocks. However, limited female role models in the highest positions of leadership in academic medicine may give women the perception that they have limited opportunities to find mentors or sponsors. If there are not enough female leaders in the highest ranks, there can be less opportunities to appoint future leaders to these positions.

2. Focused Pathways for Scholarship and Promotion

In order to advance individual success, clear pathways for promotion should be outlined for women faculty. Instead of being encouraged to focus on research and writing when not involved in clinical duties, women and UIM are often asked to participate on committees, community service, and student mentoring. They tend to have more divergent responsibilities but less support. They often spend excessive time and energy in activities that are not traditional pathways to promotion [51, 52].

Woman also must be supported with protected time for research and given access to equal funding opportunities. Gender affects funding and publication [53]. To level access, women need aggressive mentorship and sponsorship to help establish a strong foundation of scholarship.

Creating focused pathways includes realistic goal setting, planning, and feasible time allotment to accomplish goals. This should be done early in the academic career, with the guidance of senior faculty. In addition, personal life responsibilities, such as child care, should be taken into consideration to allow flexibility in promotions and advancement criteria to reflect the range of work that women accomplish [54].

Equally important to the establishment of a focused pathway to career success is keeping perspective and balance. Medicine is a profession and a calling. The passion for the work and the volume of the work can easily make it possible to let other aspects of life be minimized. It can consume all space without proper boundaries. Maintaining overall life balance defined as achieving the proper balance of work and self and others should also be taken into consideration [55].

3. Constructive Comprehensive Feedback

Constructive comprehensive feedback may be challenging in academic medicine, for a number of reasons, including lack of proper training by department leadership in providing appropriate feedback [56]. Traditionally, feedback does not encompass the full scope of what physicians do in the academic setting. However, feedback is an important element in promoting the success of women faculty; prior research has shown that women are actually more likely to seek feedback than men [57]. If done incorrectly, feedback may perpetuate the professional isolation that may already exist among women faculty members. While assessment is an important step toward improvement, it is often based on limited clinical narratives and not fully representative of the full spectrum of academic work. For example, feedback has tended to focus on the areas of patient experience and clinical productivity.

Patient experience information collected through various survey measurements usually have poor compliance so are often an unreliable measure to use for faculty feedback. Often the responses that are obtained give voice disproportionately to negative patient experience perspectives based on patient expectations [57]. Too often are the system shortcomings packaged into the overall impression of the visit disconnected from the merit of the physician work. Since women provide a large proportion of the clinical workforce, the negative patient experience feedback can have a large effect on career perception. Clinical productivity is another primary driver of feedback but is not a driver of promotion. Productivity is not a direct measure of quality but often physicians feel substandard in their ability to be good doctors based on the message that they are not working hard enough or that quantity is the marker of quality.

Constructive feedback involves taking into account the full spectrum of contribution of a faculty member, including those activities in which women faculty have traditionally been more involved. Mentoring peers and learners, institutional, regional and national committee work, community engagement, and institutional emergency response in times of coverage shortages or urgent cases should all count toward stewardship of the institution. Each institution however has their own metric of how these contributions are valued and some factors may rarely count toward promotion strategy.

At least, annual review of academic progress should be conducted with the senior leader plus more frequent checkpoints with mentors or sponsors. Balanced feedback should be provided that includes the full scope of practice, including clinical productivity as well as institutional stewardship with committee, mentoring, and community activities. Promotion trajectory with clear expectations should be reviewed regularly. Faculty should not only discuss more clinical measurements of achievement (such as RVUs) but other contributions. Feedback is linked to the career pathway and both require accountability from all parties involved. If the junior faculty incorporates feedback and stays on the proposed pathway, then the leader should be compelled to deliver on the promise of progression.

4. An Inclusive Transparent and Equitable Organizational Structure

To end professional isolation the work environment must change. The focus areas listed in 1–3 can be achieved on a micro level with individuals or on a macro level across an organization. Real sustained change requires these steps to be imbedded in the organizational and society construct. This is to ensure not only individual gains but widespread shifts toward transformative change for all faculty.

In a study of faculty representatives from 24 medical schools, 40% reported no special programs for recruiting, promoting, or retaining women in medicine, primarily because these initiatives were deemed unnecessary [58]. This may be an important barrier to overcome in order to advance women in medicine substantially. It is important to note that changes in an institution's organizational framework can lead to culture change. This includes building a pipeline to promote women in academia, ending social and professional isolation, encouraging mentorship relationships, and encouraging a culture of leadership (Fig. 8.2).

A. Building a Pipeline for Women in Academia

It is important for academic medical centers to focus on building a pipeline that focuses on recruiting and retaining women faculty. This will allow medical centers to create better gender equity at the institutional level that can further expand to equity in the national selection processes for funding, publishing, and speaking engagements. Carr et al.

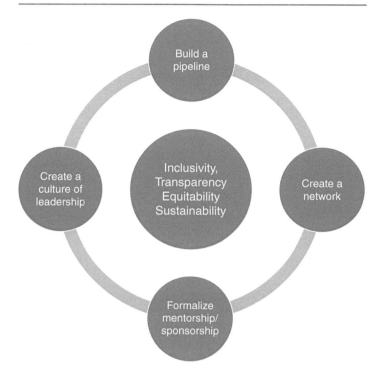

Fig. 8.2 How to foster an inclusive, transparent, equitable, and sustained structure

recommend the development of comprehensive programs for recruitment, promotion, and retention that focus on individual, interpersonal, institutional, academic community, and policy levels of intervention. This includes the provision of leadership development programs for women, either institutionally or nationally [8]. Grant writing and faculty development support should not be limited to a single seminar but instead focus on longitudinal sustained efforts to promote faculty success. In addition, women should be offered an environment supportive of work-life integration. Solutions may include changes in policies on parental leave, minimizing before and after work hour meetings, on-site child care, equitable pay, flexible work schedules, and job sharing [59, 60]. There should be customization for women's career pathways that takes into account work-life integration.

Women must also learn to aim higher than the status quo. This includes learning to be better negotiators and self-promoters. Women often take a passive approach to salary and promotion-level setting. When negotiating salaries, women frequently take offers that are below proposals that men would accept. Women seldom make competitive counteroffers [61]. Business literature demonstrates that the best effort to achieve salary equity is in the initial offer [62]. Pay inequities between men and women persist even at more advanced positions because women tend to negotiate less aggressively for better salaries [63]. In regard to promotion, both quantitative and qualitative measures should be considered. Traditional quantitative measures include clinical productivity (e.g., RVUs) and publications. Additional quantifiable factors should include educational effort including the number of lectures given as well as seminars and courses taught by faculty. Qualitative measures include team participation, committee leadership, and community outreach.

B. Ending Social and Professional Isolation

Affinity groups that bring together women in similar fields can reduce professional isolation. Such groups promote comradery and allow women to collectively work toward advancing scholarship and leadership in a supportive environment. Social networks are important for discussing challenges and sharing approaches across interprofessional and interdisciplinary groups. Common challenges may include gender-conscious experiences, workplace bias, discrimination, and gender-specific strategies. While these groups allow women to discuss common barriers, they are not always granular enough to help with the distinct challenges of promotion and publication.

Women striving for professional progress often seek more similar professional networks. Women have been shown to be more productive academically in settings in which they have a higher number of women peers. For example, those departments with a higher number of female faculty also have more publications generated by women [64]. Organizations allow women to learn from other women experiencing similar work situations but also help them develop negotiating skills to promote career advancement [65]. Encouraging such networks is a key part of creating a successful work culture for women. Networks are not just important in early career; in fact, studies show that the type of internal vs external collaborations differs by stage of career. Early-career physicians get most value from internal departmental or organization networking. Mid- and late-career faculty are less local or organizationally dependent and seek more professional networks on a regional or national level [66, 67].

C. Formalizing Enduring Structures for Role Models, Mentors, and Sponsors

Mentoring, sponsorship, and coaching are all needed for healthy academic progress. In academic medicine, most mentorship programs have focused on mentorship for junior faculty. However, it is important to recognize that women academics at the mid-career level also need mentorship. Support at all levels to encourage faculty to obtain senior leadership positions can discourage stagnation at mid-level positions [43]. Mentorship programs have been far more common than sponsorship programs at US medical schools. However, sponsorship is necessary for women to achieve high-level positions, and typically, women are less likely than men to actively seek sponsors [68]. While most mentoring relationships are organic, there is some randomness in their creation which can overlook better and more thoughtful matching. Adding a framework for more intentional matching should be done on an organizational and national level. In recommendations for expanding sponsorship programming in academic medicine, Gottlieb et al. propose that academic medical centers, medical schools, and specialty societies should launch these initiatives. They encourage system-wide inclusive formal programs that use data to facilitate matching. Clear expectations with feedback should be set. Senior leaders should become "sponsor evangelists" promoting the organizational value of formal programs including the potential for succession planning [69]. Organized programs with the explicit goal of sponsorship can help facilitate this relationship. One notable national example of a successful sponsorship program is the Society of General Internal Medicine Career Advising Program (CAP). CAP supports relationships of women with senior leaders by placing them on influential national committees as well as promotes relationships that will further advance promotion. It has supported 300 women since its inception in 2013 [7, 70]. AAMC also advocates for professional career development and sponsors a group on women in medicine and science with comprehensive resource for women [71].

D. Creating a Culture of Leadership with Equal Opportunities for Success

This requires a culture change in the organization and society. Researchers Alyssa Fried Westring and colleagues have defined a culture conducive to women's academic success (CCWAS) that includes having equal access to opportunities, support of a work-life balance, lack of gender bias in the workplace, and having a leader (such as division chief or department chair) that is supportive of success [72]. In order to encourage access to opportunities, institutions have to actively devote resources to the promotion of success of women in academic medicine. In a NIH-sponsored randomized trial to evaluate factors that would encourage productivity of women at the assistant professor level, University of Pennsylvania researchers explored a number of initiatives. These included goal-related task forces that recruited and promoted women, professional development programs that encouraged manuscript coauthorship and leadership among women faculty, and the engagement of institutional leadership in the promotion of women faculty. While there were no differences between the intervention and control groups, likely due to institution-wide changes impacted by the study, the authors recognized that these steps were still important in encouraging academic progress [73].

In addition to promoting initiatives to encourage success, it is also important that faculty leaders are aware of any implicit gender bias they may have in approaching female faculty candidates for consideration for leadership positions or promotion. These behaviors can present in varying patterns, including intermittent, pervasive, subtle, or overt, and take a toll on job satisfaction and patient care [38, 53]. All forms of discrimination and harassment should be investigated. Leaders should complete and proactively institute implicit bias training for all team members [54].

Addressing this bias also includes addressing the traditional inequities in salaries that women medical faculty have faced. Women faculty at public medical schools earn 8% less than their male counterparts, and the gender gap for physicians in clinical practice is even wider [74]. Academic leaders should encourage transparency, communication, negotiation, and compromise. Adopting transparency in compensation with a formula that is consistent and understandable to explain salary variations is important as well as sharing summary statistics of salaries by rank and gender internally [75, 76]. In addition, encouraging negotiating skills for women early in their clinical career is an important element of faculty development.

Finally, as role models, women show a pathway that is possible and provide unique insights into barriers that male leaders may not consider. Women in leadership have the power to positively affect workplace policy and lead change in national societies and regulatory agencies. With generational shifts and more women entering academic medicine, the gender gap may be closed in academic leadership as greater numbers of women enter tenure track positions. The work of developing senior women leaders in academic medicine must be intentional and strategic. Creating organizational change is difficult and requires the teamwork of all leaders regardless of gender. Women should avoid the temptation to retreat or leave academic institutions since most effective change starts within organizations. Women leaders, though few in number, must lead the change in partnership with their male associates. As more women become senior leaders, there is greater opportunity to encourage future faculty development. More women will be capable of inspiring and mentoring other women who are early in their career development, further perpetuating progress. Expanding the scope of qualifications for tenure, including taking into consideration all aspects of academic merit such as clinical excellence, teaching acumen, and administrative excellence, may expand leadership opportunities for all faculty, including women. These advances can lead national change with enforcement of policies that combat the bias and inequity that contribute to isolation and burnout. Only a systematic approach will have sustaining to break the glass ceiling for women in academic medicine.

Returning to the physician in the vignette, she would have benefitted from better department transparency. Implementation of an organized program to promote mentorship and sponsorship would help her identify a clear set of strategies for promotion, as well as open opportunities for her to be involved with activities conducive to career advancement. Transparency in the department would have made it clear about what objective components of her work contribute to her productivity. Targeted activities designed to promote faculty development skills among women in her department, which included negotiation skills, would also be helpful as guide for salary renegotiation to be on par with that of faculty of similar rank and productivity. These strategies could have reduced professional isolation and have led to a greater chance of retention in her department.

References

1. Association of American Medical Colleges. The state of women in academic medicine: the pipeline and pathways 2015–2016.
2. Association of American Medical Colleges. Women were the majority of U.S. medical school applicants in 2018. 4 Dec 2019. Accessed on May 14 from https://news.aamc.org/press-releases/article/applicant-data-2018/.
3. Association of American Medical Colleges. AAMC diversity facts and figures. Accessed on 12 May 2019 from https://www.aamcdiversityfactsandfigures2016.org/report-section/section-3/.
4. Association of American Medical Colleges. AAMC Underrepresented in medicine definition. Accessed 10 May 2019 from https://www.aamc.org/initiatives/urm/.
5. Thibault GE. Women in academic medicine. Acad Med. 2016;91:1045–6.

6. Travis EL, Doty L, Heiltzer DL. Sponsorship: a path to the academic medicine C-suite for women faculty. Acad Med. 2013;88:1414–7.

7. Travis EL. Academic medicine needs more women leaders. AAMC News. January 16, 2018. Accessed on 16 May 2018 from https://news.aamc.org/diversity/article/academic-medicine-needs-more-women-leaders/.

8. Carr PL, Raj A, Kaplan SE, Terrin N, Breeze JL, Freund KM. Gender differences in academic medicine: retention, rank, and leadership comparisons from the National Faculty Survey. Acad Med. 2018;93:1694–9.

9. Ash AS, Carr PL, Goldstein R, Friedman RH. Compensation and advancement of women in academic medicine: is there equity? Ann Intern Med. 2004;141:205–12.

10. Jagsi R, Guancial EA, Worobey CC, et al. The "gender gap" in authorship of academic medical literature- a 35 year perspective. NEJM. 2006;355:281–7.

11. Sidhu R, Rajashekhar P, Lavin VL, Parry J, Attwood J, Holdcroft A, Sanders DS. The gender imbalance in academic medicine: a study of female authorship in the UK. J R Soc Med. 2009 Aug;102:337–42.

12. Pyatigorskaya N, di Marco L. Women authorship in radiology research in France: an analysis of the last three decades. Diagn Interv Imaging. 2017;98:769–73.

13. Holliday EB, Jagsi R, Wilson LD, Choi M, Thomas CR, Fuller CD. Gender differences in publication productivity, academic position, career duration and funding among U.S. academic radiation oncology faculty. Acad Med. 2014;8:767–73.

14. Mayer EN, Lenherr SM, Hanson HA, Jessop TC, Lowrance WT. Gender differences in publication productivity among academic urologists in the United States. Urology. 2017;103:39–46.

15. Carr PL, Gunn CM, Kaplan SA, Raj A, Freund KM. Inadequate progress for women in academic medicine: findings from the National Faculty Study. J Women's Health. 2015;24:190–9.

16. Meriam Webster Dictionary. Accessed 1 May 2019 from https://www.meriam-webster.com/dictionary/isolation. Accessed 1 May.

17. Achor S, Kellerman GR, Reece A, Robichaux A. America's loneliest workers, according to research. HBR. Accessed 1 May 2019 from https://hbr.org/2018/03/americas-loneliest-workers-according-to-research.

18. Peterson OL, Stoeckle JD. Professional isolation. J Med Educ. 1977;52:1008–9.

19. Services for Australian Rural and Remote Allied Health. Professional Isolation. Accessed 1 May 2019 from https://sarrah.org.au/content/professional-isolation.

20. Aira M, Mäntyselkä P, Vehviläinen A, Kumpusalo E. Occupational isolation among general practitioners in Finland. Occup Med. 2010;60:430–5.

21. Dean of the School of Science, Massachusetts Institute of Technology. A study on the status of women faculty in science at MIT. Cambridge, MA: The MIT Faculty Newsletter, March 1999. Accessed 1 May 2019 from http://web.mit.edu/fnl/women/women.pdf.

22. Laine C, Turner BJ. Unequal pay for equal work: the gender gap in academic medicine. Ann Intern Med. 2004;141:238–40.
23. Saunders MR, Turner BJ. Unequal pay for equal work: where are we now? Ann Intern Med. 2018;169:654–5.
24. Freund KM, Raj A, Kaplan SE, Terrin N, Breeze JL, Urech TH, Carr PL. Inequities in academic compensation by gender: a follow-up to the National Faculty Survey Cohort Study. Acad Med. 2016;91:1068–73.
25. Kaplan SH, Sullivan LM, Dukes KA, Phillips CF, Kelch RP, Schaller JG. Sex differences in academic advancement results of a national study of pediatricians. N Engl J Med. 1996;335:1282–9.
26. Colletti LM, Mulholland MW, Sonnad SS. Perceived obstacles to career success for women in academic surgery. Arch Surg. 2000;135:972–7.
27. Ly DP, Seabury SA, Jena AN. Hours worked among U.S. dual physician couples with children 2000–2015. JAMA Intern Med. 2017;177:1524–5.
28. DeCastro R, Griffith KA, Ubel PA, Steward A, Jaga R. Mentoring and the career satisfaction of male and female academic faculty. Acad Med. 2014;99:301–11.
29. Jones RD, Griffith KA, Ubel PA, Stewart A, Jagsi R. A Mixed-Methods Investigation of the motivations, goals, and aspirations of male and female academic medical faculty. Acad Med. 2016;91:1089–97.
30. Kaatz A, Carnes M. Stuck in the out-group: Jennifer can't grow up, Jane's invisible, and Janet's over the hill. J Womens Health (Larchmt). 2014;23:481–4.
31. Brenner OC, Tomkiewicz J, Schien VE. The relationship between sex role stereotypes and requisite management characteristics revisited. Acad Manag J. 1989;32:662–9.
32. Eagly AH, Karau SJ. Role congruity theory of prejudice toward female leaders. Psychol Rev. 2002;109(3):573–98.
33. Kennedy JT, Jain-Link P. Sponsors need to stop acting like mentors. HBR. Retrieved https://hbr.org/2019/02/sponsors-need-to-stop-acting-like-mentors.
34. Hekman DR, Johnson SK, Foo M, Yang W. Does diversity-valuing behavior result in diminished performance ratings for non-white and female leaders? Acad Manage J. 2017;60:771–97.
35. McNulty AW. Don't underestimate the power of women supporting each other at work. HBR. Accessed 1 May 2019 from https://hbr.org/2018/09/dont-underestimate-the-power-of-women-supporting-each-other-at-work.
36. Boateng B, Thomas B. How can we ease the social isolation of under-represented minority students? Acad Med. 2011;96:1190.
37. Cropsey KL, Masho SW, Shiang R, Sikka V, Kornstein SG, Hampton C. Why do faculty leave? Reasons for attrition of women and minority faculty from a medical school: four-tear results. J Womens Health (Larchmt). 2008;17:1111–8.
38. Tolbert Coombs AA, King RK. Workplace discrimination: experiences of practicing physicians. J Natl Med Assoc. 2005;97:467–77.

39. Maslach C, Jackson SE, Leiter MP. Maslach burnout inventory manual. 4th ed. Menlo Park: Mind Garden, Inc.; 1996–2016.
40. Shanafelt TD, Noseworthy JH. CEO Executive leadership and physician well-being: nine organizational strategies to promote engagement and reduce burnout. Mayo Clin Proc. 2016;92:129–46.
41. West CP, Dyrbye LN, Shanafelt TD. Physician burnout: contributors, consequences and solutions. J Intern Med. 2018;283:516–29.
42. Patel RS, Bachu R, Adikey A, Malik M, Shah M. Factors related to physician burnout and its consequences: a review. Behav Sci (Basel). 2018;8(11):98.
43. Farkas AH, Bonifacino E, Turner R, et al. J Gen Intern Med. 2019. Accessed 15 May 2019 from https://doi.org/10.1007/s11606-019-04955-2.
44. Cummings TG, Worley CG. Coaching and mentoring. In: Organizational development and change, vol. 75. Mason: South-Western Cengage Learning; 2009. p. 491–8.
45. Ibarra H, Carter NM, Silva C. Why men still get more promotions than women. HBR. Accessed on 1 May 2019 from https://hbr.org/2010/09/why-men-still-get-more-promotions-than-women.
46. Foust-Cummings H, Dinolfo S, Kohler J. Sponsoring women to success. August 17, 2011. New York: Catalyst 2011. Accessed May 2019 from https://www.catalyst.org/research/sponsoring-women-to-success/.
47. Elmer V. To get promoted, women need champions not mentors. Quartz. 13 Aug 2013. Accessed 1 May 2019 from https://qz.com/119135/women-need-power-brokers-not-mentors-to-help-them-succeed/.
48. Pane LA, Davis AB, Ottolini MC. Career satisfaction and the role of mentorship: a survey of pediatric hospitalists. Hosp Pediatr. 2012;2:141–8.
49. Pololi L, Knight S. Mentoring faculty in academic medicine: a new paradigm? J Gen Intern Med. 2005;20:866–70.
50. Pololi LH, Knight SM, Dennis K, Frankel RM. Helping medical school faculty realize their dreams: an innovative, collaborative mentoring program. Acad Med. 2002;77:377–84. Women are Over Mentored but under sponsored Ibarra Herninia HBR.
51. Nivet MA, Taylor VS, Butts GC, et al. Case for minority faculty development today. Mt Sinai J Med. 2008;75:491–8.
52. Cohen JJ. Time to shatter the glass ceiling for minority faculty. JAMA. 1998;280:821–2.
53. Garrett L. The trouble with girls: obstacles to women's success in medicine and research. BMJ. 2018;363:k5232.
54. Butkus R, Serchen J, Moyer DV, Bornstein SS, Hingle ST. Achieving gender equity in physician compensation and career advancement: a position paper of the American College of Physicians. Ann Intern Med. 2018;168:721–3.
55. Witzig TE, Smith SM. Work-life balance solutions for physicians-it's all about you, your work and others. Mayo Clin Proc. 2019;94:573–6.

56. Lees ND, Palmer M, Dankoski M. Conducting effective faculty annual reviews: a workshop for academic leaders. Accessed 14 May 2019 from https://www.mededportal.org/publication/10270/#344134.

57. Mehta SJ. Patient satisfaction reporting and Its implications for patient care. AMA J Ethics. Accessed on 5/13/2019 from https://journalofethics.ama-assn.org/article/patient-satisfaction-reporting-and-its-implications-patient-care/2015-07.

58. Carr PL, Gunn C, Raj A, Kaplan S, Freund KM. Recruitment, promotion and retention of women in academic medicine: how institutions are addressing gender disparities. Women's Health Issue. 2017;27:374–81.

59. Mobilos S, Chan M, Brown JB. Women in Medicine. The challenge of finding balance. Can Fam Physician. 2008;54:1285–1286.e5.

60. Strong EA, De Castro R, Sambuco D, et al. Work-life balance in academic medicine: narratives of physician-researchers and their mentors. J Gen Intern Med. 2013;28:1596–603.

61. Glassdoor. 3 in 5 employees did not negotiate salary. Accessed on 20 May 2019 from https://www.glassdoor.com/blog/3-5-u-s-employees-negotiate-salary/.

62. Frank L. How the gender pay gap widens as women get promoted. Harvard Business Rev. 5 Nov 2005. Accessed on 29 May at https://hbr.org/2015/11/how-the-gender-pay-gap-widens-as-women-get-promoted.

63. Bowles HR. Why women don't negotiate their job offers. Harvard Business Review. 19 June 2014. Accessed on 29 May 2019 from https://hbr.org/2014/06/why-women-dont-negotiate-their-job-offers.

64. Sheridan J, Savoy JN, Kaatz A, Lee YG, Filut A, Carnes M. Write more articles, get more grants: the impact of department climate on faculty research productivity. J Womens Health (Larchmt). 2017;26(5):587–96.

65. Lin MP, Lall MD, Samuels-Kalow M, et al. Impact of a women-focused professional organization on academic retention and advancement: perceptions from a qualitative study. Acad Emerg Med. 2019;26:303–16.

66. Carapinha R, Ortiz-Walters R, McCracken CM, Hill EV, Reede JY. Variability in women faculty's preferences regarding mentor similarity: a multi-Institution study in academic medicine. Acad Med. 2016;91:1108–18.

67. Peluchette VJ, Jeanquart S. Professionals' use of different mentor sources at various career stages: implications for career success. J Soc Psychol. 2000;140:549–64.

68. Ayyala MS, Skarupski K, Bodurtha JN, Gonzalez-Fernandez M, Ishii LE, Fivush B, Levine RB. Mentorship Is not enough: exploring sponsorship and Its role in career advancement in academic medicine. Acad Med. 2019;94:94–100.

69. Gottlieb AS, Travis EL. Rationale and models for career advancement sponsorship in academic medicine: the time is here; the time is now. Acad Med. 2018;93:1620–3.

70. Roy B, Gottlieb AS. The career advising program: a strategy to achieve gender equity in academic medicine. J Gen Intern Med. 2017;32:601–2.
71. https://www.aamc.org/members/gwims/. Accessed 10 May 2019.
72. Westring AF, Speck RM, Sammel MD, et al. Culture conducive to women's academic success: development of a measure. Acad Med. 2012;87:1622–31.
73. Grisso JA, Sammel MD, Rubenstein AH, et al. A randomized controlled trial to improve the success of women assistant professors. J Womens Health (Larchmt). 2017;26(5):571–9.
74. Jena AB, Olenski AR, Blumenthal DM. Sex differences in physician salary in US public medical schools. JAMA Intern Med. 2016;17:1294–304.
75. Committee on Maximizing the Potential of Women in Academic Science and Engineering; Committee on Science, Engineering, and Public Policy; National Academy of Sciences; National Academy of Engineering; Institute of Medicine. Beyond biases and barriers: fulfilling the potential of women in academic science and engineering. Washington, D.C: The National Academies; 2007.
76. American Association of Women Surgeons. 2017 AWS gender salary equity statement. Accessed on 13 May 2019 from https://www.womensurgeons.org/page/SalaryStatement.

Going It Alone: The Single, Unmarried, Unpartnered, Childless Woman Physician

9

Kirsten S. Paynter

Vignette

It was 2003; I was in my mid-30s and taking that exciting and long-awaited adult rite of passage of purchasing my first home. For the fifth time since I had left home at age 18, I was moving across the country for the purpose of pursuing my education or a work-related job change. I had moved a total of 14 times since I had left home for college. Some of those moves were done simply with my car or with a friend's borrowed truck; but mostly I moved myself. I kept life simple with a minimalistic lifestyle. I had grown up in a small town of about 1200 people and was one of only four in my class of 32 who went directly to a 4-year university. At university I had worked hard to catch up academically, as a small rural school had left gaps that I needed to fill in order to even try to aspire to my ambition and dreams. I did not know if I was good enough to get into medical school or to become a doctor. My parents were always supportive of my pursuing an education; it was the means to a life of opportunity and possibility.

K. S. Paynter (✉)
Department of Physical Medicine and Rehabilitation (PM&R),
Musculoskeletal Longitudinal Course, Mayo Clinic Alix School
of Medicine, Scottsdale, AZ, USA
e-mail: Paynter.Kirsten@mayo.edu

© Springer Nature Switzerland AG 2020
C. M. Stonnington, J. A. Files (eds.), *Burnout in Women Physicians*,
https://doi.org/10.1007/978-3-030-44459-4_9

My female role models had been mostly teachers and secretaries who were always supportive and helpful. Male role models, like our local Family Medicine doctor who lived across the street and the PhD agronomist who worked at the United States Department of Agriculture research station in town, made me feel that they saw potential. This gave me courage to explore and dream in an era when women were moving into the workplace. I was allowed to be curious and encouraged to do what I wanted. New places, new faces, new homes, new roles, and new jobs were my paths through undergrad, during which I was fascinated by the brain, the mind, and the spirit; at the end of which, I received a degree in Psychology. On one particular day I had a spiritual, existential experience in which I was spiritually guided, or "called" if you will, to be a healer, medical school being the path, and I was also "called," at least "for a while," to be single. The medical school part I was ready for; the being single for a while part, I knew was going to be even more challenging. Medical school, a medical mission trip to Africa, a 4-year residency, a one-year fellowship, and securing my first official job as a physician all followed. I was a SINGLE woman following her dream, leaving the small town and pursuing her calling to serve as a healer/physician. With debt from medical school and my undergraduate degree, finances were tight. During my first 2 years in practice, I rented a condominium with the hope and dream of 1 day being able to purchase a home of my own. I was determined to lay down some adult roots and build a more lasting community, to perhaps meet someone and "settle down." Debt was a big chunk of my budget, costing more than my rent, but with frugal living and a financial plan, I had managed to save enough, for a down payment on a home, and I was determined to find a place that I could call my own.

Well-meaning people, friends, and even family members, however, would question, "Are you sure you want a whole house, all by yourself?" "Don't you want to wait until you are married to buy a home?" And "Oh, by the way, when are you going to get going with the getting married thing, you know time is running out?" As if being in my early 30s time had run out for me in the love department and as if having a home was reserved for only those who had partnered or lived with someone and making it clear that my lack of a romantic life partner had something to do with my worthiness, my deserving of a place of my choice to call home. I was in my mid-30s and "no spring chicken" anymore. Yet, in some ways, I was just getting started, 10 years behind my high school peers. I did not know anyone, nor did I have family in the new city I was moving to and I would be living alone. From my perspective, I had been living on my own and paying my own way in life since I was 19, so it did not seem like anything new to me. I paid my bills and was financially responsible. In fact, buying a home was something I saw as a long-awaited reward for all the years of living in various student housing situations, bug-infested apartments, and an apartment where the single male neighbor made it clearly known through the paper-thin walls that he was partnered and then there was the condo with toxic mold. Yes, this move was a well-deserved reward for my hard work and all the times I had kept things simple, frugal, and easily mobile. I was proud of all I had accomplished and the opportunities I had given myself especially the new position that I had secured. I was ready to settle down and grow some roots.

The moment I walked into the three-bedroom, three-bath house in a safe, gated community, with nice sidewalks for walking, a coffee shop, and shopping close by, I knew it was for me. It was not the multiunit apartment or condo with thin shared walls or the house I shared with two housemates in prior years as a student. It was all on one level, which was important, as my father uses a motorized wheelchair and I wanted my home to be accessible for my parents when they would come to visit. There were actually two master suites, which was perfect for them, or other friends or family that I hoped would come to visit and stay with me now that I had a home. There was a room for my home office too. It was lovely. My realtor felt it too, and I confidently put in a full price offer, having been preapproved and working out my end of the finances ahead of time. I was grateful that I could give myself, the woman in me, this special place to nest and finally call home.

It was my realtor who first had the pleasure of confronting the gentleman who was selling the home. Through his realtor he began posing many questions about me as the solo buyer. "Who is this SINGLE woman?" "Where is she from?" "Who is her family?" "Where is she getting the money for this, is she good for it?" "How can she be doing this alone, has her husband died?" He questioned everything, including my personal "ability" and "integrity" to purchase the home and especially questioned whether I, as a SINGLE woman, could really afford the home. He was told that I was a legitimate buyer. The interrogation continued, and eventually he was told that I was a newly hired, salaried, physician at Mayo Clinic. He again questioned whether on my SINGLE salary that I would be able to afford the home. With much ado and reassurance, he finally agreed to the sale of his home to me. I was overjoyed to have navigated the purchase of my first home, where I would stay for the next 15 years.

Approximately 3 years after moving into that home, one bright and cheerful spring morning, I came out the front door and to the driveway to pick up the newspaper. A man sitting in a red convertible parked along the sidewalk, with the top down and wearing a baseball cap and sunglasses, seemed to watch me the entire time. It was unusual, as I did not recognize the car and it was a gated community, "so why would he be parked in front of my home," I thought. I picked up the paper and as I turned to head back inside, he yelled out at me, "YOU must be THAT SINGLE LADY who bought this house from me three years ago." I turned and said, "Excuse me." I was not sure that I had heard him right and while he did not seem particularly threatening sitting in the car and making no move to exit the vehicle, he certainly wanted my attention. He repeated, yelling a little louder from the seat of his car, "You must be that SINGLE LADY DOCTOR who bought this house from me." I said, "And you are?" He mumbled his name and something about being the prior owner and being curious about "his old place and the LADY who bought it." Recalling my realtor's interactions with him and his realtor during my purchase process, I did not give him much to go on and he did not seem to like that I was not playing the game he wanted to play, so he started his engine and drove off, leaving me creeped out and wondering exactly what his intention had been and what it was about a SINGLE LADY DOCTOR that so irked him and why he had the need to sit and yell out at me in order to "check-up on the place." What or why was it for him that he would portray me in such a negative way, suggesting that I could not or perhaps should not own a home of my own. Was it simply a matter of "sexism?" But why then did he emphasize the "SINGLE" nature of how he identified me? Was a SINGLE woman not deserving of a "certain lifestyle?" Or perhaps it was just too much of a leap that I was all three – a SINGLE WOMAN PHYSICIAN, just a country girl grown up and now in the city living out her spiritual calling as a healer. Perhaps even more importantly after this, I had to ask myself, "what was I making all this to mean about me, and what did I believe about who I am, my value in the world, and my worthiness as a single, woman physician; among all the other ways that I could potentially be labeled?"

The Single, Professional, Woman: The Cultural Landscape

The women's liberation and feminism movements have been defined in part by postmaterialist values of independence and freedom, as well as a desire for self-actualization [1]. Prior to the 1960s, the women's movement was focused on the legal status of women, but still perceived women as part of the family unit. In the 1960s, an emphasis on the greater empowerment of women occurred, but culturally it was still within the family unit. This was followed in the 1990s by the fuller liberation and reconstruction of gender roles, allowing women to live as they wished in terms of their roles within the family, in regard to their sexuality, and in the division of labor [2–4]. This fundamental shift toward a more gender-equal society places less pressure on women to get married and have children while also providing them opportunities to advance professionally and academically. This shift has allowed more women to flourish outside of the traditional marital relationship status and has led to a decline in relationship formation and sometimes even to prioritizing career over family [5, 6].

The US Census Bureau reports that in 2016, 110.6 million adults (45.2%) were divorced, widowed, or never married, out of 252 million people over the age of eighteen. In addition, the typical adult spent more years unmarried than married, and more than

35 million lived alone. 53.2% of unmarried US residents age 18 and older were women, 46.8% men. Those who had never been married were 63.5%, divorced 23.1%, and widowed 13.4%. There were 88 unmarried men age 18 and older for every 100 unmarried women in the United States. 59.8 million households (47.6%) were maintained by single women and men and of these 35.4 million (28.1%) households were maintained by those living alone. The number of unmarried-partner households in 2015 was 7.3 million, of which 433,539 were same-sex households. Perhaps of interest also is that 39.6% of voters in the 2016 presidential election were unmarried, and 87.5% of those 25 and older who were unmarried had completed high school or more education [7].

A 2017 Pew Research Center survey showed that only 23% of previously married adults, and 58% of those who never married, expressed a desire to marry [8]. In other words, a substantial proportion of never-married adults do not want to marry, and even more divorced and widowed individuals do not want to remarry. Culturally, around the world today, a greater number of adults are intentionally choosing to remain unpartnered and single. These singles are a growing demographic with unique challenges.

Interestingly, it has been traditionally thought that those who marry are happier. However, Bella DePaulo, PhD, in a review of 18 studies, found that people generally become no happier after they get married [9]. They may at best become a bit more satisfied with their lives around the time of the wedding, but then go back to feeling about as satisfied (or dissatisfied) as they were when they were single. This pattern is the same for men and women. Marriage does not, therefore, result in significant increased benefit in long-term measures of well-being over those who remain single. Similarly, her review also found that both married men and women become more and more dissatisfied with their relationship over time [9]. The cultural idea that married persons are happier may be simply a myth. People who have always been single are not very different in health or happiness from those who have been continuously married. The globally growing number of singles, both men and women, especially those leading fulfilling lives, is challenging traditional cultural belief systems around the topic of marriage.

Women physicians are among those challenging traditional relationship norms. Along with others who pursue professional levels of education and compared to nonprofessional women, they are known to often experience a delay in or be of older age at the time of marriage [10, 11], thus remaining single for a more extended period of time. The emphasis on obtaining an advanced level of education influences the balance between relationship building versus career development [10]. In a follow-up to a study showing that three times as many female plastic surgeons were unmarried compared with their male colleagues, a 52-question survey was sent to all female members of the American Society of Plastic Surgeons. Seven hundred and twenty-nine questionnaires were sent via e-mail and responses were anonymous. Response rate was 34% (n-250) [11]. Respondents were either married (64%), engaged (2%), in a "serious" relationship (11%), or not in a committed relationship (23%). Of unmarried respondents, 56% wanted to marry, 44% did not wish to marry, and 42% had deliberately postponed marriage. The most frequently cited reasons for being single were perceived lack of desirable partners (45%), job constraints (14%), and personality differences (13%). Female plastic surgeons who married later than 36 years of age were more likely to choose a spouse with a lower income, less education, and lower financial success compared with those who married at a younger age, thus going against the traditional roles within marriage. This demonstrates that even women physicians who do marry, but at a later age, often defy social norms of culturally traditional relationships [12].

The Medscape Physician Lifestyle and Happiness Report 2019, a survey of 15,069 physicians across 29+ specialties who practiced in the United States between July 27 and October 16, 2018, indicates that 7% of physicians are single, 81% are married, 4% live with a partner, 6% are divorced, and 1% are widowed [13]. A retrospective analysis of surveys conducted by the US Census 2008–2013 comparing the probability of ever being divorced among US physicians with other health-care professionals, lawyers, and non-health-care professionals is shown in the table below (Fig. 9.1). It indicated that physicians had the lowest prevalence of divorce among the professions studied, but still a 24.3% prevalence of divorce. In addition, physicians were found to be less likely than

Prevalence of Divorce Among Various Professions (US Census 2008-13)

Physicians	24.3%	(CI 23.8-24.8%)
Dentists	25.2%	(CI 24.1-26.3%)
Pharmacists	22.9%	(CI 22.0-23.8%)
Nurses	33.0%	(CI 32.6-33.3%)
Healthcare executives	30.9%	(CI 30.1-31.8%)
Lawyers	26.9%	(CI 26.4-27.4%)
Other non-healthcare professionals	35.0%	(CI 34.9-35.1%)

Fig. 9.1 Prevalence of divorce among various professions [14]

those in most other occupations to divorce in the past year. Among physicians, divorce prevalence was higher among women (odds ratio 1.51, 95% confidence interval 1.4–1.63). Stratified by physician's sex, greater work hours were associated with increased divorce prevalence only for female physicians [14].

Single: Why Does It Matter?

One can be legally single or socially single, though the two often overlap. To qualify as being legally single, one can have never married, be divorced, or widowed. Being socially single or coupled, however, is often what matters most culturally, especially in a culture where being partnered or married is glorified, and in fact where those who are married have been shown to be perceived quite differently from those who are single [15]. Evidence of this bias can be seen in a study of 1000 undergraduate students, who rated married people more likely than the single to be mature, stable, honest, happy, kind, and loving. Married people were described as caring, kind and giving almost 50% of the time, compared to only 2% of the time for singles [15]. Singles were more often called immature, insecure, self-centered, unhappy, lonely, and ugly. On the positive side, the singles were also noted to be independent. When undergraduates and community members were asked to rate descriptions of single and married people that were otherwise equal in their description, other than for the single/married status and age of either 25 or 40, all groups rated the singles as less socially mature, less well-adjusted, and more self-centered and envious than the married people (though again more independent and career oriented). The differences were even more accentuated when the targets were described as 40 years old versus when described as 25 years old [12, 16].

Singlism: Stereotypes, Stigmas, and Discrimination

Singles today face a cultural perceptual stereotyping and stigmatizing, which when internalized and normalized in the culture can lead to negative social, educational, economic, and legal connotations for going solo, whether after divorce or death of a spouse or simply in the setting of choosing to or remaining single in the first place. Marriage is culturally glorified and hyped up – a phenomenon termed "matrimania." It is a cultural assumption that coupling is the key to happiness and is the path to a rewarded, rewarding, and meaningful life.

Bella DePaulo, PhD, over a decade ago, coined the term "singlism," which has yet to appear in the Merriam-Webster dictionary. Singlism refers to the stereotyping, stigmatizing, and discrimination against people who are single. It does not mean simply being single.

- Stereotype = a widely held but fixed and oversimplified image or idea of a particular type of person or thing
- Stigma = "blemish" or "mark" in ancient Greek culture, a visible tattoo or burn on the skin of traitors, criminal, or slaves that readily identified them as morally inferior, to be avoided or shunned
- Stigmatized = to be described or regarded as worthy of disgrace or great disapproval, to set some mark of disgrace or infamy upon, or to be marked with stigmata
- Discrimination = the unjust or prejudicial treatment of different categories of people or things, especially on the grounds of race, age, or sex. Recognition and understanding of the difference between one thing and another

"Singlism" is interesting in that it is a "non-violent, softer form of bigotry than what is often faced by other stigmatized groups such as African Americans or gay men and lesbians" [3]. Its impact however is far reaching, in that most people, even singles themselves, are unaware of the prejudice, or that singles are stigmatized at all. It is often considered acceptable and not meriting protection, or is in fact officially sanctioned, when a single person is targeted [12, 17–19].

An example of the way current cultural perceptions promote stereotypes and stigmatize women is in the use of language. Traditional linguistic labels or archetypes used to describe women are noted in Table A and those specifically reserved for the single woman are in Table B below [20–24]. These terms, when used, can be meant to, and have the intention of, placing the woman or single woman in a negative light.

Table A: Archetypes of the feminine
- The victim
- The maid
- The martyr
- The diva
- The slave girl
- The princess
- The prostitute/whore/ho
- The wild woman
- Wonder woman
- The Amazon/crusader
- The father's daughter/daddy's girl
- The nurturer
- The good wife
- The librarian
- The butch
- The dyke

- The sweetie, sweetheart, honey
- The good girl
- The girl next door
- The waif
- The free spirit
- The damsel in distress
- The lady
- The maiden
- The sophisticate
- The ingenue
- The gamine
- The bohemian
- The coquette
- The seductress
- The femme fatale
- The sensualist
- The siren
- The matriarch
- The mother
- The matron
- The boss
- The huntress/warrior
- The wise woman
- The sage
- The mystic
- The lover
- The cosmic goddess
- The enigma
- The prophetess
- The inspirational muse
- The survivor
- The queen
- The empress

Table B: Archetypes of the single woman
- The bachelorette
- The spinster
- The old maid
- The cat lady
- The cougar
- The bachelor girl
- The unattached female
- The goody-goody
- The lone woman
- The lonely woman
- The prig
- The prude
- The unwed
- The unmarried woman
- The unpartnered woman
- The childless woman

Singlehood is frequently viewed negatively by society and individuals, especially singleness among women [25–27]. Negative images of singles in media and literature perpetuate the "undesirable" nature of singles [28]. Children are socialized and educated to marry and build stable family units [29, 30]. The internalization of this discrimination, stigmatization, and stereo-typing creates negative social, educational, economic, and legal connotation for those considering going solo after divorce or death of a spouse or simply choosing singleness in the first place [18, 19, 31]. By analyzing data from the European Social Survey, Elyakim Kislev, PhD, was able to determine that unmarried peo-ple experience 50% more discrimination than married people [32]. He states that "unlike other disadvantaged groups, singles often go unprotected from prejudice, frequently because single-hood is not viewed as meriting protection." Additionally, "the expectation that others are either married, or if not, do not want to be single are two assumptions so heavily normalized that those guilty of singlism are unaware they are abusing singles." Stigma is increased for the single woman compared to the single man [33, 34] and is also more prevalent among traditional, religious, and socially conservative individuals who place high importance on family formation [35]. Single mothers, the single woman combined with child-rearing, is the most extreme deviation from the traditional family norm [36].

The single, woman physician values independence and individualism, which along with an advanced education and the financial means, allows today's single woman to support not only herself but also a potential partner or spouse, children, or even other family members. The stigma associated with being a single, "spinster," outcast, or outsider is certainly not as strong as it once was. It nonetheless remains present and does come with its own unique set of cultural challenges and need for strategies and solutions in order to create, develop, and maintain a happy, meaningful, and fulfilling life.

Going It Alone: The Solo Life

Work–Family–Life for the Single

Work–life balance, or the updated term work–life integration, is still in many ways thought of as work–family balance. The phrase implies that the busy and overburdened, emotionally, physically, and mentally exhausted worker has to balance work with family responsibilities. The concept however takes on a much different character when the single person/employee is considered. This individual faces the responsibility of managing house and home, perhaps parenting and coordinating the care of children or the care for a parent or other extended family member, without the help of a partner. They in fact "do it all," and they do it all alone. In fact, because of their role within traditional families, singles are actually more likely to be seen as the "flexible" member of the family or asked to take on the role of caregiver within their extended family. They are subject to these added perceptions and demands and thus have greater potential for overwhelm and burnout at the hands of the multiplicity of roles and responsibilities they are asked to or volunteer to take on.

Along with being perceived as able to take on additional responsibilities within their immediate or extended families, singles are also perceived by their workplaces as having more flexibility, ability to contribute, and potentially fewer distractions from work or career responsibilities. This perception of singles by the workplace can lead to discrimination for men or women, related to their marital status, or singlism, at work. For instance, the perception or assumption that the singles' life is more flexible may manifest as being asked to work overtime more frequently or expected to travel more often and take vacation at times when colleagues with partners or families wish to be with their families for holidays or religious celebrations. In the context of the practicing physician and healthcare, these examples can translate into being asked to perform additional shifts or on-call responsibilities, performing coverage for holidays or days of religious celebrations. The assumption again being that those that are partnered, those with "families of their own" (i.e., children), and other child-care-related responsibilities take precedence over a single adult employee's need for leisure time, vacation time, or time with their own "family." Singles may feel pushed to abandon their own personal priorities, work harder, and surrender their own leisure activities, which in light of the data regarding what actually helps the single person find well-being and happiness, as described later in this chapter, serves as a direct inhibitor to finding work–life balance.

The Solo Experience

Psychologist Abraham Maslow's paper entitled "A Theory of Human Motivation," published in 1943, relays a theory describing a hierarchy of human needs (Fig. 9.2). The theory describes the pattern through which human motivations generally move and implies that in order for motivation to occur at the next higher level, each lower level must be satisfied within the individual themselves. The most basic of needs are those that are "physiological," which when met allow for the development of "safety," followed by "belonging and love," then "social needs or esteem," and finally "self-actualization" [37].

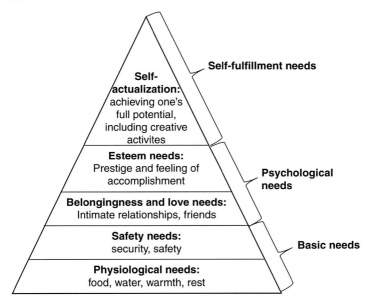

Fig. 9.2 Maslow's hierarchy of human needs

When individuals feel secure (safe, financially stable, supported in culture/community), they desire to try new things, express their unique voice, and self-actualize by fulfilling their potential [38, 39]. Postmaterialism, a term coined by Ronal Inglehart in his book The Silent Revolution: Changing Values and Political Styles Among Western Publics, outlines a shift in values from those of physical security and economic growth, identified as materialist values, to those of high quality of life, creativity, environmental protection, freedom of speech, and human rights in the 1970s [39]. This coincided with the shift in the legal status and role of women within the family unit and later the ability of women to live as they wished and to challenge the roles of family, sexuality, and labor division [4, 40].

Postmaterialistic values of fun, freedom, creativity, and trying new things correlate with levels of education, health, wealth, secularism, and social activity. Singles, cohabitators, and divorced people score higher on all these variables, while the never married are a mixed bag: they value fun and freedom more but score similarly to the married group on creativity and trying new things [41].

Postmaterialism values, while more commonly held by single people, do not necessarily lead those individuals to a higher state of happiness. The emphasis on freedom actually increases competition, stress, and inequality. There can be a constant focus on or consumption with the instability of solo life and the desire to relentlessly experience new things. The stigma surrounding singles remains, with their individualistic values being seen as selfish, desperate, and sad, but also immature, self-centered, and unhappy. They continue to face more harsh social exclusion and discrimination, being perceived negatively by both social institutions and individuals, even if they overcome the economic, psychological, and behavioral difficulties associated with being unmarried and the cost of freedom and uncertainty [9, 26, 42, 43].

Singles who are happy with their single status have been shown to be more negatively perceived than singles who are unhappy with their singlehood and who would like to become coupled [44, 45]. Singles by choice are seen as individuals who are rebellious and go against tradition or mainstream society, drawing criticism as a result, while those who are single by circumstances are typically seen as unfortunate and in need of help in order to find their sole mate. Evidence from multiple sources also suggest that choosing to go solo comes with significant negative costs in terms of economic, psychological, behavioral, and physical aspects of life [46–48]. In what remains a traditional culture, significant advantages and benefits remain for those who choose marriage when it comes to finances, mental health, physical health, and general well-being [49–57].

In this postmaterialistic values system where the pursuit of freedom and self-actualization is of greater priority for solo individuals, there may come a point where unless they have also met their lower needs of human interaction and emotional satisfaction, that they may experience an imbalance. The constant pursuing of self-actualization through pursuit of new experiences, while neglecting the need or the nurturing of their elementary emotional needs, similar to the workaholic, leads to an imbalance and a decline in well-being.

To the opposite effect however, the postmaterialistic values benefit singles in the sense that they are free to create more joy in their lives, on their own terms, and without relying on someone else to provide it for them. The happy single person (widowed, divorced/separated, or never married) appears to be happy in part because of their placement of high value on freedom, fun, creativity, and trying new things. These values do appear to help protect the single against the stereotypes, stigmatization, and discrimination they encounter. They are less likely to compare themselves to others and society and free themselves from the negative judgment by others [42, 57]. Singles who are successful embrace the concept of being in integrity with one's self, creating a safe, belonging, worthy, and loving relationship with one's self that minimizes or eliminates the need for external validation, attention, or affection. They reinvent for themselves what it means to be loved, to have companionship, via the curation of "alternative families" and arrangements [57, 58]. Evidence also indicates that singles may improve their well-being by engaging in leisure activities, such as running or other solo sports, as a means to develop themselves as well as to foster social connections [59, 60]. Outside of work, singles can also try new things such as joining social clubs, taking classes, adventure travel, or even participating in coaching, counselling, or psychotherapy in order to foster a greater level of happiness and build their own network or culture that promotes a sense of well-being for themselves.

Doing Life Alone

The increasing population of adults that are single and the new and increasingly popular choice of intentional singlehood are becoming more apparent. Many singles thrive as they take themselves by the hand and navigate life and sometimes even rebelliously confront the traditional cultural stereotypes, stigma, and outright discrimination they encounter as a single person [12, 58, 61, 62]. The strategies and practices singles use to "thrive" have yet to be fully explored, but the following strategies provide some insight into how singles successfully navigate their journey through life.

Awareness Singles are themselves becoming more aware of their own stigmatization, by society, whereas in the past they have been largely unaware of how traditional perceptions and values, which they too have believed, have led to decreased self-esteem, diminished sense of self-worth, and decreased levels of happiness. Happier singles are those who are aware of the social pressure they experience, which can come from even within their own families, let alone from the sociocultural system at large [63]. Creating greater awareness by sharing their experiences, both positive and negative with family, friends, communities, and workplaces, will help others to understand the special experiences, challenges, and obstacles that singles face.

Positive self-perception, self-confidence, optimism and feeling valuable For those who are or who have made the choice to remain single for longer and who tend to be more individualistic than others, the construction of a positive self-perception and interpersonal self-perception results in a hopeful outlook and increased well-being [64–66]. Feeling good about oneself, via a positive self-image, self-confidence, and having assurance in the choice to be single, melds one's positive self-perception and one's reality. For the unmarried person, having a positive self-perception improves one's measure of happiness by close to 30% and includes those who have been divorced or widowed [67]. This helps to combat the many people around singles who offer criticism, undermine self-confidence, and contribute to negative self-image, sometimes without an understanding of the consequences of their words or actions.

In research performed by and reported by Elyakim Kislev, PhD, in his book, Happy Singlehood, The Rising Acceptance and Celebration of Solo Living, singles who feel secure, less worried, valuable, and accomplished (through work, hobbies, or friends) also tend toward improved levels of happiness [68]. In addition, he finds that holding an optimistic view offers the single person about 35% more happiness than those without it. His studies indicate that optimism actually plays a greater role in producing measures of happiness experienced by the single, in comparison to that of the happiness experienced by married individuals [68]. He notes that singles have a greater likelihood to be friendly, less materially focused, receive more meaning from their work, and gain more from participating in interesting or challenging work than married persons. Feeling accomplished and valuable helps all singles gain in the scale of happiness compared to married people, because singles largely derive meaning from outside of the nuclear family and it increases their self-worth. Income, level of education, and family support also contribute to increased levels of happiness, while religiosity has mixed effects on the single person's experience, sometimes boosting and sometimes lowering it [68].

Choosing single-friendly environments An obvious way that singles will self-protect is to avoid negativity and situations or surroundings in which singlehood is singled out, stigmatized, or discriminated against. Surrounding oneself with friendly environments, workplaces, and networks that provide opportunities to connect with others is especially important to the single person. Singles supporting other singles within these networks and self-chosen "families," and even in more communal living spaces where people gather to share, engage in meaningful relationships, and gain social capital, are also challenging the culturally traditional marriage-family-centered lifestyle.

The traditional "family values," of many religious institutions, can also marginalize singles. This can result in many of them abandoning their participation in the corporate activities of their local faith community. Among various religious communities in the United States, how to address the single life has been a pressing topic for which specific action plans aimed at addressing the needs of singles have been aimed [69]. For singles who place a high value on developing a higher spiritual connection and who have an active spiritual life, finding a community that normalizes their single lifestyle and minimizes singlism and matrimania will improve their self-esteem and overall level of well-being [12]. Others may focus their spiritual energy in other ways, such as volunteer work, launching ministries or nonprofit organizations, obtaining further education, or helping in the finance of neighborhood or community efforts and supporting others by prayer.

Directly pointing out the presence of singlism Pointing out when people (family, friends, colleagues) say things like, "Oh, are you still single? Haven't found anyone yet?" is a good first step. The appropriate response will depend on the relationship that exists with the person making the offensive comment. Unless we bring awareness to the cultural perception that assumes that everyone "should" strive toward being partnered in some way, then the stigma will continue. Everyone should take personal responsibility to reduce the stigma aimed at singles, working to build a culture that no longer excludes or opposes the interests of single individuals. After all, in this life, we are solo travelers. As one woman in her blog states, "As singles, we know more than anybody else that the true independence is actually interdependence. We can use this to work for a more compassionate society – and ensure that the increasing numbers of singles are taken care of no matter what they do for a living or how old they are, even when they choose to remain single for their whole life" [70].

Empowering oneself Empowering oneself by the adoption of a positive view about one's single status as a situation, learning to be comfortable single, and viewing the single relationship status positively, versus perpetuating the thoughts and feelings of being neglected or unattractive, is of significant benefit to the single person. This attitude may also be a useful reframing for the single person who desires to be partnered, but for singles who are single by choice, happy with their single status, and not currently looking for a partner, self-empowerment also buffers the social scrutiny that they typically face. As they defy social norms, singles by choice are deemed to be more miserable and lonelier than those who are single by circumstance, the latter being viewed as more mature and sociable [44, 71, 72]. Empowerment for singles in the form of reading books promoting positive thinking, attending a course, participating in a workshop, taking a consulting session, and establishing a support network shows evidence that they can improve the single person's happiness and enable them to face social tensions and discrimination [73].

If today's children are less likely to see marriage or partnership as a relationship aspiration and will likely spend a longer portion of their adult lives single, education and empowerment of our children should include the basic survival skills for how to be, thrive, and live happily in a state of singlehood.

Beyond Going Solo: What Makes Being Single Hard?

The Challenges, Obstacles Beyond the Social Stereotyping, Stigmatizing, and Discrimination

Isolation, Loneliness, and Solitude

In 1965, 72% of all adults aged 18 and older were married. Today it is about 50% [74]. Being and living life as a single person does present certain challenges. Most studies show that one of the prime reported advantages of being married is the human company and reliance found in a marriage. The institution of marriage is seen as a means to prevent long bouts of isolation which are also known to reduce any individual's well-being [75, 76]. It is in this realm of the emotional challenge of singlehood that we find one of the biggest obstacles to curating a happy single life. The feelings of isolation and of loneliness can grip the single in times such as waking up alone on a weekend morning or going to bed alone at the end of a busy week; going to a movie alone; going to church, synagogue, or other communal social event alone; repeatedly sitting at a table meant for two or more alone for a meal; celebrating a birthday, work, or personal achievement alone; or simply sitting in front of the TV alone without the presence of another to help pass the time or to fulfill that basic desire and healthy need we all have from our infancy for human contact. Other emotions that singles may commonly express include fear of being alone, inadequacy, and vulnerability. How does a single person address the fears of and the actual reality of being alone, the feeling of isolation or loneliness that inevitably shows up from time to time, or perhaps is a more constant companion for those who are in-waiting and truly desire to be partnered?

Studies show that it is actually the fear of aging alone and dying without anyone at our bedside that is one of the most common and deeply ingrained reasons for getting married [77, 78]. Being alone versus the emotion of loneliness is certainly a dynamic experienced in the single person's life. Loneliness is defined as "a discrepancy between one's desired and achieved levels of social relations" and "may concern the number of relationships or the level of intimacy in the relationship" [79, 80]. Loneliness must be separated conceptually, however, from social isolation. Social isolation refers to the objective state of having minimal contact with other people, whereas loneliness is the perception of isolation or neglect and is not reality [81, 82].

Four strategies, identified through his interviews with older singles, are described by Elyakim Kislev, PhD, as being used to adapt to being single and the mechanisms behind their happiness [83]. These include:

1. The ability to look back and gain control over the circumstances that led to being single
2. Making effort to shift from the fear of being lonely when I am old to making a clear distinction between solitude and loneliness and patiently curating a practice of enjoying solitude
3. The ability to foresee possible emergencies and to prepare accordingly, taking control of such unpredictable situations, such as the practical measures of managing physical, fiscal, and other responsibilities
4. Adjustment in self-identity in order to deal with the societal pressures and prejudices, especially as they relate to the stigmatization of long-term singleness. The development of positive self-identity, a practice of optimism, focusing on their equality, and building strong social networks
5. The construction of alternatives to intimate relationships, through building social capital and alternative "family"

The internal, mental dialogue of thoughts with which one speaks to or questions oneself, as a single person, can be a battleground that must be mastered. Thoughts or beliefs that reinforce the traditionally held stigma and stereotypes about singles are often part of the single person's internal dialogue, having been conditioned by culture over long periods of time. Recognizing when these beliefs arise, shedding light on them and calling them out for what they are, is the first step to creating awareness. Changing those thought patterns and replacing them with new beliefs about what it means to be single is a powerful process. The transition from thoughts and fears of being or going it alone, being lonely, and not good or worthy enough can be changed into thoughts in which the single person develops an appreciation for their privacy and time to devote to solitude or to meaningful and fulfilling activities of their choosing. These new mental frameworks and beliefs have a powerful downstream effect on the emotional experience of the single person, having great power to affect the ways in which the single person shows up in the world and the way in which their life either thrives and flourishes or not.

The Importance of Social Capital

Social capital is understood as "the norms and networks facilitating collective action for mutual benefit" [84]. It refers broadly to effectively functional social groups and includes interpersonal relationships, a shared sense of identity, a shared understanding, shared norms, shared values, trust, cooperation, and reciprocity [85].

Social capital is of particular significance for singles [86], as outlined in the following five reasons:

1. Singles derive more happiness from social capital because they meet more diverse people and engage in a wider variety of activities. They have a diverse set of confidants and create stronger core networks in which they experience less isolation than married peers [87, 88].
2. Whereas couples participate in increasingly uniform and conformist social activities, singles are more flexible and become ever more adept at constructing social frameworks that cater to their needs, while remaining flexible and open to change [89].

3. Singles are more attentive to social relationships and make them central to their lives. They focus on a wider sphere of family and friends [90].
4. Singles utilize modern technology to facilitate and maintain their social capital and to make it more efficient [91].
5. Markets have adapted to the rise of singlehood and new products, services, and living arrangements targeting singles, such as community spaces in condominiums to facilitate the development of social ties [92–94].

Maintaining social capital has been found to be a direct predictor of well-being and has strong correlation with greater life satisfaction, involvement in clubs, nonpolitical societies, and noneconomic organizations [95–99]. Religious social capital, such as measured by attendance at church, is also positively associated with well-being [100]. Social capital has been shown to contribute to the development of greater awareness, improved health via physical training, increased economic support, and an improved ability to deal with stress [101, 102]. Additionally, it has been shown to decrease anxiety and increases motivation to lead an active and healthy lifestyle [103].

Singles who proactively and creatively pursue the development and maintenance of social networks and who intentionally cultivate social capital via participation in social activities (volunteering, social clubs) and social meetings (visiting friends or family) do so to the benefit of their happiness, life satisfaction, and well-being [104]. In addition, they enjoy greater resilience in the face of adversity and receive support found in the midst of and after divorce, or in the midst of single parenthood [57, 105, 106].

Singles do not all want to be partnered, but they do want to be included and are willing to extend themselves to others in recognition of our common human condition. Singles spend time and energy building their own social networks by participation in social meetings and activities (volunteering, civic organizations, charities, clubs), nurturing these relationships as central to their lives, much like couples turn inward and focus on their relationships. Singles often form more diverse, flexible, sophisticated, and efficient networks. Their wider sphere of confidants is held in high esteem, like a nonromantic, nonsexual network of people who serve as the safety net of connection singles desire and that can be relied on.

The Physical and Material Challenges of Singlehood

It is not just the emotional, mental, or social challenges that singles navigate, but also the actual physical and material challenges of living life solo. As a Physical Medicine and Rehabilitation physician, I am routinely using physical functional assessment tools, such as the Functional Independence Measure (FIM) (Fig. 9.3), to assess a patient's level of function as it relates to various activities of daily living (ADLs) and instrumental activities of daily living (IADLs) [107–112]. These physical, cognitive, communication, and behavioral realms are assessed in the setting of a patient's specific medical diagnoses. These measures provide a more

Functional Independence Measure - Activities of Daily Living (ADLs)	Instrumental Activities of Daily Living (IADLs)

Self-Care
    Eating
    Grooming
    Bathing
    Dressing –Upper Body
    Dressing –Lower Body
    Toileting
Sphincter Control
    Bladder
    Bowel
Transfers
    Bed, Chair, Wheelchair
    Toilet
    Tub, Shower
Locomotion
    Walk / Wheelchair
    Stairs
Communication
    Comprehension
    Expression
Social Cognition
    Social Interaction
    Problem Solving
    Memory
	Cleaning and maintaining the house
	Managing finances
	Community Mobility
	Preparing meals
	Shopping of groceries and necessities
	Taking prescribed medications
	Using the telephone or other form of communication
	Care of others
	Care of pets
	Child rearing
	Communication management
	Health management and maintenance
	Home establishment and maintenance
	Religious observances
	Safety procedures and emergency responses

Fig. 9.3 Functional Independence Measure (FIM)

objective description in regard to a person's capability to perform various tasks. In rating the task, the level of function is described as independent, independent with some type of aide or equipment, or some version of dependent, which can vary from requiring only supervision for safety to completely dependent on the assistance of another in order for the task to be completed. Some activities are deemed necessary for fundamental functioning in life and other tasks are not necessary but if able to be performed allow an individual to live independently in a community. These are the essential tasks for living, and when the busy professional, who dedicates their time to the care of others or their business, is unable to do these tasks on their own, they will need to at least be able to manage or delegate them in a way that allows for their completion.

Vignette: At this very moment, on a Saturday morning, I am not only sitting at my dining room table working on writing this chapter, but also am processing a third load of laundry through the separate/wash/dry/fold/put away process. My workout this morning was followed by my centering prayer/mindfulness/ meditation practice. I have made arrangements with my parents to have dinner with them tonight, necessitating travel 20 min in each direction. My dog sitter is out of town next week, so I have also coordinated with my mother to watch my dog through that time, and I need to make sure that I pack up everything she will need to spend a week away from home. I sent a message to a friend regarding an exciting event she had planned for her business this weekend, offering my support, encouragement, and congratulations. I spoke to a family member with a recent medical issue. I called my 98-year-old grandmother and bought and sent birthday cards/gifts to my two nieces who live out of state, for their respective upcoming birthdays. I turned down an invitation to a social event for tomorrow, choosing instead to honor my spiritual practice of attending church and participating in my faith community. Tomorrow, I will also stop at the grocery store to purchase food and supplies in preparation for the next week and put those items away upon returning home along with doing some food prep work so that healthier meals are more readily available. I will attend to the delivered mail, the monthly finances, and e-mail communications. The air conditioner in my home has been not working well, necessitating a total of 12 phone calls and 4 in person visits thus far in the last 2 weeks and is still not working correctly and for which I tentatively have a service appointment for early next week, which will require that I coordinate with someone to be available to let them in, as I have a full schedule in the clinic and hospital coverage. I need to make flight and hotel reservations for an upcoming work trip and find someone who can sit and wait and drive me home after an upcoming colonoscopy. The plants in my house look droopy, as I look at them now, and at some point, they will need some "TLC" (i.e., water) this weekend too. Whew, so much for the weekend.

Time and Energy

We all have time (24 h, 1440 min, 86,400 s per day) and energy to give to each day. The way we think about, organize ourselves around, and prioritize our use of time and energy will depend on many factors. For the single, woman physician with extended and often irregular work hours, overnights, weekends, and on-call responsibilities, and limited time for out of work activities, the time and energy spent managing and engaging in life has to be strategic. Can I also give a special shout out to and special recognition for the single physicians (women and men), whether by choice or by circumstance, who are also parenting children or caregiving for a parent or another extended family member or even perhaps caring for a friend in a time of need?

While it would be nice to have a personal chef and personal assistant or concierge service to help in our personal lives, and this type of service is becoming more readily available and frankly more necessary, single women physicians have typically had the responsibility of doing it all and doing it all alone. A list of activities and responsibilities on the home front, each requiring management to make the rest of life and going to work even feasible, is noted in the table below [112]. For the single, there is no partner with whom to split or share the tasks of running a home or having the semblance of a social calendar. While one may not perform the actual tasks themselves (i.e., pool care), these tasks require at least a measure of time for supervision, monitoring, and management. In my personal experience, it is amazing sometimes how challenging it is, and what a special effort it takes, to be able to enjoy the simple act of sitting down at a table to eat a healthy home-cooked meal, even if that meal is just for me.

A Single's Work (at Home) [113]
- Child care, parenting, school events/parties, athletic or club activities
- Pet care
- Laundry
- Grocery shopping
- Food/meal preparation
- Housekeeping
- Yard care
- Pool care
- Exterminator (monthly)
- Termite inspector (yearly)
- Car care
- Appliance maintenance (i.e., A/C filter changes)
- Appliance repair service appointments (i.e., twice-yearly A/C – heat systems service)
- Management of finances
- Time for personal shopping
- Houseplant care
- Gift and card buying
- Travel planning and associated coordination
- Celebration and social event planning and associated coordination

These necessary tasks can end up taking a majority of the single person's time when away from work. Some tasks may even need to be attended to during work hours. The time and energy required for management of these activities can end up leaving very little actual time to engage in true restorative, leisure activities, limiting the time to relax or the energy to enjoy the important process of building a supportive social network. If supportive and helpful extended family are available, keeping these relationships close is vitally important for the single person, as it is these individuals on whom the single will call for help when in times of need. Those singles who truly are living solo without the support of family locally, must strategically prioritize their time and energy in order to attend to these tasks. They must also prioritize time for self-care and for nurturing trusting relationships that become "like family" in order to achieve at least a measure of work–life integration.

When the Single Is Sick

What happens when the single person gets sick, has an accident, needs a surgery, or suffers immobility, disability, or job loss? Who helps the single person in their time of need? Those in partnered relationships, and even more so those with a partner and children, are culturally assumed to be better off when it comes to times when one needs physical assistance in the setting of illness, immobility, disability, or job loss. There is an assumed "safety net" of guaranteed help in times of need. Marriage doesn't necessarily fix this problem as it is noted that following the loss of a job, there is an increased risk of also losing a marriage. It is also well noted that people with a disability are 42% more likely to be divorced than those without a disability, perhaps for the burden that a disability puts on the relationship and the ability of the spouse to provide the expected support and attention required [95, 114, 115].

Single or married, we all need a little help from our family/friends, at least every once in a while. The simple act of opening a jar needed for the evening meal's recipe, which if unable to be opened and necessitating and block long search for a neighbor to help, can make a single woman feel completely frustrated, isolated, alone, and even helpless, when all she wants to do is make dinner after a long day at work. Packing up and moving out of your home and the comfort of your own bed and into your parent's house for a period of time, because you needed surgery and a place to recover, where you have someone to look out for you, are some straightforward examples of how the single adapts to their life circumstances, and demonstrates their being available to ask for help, to include others and to nurture the kind of relationships in which trusted help is found. When a person who is single gets sick and needs help, who do they call for help? Who's available to help them? Often singles are left to fend for themselves. The feelings of inadequacy, isolation and helplessness can be paralyzing; the vulnerability and the fear of being stranded are real.

It would certainly be nice if we could predict and plan for our physical needs as it relates to illness, disability, and our care leading up to the time of our death, but we can only prepare to a certain extent. For the single person, this means that preplanning often includes not only the traditional legal paperwork and preplanning, but also consideration of a network of non-immediate family and friends; individuals outside of the traditional immediate family become potentially all the more important. A strengthened role of friendship, which is likely even stronger among those that are mutually single, may be relied upon for emotional, social, material, and even financial support that was once traditionally provided by the family.

Help in times of need comes from within this community or network with which the single person has forged deeper relationships and accountability. The richer, more diverse social lives of singles versus married partners, who spend most of their time investing in their mutual relationship, seem to be the key to allow for this type of networked support to be created and leveraged in times of need. Singles are also more poised to be of help to their extended families and friends and can benefit in return. These networks, however, take time and effort to develop and sustain, which for the busy practicing single professional can be an obstacle and challenge to their finding a satisfying and reliable social support system outside of the workplace.

Singles and Burnout

Integrating Work and Life

- *A job* = work that provides financial reward and is necessary for subsistence and paying the bills.
- *A career* = work that fulfills the necessity of earning an income, with the added value of permitting one to seek advancement, to feel successful and capable.
- *A calling* = work in which workers choose their profession for reasons of personal enjoyment and fulfillment, or with a focus on creating change and/or contributing to a wider cause [116]. Self-fulfillment, whether having to do with meeting personal goals, seeking deeper meaning in life, or the fulfillment of one's hopes, dreams, and ambitions is now a direct measure of our happiness [117–119].

In comparison to married persons, for singles, and especially the long-term, never-married single, the pursuit of a career and job satisfaction versus the creation of a nuclear family often serves as a means to self-fulfillment and happiness [120]. In particular, highly individualistic singles tend to value meaningful work because it actualizes their capabilities, brings them a sense of freedom, and makes them feel worthy, thus gaining for themselves more life satisfaction [121, 122]. Singles, therefore, stand to gain more from investing in their career than married individuals do [123]. Never-married singles have freedom to choose a potentially less secure career path, or ones that may be more emotionally rewarding, than those who are married and/or have family who select jobs with more security and financial stability [124]. Many singles are happier with their singleness and find their lives enriched, when they are unbound by family responsibilities and can fully invest in their careers, even choosing not to enter relationships because they want to avoid the work–family conflict [125].

One can see then that the single person, in general, might make for a loyal, committed employee, having great capacity, ability, and desire to commit to meaningful and fulfilling work. However, in the absence of integrating the other realms of life, being "married" to work puts the single person at increased risk for job burnout. In fact, there is evidence that unmarried individuals, especially men, are more prone to the symptoms of job burnout compared to those who are married [126–128]. Singles (never married) seem to experience even higher burnout levels than those who are divorced (previously married) [128].

Job burnout is a type of stress characterized by elevated levels of exhaustion, cynicism, and inefficacy. Singles do not wish to neglect friends and family, but they may experience job burnout when they place high importance on their professional lives, along with a driving need to be perceived as a successful and dynamic professional at the expense of supportive networks [129]. According to Elyakim Kislev, PhD, "…by placing such high value on their careers, single people have more at stake in their jobs. Challenges in this sole realm of focus can prove daunting. The pressure to succeed is greater and the risk of losing one's sense of self-fulfillment because of underperformance is higher" [130]. In comparison, married couples have a "safety net" of sorts, in that they place high importance on their roles as spouses and parents; thus, work is not their only source of satisfaction.

On the other hand, the safety net that the single person attempts to create for themselves through involvement in a wide variety of activities (sporting, volunteer, community, and family–/friend-related activities may divide their social lives into far more pieces than coupled individuals) [12]. This multiplicity of roles played by singles can in turn become a source of imbalance and additional conflict, thus contributing to the development of burnout [131]. In his book, *Happy Singlehood*, Dr. Kislev also explains that the "emotional and physical exhaustion among singles is evident in today's workplace because of ignorance, about their needs, and because of pervasive, yet seldom scrutinized discrimination against singles" [130]. As discussed earlier in this chapter, singles may be prone to place excessive pressure on themselves to perform in order to perhaps compensate for their self-perceived lesser value or in fact the actual external expectation that singles will work harder than their married colleagues. These sources of overwork without a net gain of benefits have an effect on work–life integration that is a direct result of the workplace itself, employers, and policies [132]. Unmarried people without children are at particularly high risk. The cultural "assumption that, since singles do not have traditional familial responsibilities, they can meet higher work expectations" overlooks the notion that many singles are balancing numerous social roles outside of work and are often leading much more involved and complicated lives than coupled individuals [133]. In contrast to the assumption that married individuals are the ones for whom the balance is difficult because of family responsibilities, it is actually singles who suffer more from the difficulties of work–life integration, as evidenced by widowed or divorced singles, who are 31% and 22%, respectively, more likely to think their work and lives are out of balance compared to married people [133].

The overattention in "work–life balance" directed to "life" as "family," and as such the nuclear family, is unfair to the single worker [134]. "Life" includes, among other things, the pursuit of leisure, educational activities, community involvement, household management and maintenance, and friendship development [135]. Family is but one of many domains of "life" that deserves cultivation by the application of our attention, time, and energy.

Work–Life Integration Strategies for the Single Female Physician

In his book, Happy Singlehood: The Rising Acceptance and Celebration of Solo Living, Elyakim Kislev, PhD, identifies 6 ways that happy singles broaden their understanding of the work–life integration [136]:

1. Complement work with a healthy array of leisure activities (casual leisure time activities or serious hobbies).
2. Foster enriching educational activities (learning outside of the formal work environment). Highly individualistic singles are

especially interested in noncompulsory learning, reading, or taking a course. Others pursue extra degrees, certificates, or other general self-improvement.

3. Make time for health and appearance needs (exercise, cooking and eating healthy meals, and spiritual practices, prayer, or mindfulness). Mindfulness, spirituality, and, in some situations, religion can be used to increase singles' happiness at work [137–140]. Several studies show a strong positive relationship between mindfulness and job satisfaction and a strong inverse relationship with work burnout [141, 142]. Mindfulness-based cognitive therapy for the divorced single reduces anxiety and depression [143, 144]. Prayer or meditation calms and improves spiritual health for those who practice Islam, and in India, the practice of dharma is an important predictor of stress reduction and increased well-being [145, 146]. Loneliness and depression among older singles were found to be moderated by one's spiritual practice and religious beliefs [147].

4. Creative attention to household management (housekeeping, yard care, bills/finances, food shopping/meal preparation, home improvements/services, car care, and social responsibilities). Singles, who live alone and who work long hours that eat into the time required for housekeeping tasks, let alone their other multiple social responsibilities, can find this to be a very challenging aspect of work–life integration. Even if money is not an issue, finding the time to complete these tasks can prove to be a burden. Being organized and yet flexible, hiring or asking for help, exchanging services, and keeping a positive attitude for getting tasks done are helpful strategies.

5. "Selecting" a family for oneself (family, friends). The idea that your friends are the family you choose for yourself is of benefit to the single person. Singles, and particularly those who live alone, are very likely to be solely responsible for their time outside of work, so purposely investing more in their chosen relationships is even more important for their well-being than for married couples, cohabitators, and parents, all of whom are naturally consumed by their nuclear family.

6. Turn the work environment into a social one (find connection and community at work). Singles are constantly finding and making new friends, both in the community and at work.

Making friends at work helps to diffuse the alienation that can be felt in the workplace, eliminate the emotional distance between colleagues, and even disrupt the hierarchy within an organization. Singles who find personal connections in their work environments are happier by virtue of their tending to their need for work–life integration.

The Workplace

Income

Another area of concern for singles that can tie into burnout is equality in pay, which is also associated with ratings of job satisfaction among singles. This is especially so, considering the effort some singles give to their work when compared to married colleagues. Married individuals in the workplace (both men and women), in one study, were found to earn approximately 26% more than singles performing equivalent jobs [148]. Another study suggests that there is a correlation between marital status and wealth level for men and that married men between the ages of 28 and 30 make $15,900 more than their single counterparts, whereas the difference becomes $18,800 for men between 44 and 46 years of age [149]. They also found that married men were working 400 more hours per year than single men of comparable educational achievement and similar economic classes, concluding that married men are motivated to maximize their income and benefit from the advice and encouragement of their wives. But what about the extra burden that the single man has in managing life outside of work? Is that perhaps what keeps him from working the extra hours and receiving the added benefit of social support he needs in order to rise to greater success?

Singles who choose to invest themselves in their work, over-deliver value, and go beyond the contribution of their married colleagues should be acknowledged and financially rewarded accordingly. In healthcare, this might look like the physician or employee who takes extra shifts or coverage for colleagues, takes more overnight calls, does more travel, or covers holidays. In contrast, for those seeking better work–life integration, one may choose to work less and sacrifice income in order to have time off every day for oneself, to manage life outside of work, to pursue time with family and friends, or to pursue hobbies or other interests. If a nontraditional work schedule is an option and helps one to promote and preserve a positive work–life integration, then it should not be judged and perhaps even encouraged.

Healthcare and Other Benefits

Employers subsidize the cost of healthcare and other benefits for an employees' spouse, children, or domestic partner, but offer no such benefit to the single person's parents, siblings, or close friends [150]. The single who might wish to take time off to provide needed care to someone within their close network of social support, often consisting of other singles, is not supported. When the single employee is sick, they are potentially in a much more vulnerable position than their married colleagues, because they may not have anyone to provide needed support or assistance. Their closest support system may consist of other singles, who are employed and do not have the ability to take time off to help. Whereas for a married couple, when one individual is ill, their spouse is granted time off or leave through the Family Medical Leave Act in order to help provide care for their ill spouse.

For singles who also have the responsibility of parenting children or who oversee the care of a parent or other family member, having access to a work environment that is understanding and supportive of these additional roles is vitally important. Workplace support services that provide day care or elder day care might be an important benefit that allows an employee to go to work, knowing that their child or loved one is being cared for in a safe, stimulating, supportive, and caring environment. If not on-site, then employee programs that provide support or assistance in finding quality at-home or community-based childcare or elder care services are helpful. Quality day care, after-school care, or care for children or adults that includes off-hours or overnights is essential for the busy working single physician. If this type of care and supervision cannot be arranged through coordination with other family members or friends, then having assistance to connect with quality services either through the workplace directly or via recommendations of community providers is a benefit that helps meet the most basic of work–life integration needs of the single physician parent or single physician who is responsible for the care of one of their own immediate or extended family members.

Choice of Specialty

It is well known that women, more often than their male physician colleagues, who have or expect to have children, consider current or future family obligations, among other factors, when choosing either a particular specialty or a particular job [151–153]. Those who are single or who expect to remain single may make specialty choices and career move decisions with regard to their expectations of current or future family obligations and their perceived ability to find work–life integration. There is no data specifically looking at this and more research is needed to define how singleness for the female physician plays a role in specialty choice and opportunity.

The Medscape Physician Lifestyle & Happiness Report 2019, a survey of 15,069 physicians across 29+ specialties who practiced in the United States between July 27 and October 16, 2018, indicates that there is a similar percentage of men and women physicians who rate themselves as having a low or very low self-esteem, 7% versus 9%, respectively [13]. However, men reported having very high or high self-esteem at a much higher rate than their female colleagues (61% versus 47%, respectively). Carol A. Bernstein, MD, a professor of psychiatry and neurology at New York University School of Medicine/NYU Langone Health, says that she believes "that the major causes for the discrepancy are ongoing cultural issues in medicine and in our culture overall. While women and men are entering medical school in equal numbers, male physicians are more frequently promoted and advanced in their careers than are women [13]." Additionally, "there is also the impression that women are more likely than men to acknowledge their insecurities. Women will more frequently admit that they lack confidence and state that they are struggling." Does this have an effect on their own perceived capability to pursue a particular specialty? Does this affect how they are perceived by others as potential candidates for a specific specialty training or promotion? Does the added social burden of being a single woman contribute to any more or less of a difference from their married or partnered female colleagues? More research is needed to understand these influences.

Mentorship, Sponsorship, and Promotion

Singles, both men and women, may encounter marital status bias in the workplace [154, 155]. Marital status bias has been shown to be present in the workplace in regard to employees and employment decisions. A study consisting of three survey experiments was performed to look at different aspects of marital bias and the perceptions of employees or job applicants [156]. In the first experiment, participants were asked to report their perceptions of a prospective female employee (e.g., her willingness to work long hours) whose purported marital status varied by condition. The findings showed that participants rated a married female job applicant as less suitable for employment than a single counterpart. The second survey looked at how perceptions of prospective employees varied by marital status for both women and men. Participants again perceived a female job applicant less favorably when she was married; in contrast, a male applicant was perceived more favorably when married. The third survey experiment asked participants to predict how a male or female employee's suitability for his or her current job (e.g., dedication and work performance) would change following his or her recent marriage and whether these predictions affected participant's willingness to lay off the hypothetical employee. In this experiment, participants predicted that a recently married woman's job performance and dedication would decline, whereas a recently married man's dedication was predicted to rise; this difference made participants more willing to lay off the woman than the man. This form of marital bias, whether conscious or unconscious, may play a role in the way that women are evaluated for employment or perhaps even within the context of their ascension and promotion. More needs to be done to study this form of bias and the ways in which to create greater awareness of its presence and methods to prevent it from keeping employers from allowing these biases to influence employment and promotion decisions.

Despite the fact that there are 50% women graduating medical school, the number of women in leadership positions are far less, with only 16% of medical school deans being women [157]. A study looking at the process of professional identity formation (PIF) for women physicians found that professional identity was profoundly affected by gender stereotypes. It further revealed the existence of conflict between married and unmarried women physicians, creating a considerable gap between them [158]. "Female physicians lived with conflicting emotions in a chain of gender stereotype reinforcement," suggesting that in addition to being a woman physician, being a single woman physician carried an additional burden of stereotyping. The study proposed that "it is necessary to depart from a culture that determines merit based on a fixed sense of values, and instead develop a cultural system and work environment which allow the cultivation of a professional vision that accepts a wide variety of professional and personal identities, and a similarly wide variety of methods by which the two can be integrated."

Due to the earlier noted culturally held stereotypes and stigmatized perceptions that those who are single are less capable, less socially mature, less well-adjusted, and more self-centered, singles perhaps are less likely to be mentored or given opportunities to grow in their leadership skills. This may be reflected in the current difficulty early career women encounter in obtaining mentorship and sponsorship, especially in specialties where there are few women and the ones who do choose these specialties rely on and must forge relationships with their male colleagues.

Mentorship refers to someone who imparts wisdom and knowledge and can be at any level in an organization. Mentors are selected for their content expertise and often work behind the scenes to support their mentees. Sponsorship involves action on the part of a highly placed individual within an organization, who provides public support for the advancement and promotion of an individual within whom they see untapped or underappreciated leadership potential. The challenges or barriers to obtaining adequate mentorship and/or sponsorship may also influence a woman's ability to pursue leadership training and contributes to her ability to otherwise achieve future job promotion and self-actualization of her full potential.

Part-Time and Other Work Models

The esteem doctors hold in the eyes of their colleagues has often been linked to their dedication to work [159–161]. This dedication used to be regarded as being synonymous with the number of hours worked: the more hours you worked, the more doctor you were. Given the multiplicity of outside of work demands that the single must also attend to, having flexibility and control in schedules and the option for part-time work are often considered as one way of dealing with the incompatible demands of work and life [159, 162].

Income inequality is yet another barrier to working part-time. If a woman is being paid less for full-time work to begin with, there is an additional financial loss to consider when contemplating the possibility of working part-time in an effort to create better work–life integration. In one study, although almost one-third of women indicated they were working or had in the past worked part-time, those aged <35 were least likely to do so and 86% of the women physicians responded that there were barriers that prevented them from working part-time [151, 152, 163]. In another study of part-time radiologists, comparing them to their full-time colleagues, the part-time employees had disproportionately fewer benefits, were less likely to be partners, and had lower academic rank [153, 164]. In addition, there were statistically significant differences in part-time versus full-time benefits in regard to health insurance, disability insurance, vacation time, sick leave, and time for educational meetings.

The single, woman physician wishing to work part-time in order to achieve greater work–life integration needs to be aware of the potential barriers to doing so. Evaluating the standards for or the actual negotiation for an equitable income, schedule, and benefits portfolio will go a long way in helping to craft a meaningful integration of work and life. With the advance of technology and telemedicine, work from home options may be an appealing consideration for the single physician, who perhaps can design a more flexible work schedule allowing them to be creative in achieving a fulfilling work–life integration.

Work Policy and Benefits

Vacation benefits: The amount of time taken by physicians as assessed by the Medscape Physician Lifestyle & Happiness Report 2019 indicates that the average number of vacation days taken by Americans in 2017 was 17. Nearly a quarter of all physicians reported taking 5 or more weeks of vacation, yet the majority takes less. Forty-three percent of doctors reported taking 3 or 4 weeks of vacation annually, while 28% take 1 or 2. The importance of time off and employers who encourage physicians to take their available time off is not to be underestimated as it pertains to the discussion regarding work–life integration, burnout prevention, and burnout recovery.

When the Single Is Sick: Legislation systematically advantages married individuals, without also offering assistance to singles. One example of this includes the rules and regulations of the Family Medical Leave Act (FMLA), which are not universal and are not necessarily implemented effectively, but which are designed to allow protected time away from one's work for the purpose of caring for a spouse or immediate family member, whereas the single person does not enjoy the same freedom to care for someone equally close, say perhaps another single friend with whom they share a mindset of "adopted" or alternative "family," for the purpose of providing that basic level of needed human support.

When a single person is sick, a tremendous sense of perceived or actual vulnerability can arise. A straightforward case of the flu or a passing gastrointestinal bug can be of great challenge for the single, let alone a more protracted or serious illness requiring care over a more extended period of time. When simply navigating from bed to bathroom is a challenge, making it to the kitchen to make a bowl or pot of soup, or to let the dog out, is an extra stress and sometimes simply not feasible. Having a plan and the supplies needed ahead of time helps, but there is no going to the store when one is ill. A grocery delivery service may be of help, but for the single it sometimes means calling in a favor from a local family member (if you have one), a neighbor or a friend, or a church or social group that you are a part of, letting them know of your need and placing trust in "the universe" and human kindness to help meet ones' needs. These types of situations for the typically highly independent single can be particularly humbling and challenging, sometimes reinforcing a sense of isolation and loneliness, even provoking feelings of helplessness. It raises the questions: Who can take time off to care for the single person when they experience their time of need? Who can "be there," providing moral support when one is given bad news? Who is available to give a ride home after a medical procedure performed in the outpatient setting with sedation, and who will stay with them at home to ensure their expected recovery? In my personal experience these have been some of the most isolating and humbling experiences as a single person living alone and sometimes far away from all immediate family.

Policy and employment contracts should be designed in such a way that takes into account the single physician, woman or man, who is juggling work and life; they should promote a fair, equitable, or prorated (for those working part-time) sharing of work (patient care schedules, cross-coverage, on-call duties, travel, overnight, or holiday coverage), access to benefits (health insurance, disability insurance, vacation time, sick leave, time for educational activities), and opportunities to grow and mature professionally (attendance at professional educational activities and academic advancement) in one's career.

I was the only woman in my department for the first 8 of my now 16 years with my department. For most of that 16 years I have also been the only woman in the department working as an outpatient PM&R musculoskeletal and sports medicine specialist. I also have training as a life, health, and weight loss coach and have a certification in acupuncture. I have a skewed patient population as a result of this. I receive referrals that are different from my colleagues and I have chosen to allow patients to "request" the female doctor. My patient portfolio is therefore different from my male colleagues. My practice includes patients that, while I have no additional or special training above or beyond that of my male colleagues, simply prefer to be seen by the "woman," in the department. These cases, while not always unusual or extraordinary, have been some of the most clinically challenging cases I've ever encountered. Fortunately, I work with colleagues who understand this dynamic and have been supportive, perhaps in part because they know that if it were not for me, they would be seeing these cases.

Legislation

As stated in an article entitled, The High Price of Being Single in America, "over a lifetime, an unmarried person can pay as much as a million dollars more than a married one for health care, taxes, IRAs, Social Security and more." The authors "found over a thousand laws providing overt legal or financial benefits to married couples that are unavailable to singles. This is despite US Federal Code, which, in title 5, part III, says 'The President may prescribe rules which shall prohibit discrimination because of marital status'" [165].

Marketplace Economic Interactions

Healthcare: Single, women physicians can even experience challenges or discrimination at the hands of their own health-care colleagues and institutions in which they receive their own health-care services. Bella DePaulo, PhD, describes that health-care providers, upon knowing that a woman is "single," may make certain assumptions in regard to their patient's health-care values and her ability to have the support needed to endure certain treatment protocols [166]. A treatment considered the best and most recommended for a certain type of cancer, but also associated with a greater risk of side effects thought to be more difficult to endure without the assistance of a spouse/family member, might sway the practitioner to offer a lesser effective, but possibly better tolerated therapy or surgical procedure. The practitioner may offer only what he/she believes would be the best option considering their patient's single status and not the patient's preference for a particular approach to treatment. This can occur even in the face of singles who, while they may not have immediate family support available, may have an extensive and supportive, network of friends and "extended family." Thus, training health-care practitioners to enquire about the single person's health values, life, and support system may help optimize outcomes in their care.

Housing: When otherwise presented with potential residents of equal education, job, age, and interests, there has been shown to be a clear preference by realtors to rent a property to a married couple (61%) versus a cohabitating romantic couple (24%) and lastly a man and a woman presented as "just friends" (15%) [12]. When asked why the realtors had a preference, the answer was that singleness was reason enough and their judgement of the singles was not self-identified as overtly discriminatory. As in my own personal story at the beginning of this chapter illustrates, "singlism" is a cultural phenomenon, often unrecognized, and affecting all aspects of the marketplace and economic interactions of the daily life of the single person. Marketing targeting couples or family travel, special offers on memberships and discounts for couples, special deals like 2 for 1, and discounts for families all serve as a constant reminder and sometimes an affront that being single is not seen as equal or as valued.

Putting It All Together, The Single, Woman Physician in Perspective

Single, women physicians, who are either single by choice or by circumstance, are a phenomenon to which the greater culture and the workplace is still adapting. While the feminist movement has allowed women to become legally single, it is still whether a woman is socially single (i.e., married or not) that culture deems as mattering most. By pursuing high levels of education, careers which demand greater time and energy to perform than the average worker and challenging or even defying traditional relationship norms (single mothers and those who never marry or never partner), single, women physicians face their own form of being misunderstood. They encounter stigmatization, stereotypes, and discrimination, both inside and outside of the workplace that go beyond that of even their female married physician colleagues. "Singlism" is often not even recognized by singles themselves, but like discrimination in all forms is damaging and has consequences. Measures of psychological distress, psychiatric disorders, feeling life is harder, and sensing interference with life are some of the perceived ways that discrimination exerts its effects [167–169]. In addition, there are strongly associated physical heath markers in which perceived discrimination has influence, including weight gain, obesity, higher blood pressure in minorities, and elevated levels of smoking, alcohol use, and substance abuse [170–173].

Single, women physicians, while misunderstood, have great capacity, in part due to their greater freedom to pursue work that they find meaningful and which provides them a sense of fulfillment or self-actualization. They, in addition, have the financial ability to support themselves and perhaps too their families and even their closest of chosen non-intimate, non-romantic friends. Because they are able to commit themselves to, and find great meaningfulness in, their work, they can fall into the trap of overwork or in some cases are actually inequitably singled out to work in ways such that they become "married to work." The work of an in-demand highly trained physician within the context of the current health-care system requires the single, woman physician to be awake and aware of the potential pitfalls that lead to being "married to medicine."

The cultural, and even workplace-generated, perception that the single person has more freedom and flexibility to do more at work is a myth. Singles, and especially those who are unpartnered and do not have children, while they can make fabulous, loyal, committed workers or employees with great capacity to produce value, can actually fall more easily into overwork, isolation, loneliness, vulnerability, and burnout. Doing it all, and doing it all alone, is simply not possible. Singles require adequate time and energy to attend to the areas of life that make work and life possible. The management of one's home and social capital including family, friends ("the family we choose for ourselves"), and other social networks takes time and energy, but serves the purpose of providing social company, emotional support, intellectual stimulation, and even physical and financial assistance.

The single, woman physician's abilities to maintain perspective, create awareness and a positive self-perception, choose single-friendly environments, directly call out singlism when it occurs, empower oneself, and build social capital and networks of support are essential work–life integration skills. Time and energy are the limiting resources that make work–life integration challenging. Personal strategies that can be used by single, women physicians to prevent or combat burnout include engaging in leisure activities, participating in educational activities, making time for health and appearance needs, managing household tasks, "selecting" a family for oneself, and turning the work environment into a social one. The irreplaceable time and energy, which the single person needs for the management of their personal at-home life and for the development and maintenance of a robust and supportive network of deep, personally satisfying and accountable personal and social, "family, and family-like" relationships, is vital to the health and wholeness of singles.

Single women physicians can and should be educating workplaces and employers regarding not only their desire for and ability to pursue fulfilling and meaningful work, but also what it takes in terms of time and energy to manage all of life outside of work, so that a better balance can be found. Workplaces need to ensure that women receive equal pay compared to their male colleagues for equal work. Work schedules, cross-coverage, on-call, travel, educational responsibilities, and vacation coverage among other work responsibilities should be shared in equitable ways among colleagues, so as to allow them each to have a measure of work–life integration. Training programs must recognize that barriers exist that inhibit women from entering certain specialties and, even once entering them, limit their ability to engage in meaningful mentorship or obtain sponsorship, and being a stigmatized single woman may even perhaps accentuate this phenomenon. Opportunities for promotions among women physicians, and especially among single, women physicians, should not be inhibited because of traditionally held cultural stereotypes or stereotypes of single women, but should be made based on their expressed interest and deserved merit. Workplace polices and benefits plans should take into account the needs and circumstances of singles. Part-time employment should not further compromise the ability of the single to maintain work–life integration. Flexible schedules and support for safe, reliable childcare allow single, physician parents to attend to both their work and parenting roles. The use of technology and alternative work sites (work from home, telemedicine) will likely appeal to and help the single who is juggling multiple roles at work and within a more complex web of social networks. Sick leave policies and resources that help singles when they themselves are sick, or that allow for the single who wishes to provide needed care to a non-intimate, non-romantic, likely also single, friend in their time of need, would be of support to the greater network of singles in the community. The workplace can also, on behalf of their single employees, advance and advocate for legislation and other marketplace economic fairness policies to be implemented.

In 2011 the World Health Organization declared July 30 to be Friendship Day and in 2015 Facebook promoted Friends Day on February 4th, the anniversary of its founding [174, 175]. Communities of singles that have nothing to do with dating or romantic relationships will likely increasingly contribute to the wellness and well-being of singles. Due to the prioritization of social capital, singles spend a larger portion of their incomes on clothes, food, restaurants, leisure, and entertainment and their expenditures are increasing [176, 177]. The trend of increasing singlehood will have effects throughout culture including change in the demands on housing and urban planning, home/housekeeping management, food preparation and delivery, medical care, other goods and services, solo travel, technology use for connection to services, and social communities.

There are more people on any given day in the building where I work now than lived in my hometown where I lived for the first 18 years of my life. The clinic and the hospital where I work are like cities in and of themselves. They each have their own physical landscape, leadership, management, city planners, smaller communities with variable qualities, and organizational and traffic patterns along with multiple social structures. I have learned to navigate not only the city within their walls, but also one of the largest metropolitan cities in the United States. I have come a long way since growing up in a rural farm town with one stoplight. I provide care for patients in one of the world's foremost healthcare systems. I work in the outpatient and inpatient settings.

I have taken first call as an attending physician, a week at a time, for 16 years. I have served as a first responder on the side of the road, on the game field sideline, in my church, while on vacation, on a hiking trail in a foreign country, on an airplane at 30,000 ft, and for my own friends and family. My calling to be single for a while and the calling to be a healer have been a gift in my life. It has not been easy and there have been times when I have resisted or buffered myself in the midst of my journey. I have become comfortable in the solitude that my singleness allows and yet I do regularly seek out opportunities to connect and grow my personal network of support and community. I continue to stay open to receive the calling and the vision for being a physician, using the masculine, logical, linear, structures, protocols, and frameworks in support of the more feminine, flexible, intuitive, empathic, and passionate means of healing. I strive to use my time well and make the most of my personal gifts, talents, and opportunities. I trust that those who cross my path are those I am meant to see and serve. I care for my patients in their time of need, in the midst of their pain and life suffering. They come with anxiety, fear, worry, resistance, and overwhelm. I see them through their time of loss and grief, their transition into a life with functional impairments or a new disability. I help them rehabilitate lost function and retrain for a new level of function, along with a new self-identity. I help them to be whole, to perform to the best of their ability, whether they are looking to lose weight and get in better shape in order to lower their cholesterol or risk related to glucose intolerance. I help the teen with an ankle sprain and trying to make their high school team, the recreational athlete who falls and has a brain or spinal cord injury. I help the elderly who present with deficits from a stroke, those involved in trauma resulting in loss of limb(s), the severely deconditioned in the setting of complex medical care, the elite athlete who needs to tweak their training or their mental game in order to achieve peak performance, or the geriatric weekend warrior who simply wants to stay active and fit and enjoy living in and moving their body while maintaining their functional independence. We talk about lifestyle, habits, sleep, nutrition, flexibility, strength, balance, agility, endurance, stress management, resilience, having fun, nurturing their closest relationships, growing their social capital, and all of what makes life for them meaningful, fulfilling, and worth living. I hope to challenge and inspire them to develop themselves to live the best life that they can. In order to do this, I must walk my walk and talk my talk, to live authentically, honestly, and within boundaries that keep me aligned with my own life values, purpose, and goals. This means that I must tend my own garden if I am going to flourish, as I strive to be at my best every day.

The single, woman physician is an empowered force; she has defied traditions and norms; she has navigated the stigma, stereotyping, and discrimination from traditional culture in general, from her workplace, and even sometimes from her own family and friends. She is free to be dedicated to her calling, the healing work that is her profession. She expends her time and energy serving others, giving of herself in ways that are in turn meaningful and fulfilling to her. She desires to self-actualize and grow and wants to see others be able to do the same. Isolation, loneliness, and vulnerability are all part of her experience at some point in time, and yet she cultivates not only her own positive self-image and an attitude of positivity as she serves others, but also cultivates a community, a network of extensive support that may include family or a "family of friends." She bears the burden of work and also the work of managing life outside of work, which may include the parenting of children or the care of other family members. She does it all. She faces the challenges of the solo journey and the potential path of burnout by taking herself by her own hand and understanding that her independence, health, and success are best supported by her interdependence within her greater social community. She is a catalyst for change, a flourishing queen and an example of what is possible.

Bibliography

1. Taylor V, Whittier N. Analytical approaches to social movement culture: the culture of the women's movement. Soc Mov Cult. 1995;4:163–87.
2. Moran RF. How second-wave feminism forgot the single woman. Hofstra L Rev. 2004;33(1):223–98.

3. Evans J. Feminist theory today: an introduction to second-wave feminism. New York: Sage; 1995.

4. Whelehan I. Modern feminist thought: from the second wave to postfeminism. New York: NYU Press; 1995.

5. Eisenstein ZR, editor. Capitalist patriarchy and the case for socialist feminism. New York: Monthly Review Press; 1979; Ferguson A, Folbre N. The unhappy marriage of patriarchy and capitalism. Women Revol. 1981;80: 10–11.

6. Barnett RC, Hyde JS. Women, men, work, and family. Am Psychol. 2001;56(10):781–96; Inglehard R, Welzel C. Modernization, cultural change, and democracy: the human development sequence. Cambridge: Cambridge University Press; 2005.

7. census.gov. 14 August 2017.

8. https://www.pewresearch.org/fact-tank/.

9. De Paulo BM. Is it true that single women and married men do best? Sex differences in marriage and single life: still debating after 50 years. www.psychologytoday.com. 11 Jan 2017.

10. Blossfeld H-P, Huinink J. Human capital investments or norms of role transitions? how women's schooling and career affect the process of family formation. Am J Sociol. 1991;97(1):143–68.

11. Ridgway EB, Sauerhammer T, Chiou AP, LaBrie RA, Mulliken JB. Reflections on the mating pool for women in plastic surgery. Plast Reconstr Surg. 2014;133(1):187–94.

12. DePaulo BM. Singled out: how singles are stereotyped, stigmatized, and ignored, and still live happily ever after. New York: St Martin's Griffin; 2007.

13. Martin KL. contributor, Medscape physician lifestyle & happiness report; 2019, 9 Jan 2019.

14. Ly DP, Seabury SA, Jena AB. Divorce among physicians and other healthcare professionals in the United States: analysis of census survey data. Br Med J. 2015;350(h706):18.

15. Morris WL, DePaulo BM, Hertel J, Ritter L. Perception of people who are single: A developmental life tasks model. Manuscript submitted for publication; 2006.

16. Morris WL, Sinclair S, DePaulo BM. The perceived legitimacy of civil status discrimination. Manuscript submitted for publication; 2006.

17. Crock J, Major B. social stigma and self-esteem: the self-protective properties of stigma. Psychol Rev. 1989;96(4):608.

18. Fink PJ. Stigma and Mental Illness. Washington, DC: American Psychiatric Press; 1992.

19. Major B, O'Brien LT. The social psychology of stigma. Annu Rev Psychol. 2005;56(1):393–421.

20. Faines AK. (blog) "An explanation of the 7 Feminine Archetypes"; 2017. www.womenlovepower.com.

21. Faines AK. (blog) "13 Feminine seduction archetypes"; 2017. www.womenlovepower.com.

22. Ellis J. (blog) "Female character archetypes and strong female characters". www.Jenniferellis.ca. 1 Apr 2015.
23. Scott AO, Dargis M. Sugar, spice and guts. New York Times (Movies), 3 Sept 2014.
24. DeVee G. The audacity to be queen: the unapologetic art of dreaming big and manifesting your most fabulous life. New York: Hachette Book Group; 2020.
25. Maeda E, Hecht ML. Identity search: interpersonal relationships and relational identities of always-single Japanese women over time. West J Commun. 2012;76(1):44–64.
26. Poortman A-R, Liefbroer AC. Singles' relational attitudes in a time of individualization. Soc Sci Res. 2010;39(6):938–49.
27. Sharp EA, Ganong L. I'm a loser, I'm not married, Let's just all look at me': ever-single women's perceptions of their social environment. J Fam Issues. 2011;32(7):956–80.
28. Greitemeyer T. Stereotypes of singles: are singles what we think? Eur J Soc Psychol. 2009;39(3):368–83.
29. Thornton A, Freedman D. Changing attitudes toward marriage and single life. Fam Plann Perspect. 1981;14(6):297–303.
30. Wilson JQ. The marriage problem: how our culture has weakened families. New York: Harper Collins; 2002.
31. Crocker J, Major B. Social stigma and self-esteem: the self-protective properties of stigma. Psychol Rev. 1989;96(4):608.
32. Kislev E. Happy singlehood: the rising acceptance and celebration of solo living. Oakland: University of California Press; 2019. p. 83.
33. Kay Clifton A, McGrath D, Wick B. Stereotypes of woman: a single category? Sex Roles. 1976;2(2):135–48.
34. Eagly AH, Steffen VJ. Gender stereotypes stem from the distribution of women and men into social roles. J Pers Soc Psychol. 1984;46 (4):735.
35. Hassouneh-Phillip DS. Marriage is half of faith and the rest is fear of allah': marriage and spousal abuse among American muslims. Violence Against Women. 2001;7(8):927–46.
36. Zongker CE. Self-concept differences between single and married school-age mothers. J Youth Adolesc. 1980;9(2):175–84.
37. Maslow A. A theory of human motivation, vol. 50: Psychol Rev; 1943. p. 370.
38. Florida R. The rise of the creative class – revisited: revised and expanded. New York: Basic Books; 2014.
39. Inglehart R. The silent revolution: changing values and political styles among western publics. Princeton: Princeton University Press; 1977.
40. Reynolds J, Wetherell M. The discursive climate of singleness: the consequences for women's negotiation of a single identity. Fem Psychol. 2003;13(4):489–510.
41. Kislev E. Happy singlehood: the rising acceptance and celebration of solo living. Oakland: University of California Press; 2019. p. 131–2.

42. Adamczyk K. Krakow, Poland: Libron; 2016. p. 145–62; Slonim G, Gur-Yaish N, Katz R. By choice or by circumstance?: stereotypes of and feelings about single. Peopl. Studia Psychologica. 2015; 57(1): 35–48.

43. Kislev E. Happy singlehood: the rising acceptance and celebration of solo living. Oakland: University of California Press; 2019. p. 133–5.

44. Bur-Yaish GSN, Katz R. By choice or by circumstance?: stereotypes of and feelings about single people. Stud Psychol. 2015;57(1): 35–48.

45. Burt S, Donnellan M, Humbad MN, Hicks BM, McGue M, Iacono WG. Does marriage inhibit antisocial behavior?: an examination of selection vs. causation via a longitudinal twin design. Arch Gen Psychiatry. 2010;67(12):1309–15.

46. Garrison M, Scott ES. Marriage at the crossroads: law, policy and the brave New World of twenty-first-century families. Cambridge: Cambridge University Press; 2012.

47. Koball HL, Moiduddin E, Henderson J, Goesling B, Besculides M. What do we know about the link between marriage and health? J Fam Issues. 2010;31(8):1019–40.

48. Dupre ME, Meadows SO. Disaggregating the effects of marital trajectories on health. J Fam Issues. 2007;28(5):623–52.

49. Gove WR, Hughes M, Style CB. Does marriage have positive effects on the psychological Well-being of the individual? J Health Soc Behav. 1983;24(2):122–31.

50. Hughes ME, Waite LJ. Marital biography and health at mid-life. J HealthSoc Behav. 2009;50(3):344–58.

51. Johnson DR, Wu J. An empirical test of crisis, social selection and roe explanations of the relationship between marital disruption and psychological distress: a pooled time-series analysis of four-wave panel data. J Marriage Fam. 2002;64(1):211–24.

52. McCreery J. Japanese consumer behaviour: from worker bees to wary shoppers. New York: Routledge; 2014.

53. Sbarra DA, Nietert PJ. Divorce and death: forty years of the Charleston heart study. Psychol Sci. 2009;20(1):107–13.

54. Wade TJ, Pevalin DJ. Marital transitions and mental health. J Health Soc Behav. 2004;45(2):155–70.

55. Power C, Rodgers B, Hope S. Heavy alcohol consumption and marital status: disentangling the relationship in a National Study of young adults. Addiction. 1999;94(10):1477–87.

56. Reynolds J. The single woman: a discursive investigation. London: Routledge; 2013.

57. DePaulo B. How we live now: redefining home and family in the 21st century. Hillsboro: Atria books; 2015.

58. Weston K. Families we choose: lesbians, gays, kinship. New York: Columbia University Press; 2013.

59. Camacho AS, Soto CA, Gonzalez-Cutre D, Moreno-Mucia JA. Postmodern values and motivation towards leisure and exercise in sports centre users. RICYDE: Revista Internacional de Ciencias del Deporte. 2011;7(25):320–35.

60. Llopis-Goig R. Sports participation and cultural trends: running as a reflection of individualisation and post-materialism processes in Spanish society. Eur J Sport Soc. 2014;11(2):151–69.

61. A table for one: a critical reading of singlehood, gender, and time. Manchester: University of Manchester; 2017).

62. Lauri, response to Bella DePaulo, Is it bad to notice discrimination?" Psychology today, on 16 June 2008. www.psychologytoday.com/blog/living-single/200805/is-it-bad-notice-discrimination.

63. Baumeister RF, Campbell JD, Krueger JI, Vohs KD. Does high self-esteem cause better performance, interpersonal success, happiness, or healthier lifestyles? Psychol Sci Public Interest. 2003;4(1):1–44.

64. Caprara GV, Steca P, Gerbino M, Paciello M, Vecchio GM. Looking for adolescents' well-being: self-efficacy beliefs as determinants of positive thinking and happiness. epidemiologia e psichiatria soiale. 2006; 15(1):30–43.

65. Schimmack U, Diener E. Predictive validity of explicit and implicit self-esteem for subjective well-being. J Res Pers. 2003;37(2):100–6.

66. Rachel, A call for single action," Rachel's Musings. 16 Sept 2013. www.rabe.org/a-call-for-single-action/.

67. Kislev E. Happy singlehood: the rising acceptance and celebration of solo living. Oakland: University of California Press; 2019. p. 91–2.

68. Kislev E. Happy singlehood: the rising acceptance and celebration of solo living. Oakland: University of California Press; 2019. p. 91–4.

69. Winner LF. Real sex: the naked truth about chastity. Theol Sex. 2015;26(1):84.

70. Anonymous. When singlutionary is "sick of being single!" singlutionary. 9 Oct 2011. http://singlutionary.blogspot.com.

71. Morris WL, Osburn BK. Do you take this marriage? perceived choice over marital status affects the stereotypes of single and married people. In: Singlehood from individual and social perspectives; 2016. p. 145–62.

72. Cohn D'V, Passel JS, Wang W, Livingston G. Barely half of U.S. adults are married – a record low. Washington, DC: Pew Research Center; 2011.

73. Bolier L, Haverman M, Westerhof GJ, Riper H, Smit F, Bohlmeijer E. Positive psychology interventions: a meta-analysis of randomized controlled studies. BMC Public Health. 2013;13(1):119.

74. Turner HA, Turner RJ. Gender, social status, and emotional reliance. J Health Soc Behav. 1999;40(4):360–73.

75. West DA, Kellner R, Moore-West M. The effects of loneliness: a review of the literature. Compr Psychiatry. 1986;27(4):351–63.

76. McKenzie JA. Disabled people in rural south africa talk about sexuality. Cult Health Sex. 2013;15(3):372–86.

77. Spielmann SS, MacDonald G, Maxwell JA, Joel S, Peragine D, Muise A, Impett EA. Settling for less out of fear of being single. J Pers Soc Psychol. 2013;105(6):1049.

78. Spielmann SS, MacDonald G, Joel S, Impert EA. Longing for ex-partners out of fear of being single. J Pers. 2016;84(6):799–808.

79. Gatz M, Zarit SH. A good old age: paradox or possibility. In: Handbook of theories of aging. New York: Springer; 1999. p. 396–416.

80. Fokkema T, Gierveld JDJ, Dykstra PA. Cross-national differences in older adult loneliness. J Psychol. 2012;146(1–2):201–28.

81. Clare Wenger G, Davies R, Shahtahmasebi S, Scott A. Social isolation and loneliness in old age: review and model refinement. Ageing Soc. 1996;16(3):333–58.

82. Jylha M. Old age and loneliness: cross-sectional and longitudinal analyses in the Tampere longitudinal study on aging. Can J Ageing/La revue canadienne du viellissement. 2004;23(2):157–68.

83. Kislev E. Happy singlehood: the rising acceptance and celebration of solo living. Oakland: University of California Press; 2019. p. 57–77.

84. Woolcock M. Social capital and economic development: toward a theoretical synthesis and policy framework. Theory Soc. 1998;27(2):151–208.

85. Wikipedia, Social capital. (July, 2019).

86. Kislev E. Happy singlehood: the rising acceptance and celebration of solo living. Oakland: University of California Press; 2019. p. 119–24.

87. Hampton KN, Sessions LF, Her EJ. Core networks, social isolation, and new media: how internet and mobile phone use is related to network size and diversity. Inf Commun Soc. 2011;14(1):130–55.

88. Solomon P. Peer support/peer provided services underlying processes, benefits, and critical ingredients. Psychiatr Rehabil J. 2004;27(4):392.

89. Amato PR, Booth A, Johnson DR, Rogers SJ. Alone together: how marriage in America is changing. Cambridge, MA: Harvard University Press; 2007.

90. Gerstel N, Sarkisian N. Marriage: the good, the bad, and the greedy. Contexts. 2006;5(4):16–21.

91. Quiroz PA. From finding the perfect love online to satellite dating and 'loving-the-one-you're near': A Look at Grindr, Skout, Plenty of Fish, Meet Moi, Zoosk and Assisted Serendipity. Humanit Soc. 2013;37(2):181.

92. Alden DL, JBE S, Batra R. Brand positioning through advertising in asia, north america, and europe: the role of global consumer culture. J Market. 1999;63:75–87.

93. Ewen S. Captains of consciousness: advertising and the social roots of the consumer culture. New York: Basic Books; 2008.

94. Yee CD. Re-urbanizing Downtown Los Angeles: Micro housing densifying the city's core. Master of Architecture thesis, University of Washington; 2013.

95. Helliwell JF, Barrington-Leigh CP. How much is social capital worth? In: Jetten J, Haslam C, Haslam SA, editors. The social cure. London: Psychology Press; 2010. p. 55–71.

96. Winkelmann R. Unemployment, social capital, and subjective well-being.

97. Helliwell JF. How's life? combining individual and national variable to explain subjective well-being. Econ Model. 2003;20(2):331–60.

98. Pichler F. Subjective quality of life of young europeans: feeling happy but who knows why? Soc Indic Res. 2006;75(3):419–44.

99. Cornwell EY, Waite LJ. Social disconnectedness perceived isolation, and health among older adults. J Health Soc Behav. 2009;50(1):31–48.

100. Hayo B, Seifer W. Subjective economic well-being in Eastern Europe. J Econ Psychol. 2003;24(3):329–48.

101. Helliwell JF, Putnam RD. The social context of well-being. Philos Trans R Soc Lond B Biol Sci. 2004;359:1435–46.

102. Rodrik D. Where did all the growth go? external shocks, social conflict and growth collapses. J Econ Growth. 1999;4(4):385–412; Zak PJ, Knack S. Trust and growth. Econ J. 2001;111(470):295–321.

103. Haber D. Health promotion and ageing: practical applications for health professionals. New York: Springer; 2013.

104. Tomas JM, Sancho P, Gutierrez M, Galiana L. Predicting life satisfaction in the oldest-old: a moderator effects study. Soc Indic Res. 2014;177(2):601–13.

105. McDermott R, Fowler JH, Christakis NA. Breaking up is hard to do, unless everyone else is doing it too: social network effects on divorce in a longitudinal sample. Soc Forces. 2013;92(2):491–519. (page 116).

106. Louis J. Single and …'#6 Parenting. Medium (blog), 22 May 2016. https://medium.com/@jacqui_84.

107. Functional Independence Measure (FIM). www.physio-pedia.com

108. Activities of Daily Living, Wikipedia 8/3/2109.

109. Williams B. Consideration of function & functional decline. In: Current diagnosis and treatment: geriatrics. 2nd ed. New York: McGraw-Hill; 2014. p. 3–4. ISBN 978–0–079208-0.

110. Bookman A, Harrington M, Pass L, Reisner E. Family caregiver handbook. Cambridge, MA: Massachusetts Institute of Technology; 2007.

111. Williams C. CURRENT diagnosis & treatment in family medicine, 3e, chapter 39. In: healthy aging & assessing older adults. New York: McGraw-Hill; 2011.

112. Roley SS, DeLany JV, Barrows CJ, et al. Occupational therapy practice framework: domain & practice, 2nd edition. Am J Occup Ter.

2008;62(6):625–83. https://doi.org/10.5014/ajot.62.6.625. PMID 19024744. Archived from the original on 2014-04-13.

113. Blair JE, Files JA. In search of balance: medicine, motherhood, and madness. J Am Med Women's Assoc. 2003;58(4):212–6.

114. Pawdthavee N. What happens to people before and after disability? Focusing effects, Lead effects, and adaptation in different areas of life. Soc Sci Med. 2009;69(12):1834–44.

115. Singleton P. Insult to injury disability, earnings, and divorce. J Hum Resour. 2012;47(4):972–90.

116. Wrzesniewski A, McCauley C, Rozin P, Schwartz B. Jobs, careers, and callings: people's relations to their work. J Res Pers. 1997;31(1):21–33.

117. Haybron DM. Happiness, the self and human flourishing. Utilitas. 2008;20(1):21–49.

118. Gewirth A. Self-fulfillment. Princeton: Princeton University Press; 1998.

119. Zika S, Chamberlain K. On the relation between meaning in life and psychological Well-being. Br J Psychol. 1992;83(1):133–45.

120. Kislev E. Happy singlehood: the rising acceptance and celebration of solo living. Oakland: University of California Press; 2019. p. 146.

121. Johnson MK. Family roles and work values: processes of selection and change. J Marriage Fam. 2005;67(2):352–69.

122. Wein R. The 'always singles': moving from a 'problem' perception. Psychother Australia. 2003;9(2):60–5.

123. Donn JE. Adult development and well-being of mid-life never married singles. PhD diss., Miami University; 2005.

124. Philipson I. Married to the job: why we live to work and what we can do about it. New York: Simon and Schuster; 2003.

125. Kislev E. Happy singlehood: the rising acceptance and celebration of solo living. Oakland: University of California Press; 2019. p. 149.

126. Sahu K, Gupta P. Burnout among married and unmarried women teachers. Indian Journal of Health and Wellbeing. 2013;4(2):286.

127. Tugsal T. The effects of socio-demographic factors and work-life balance on employees' emotional exhaustion. J Human Sci. 2017;14(1):653–65.

128. Maslach C, Schaufeli WB, Leiter MP. Job burnout. Annu Rev Psychol. 2001;52(1):397–422.

129. Engler K, Frohlich K, Descarries F, Fernet M. Single, childless working women's construction of wellbeing: on balance, being dynamic and tensions between them. Work. 2011;40(2):173–86.

130. Kislev E. Happy singlehood: the rising acceptance and celebration of solo living. Oakland: University of California Press; 2019. p. 151.

131. Herman JB, Gyllstrom KK. Working men and women: inter- and intra-role conflict. Psychol Women Q. 1977;1(4):319–33.

132. Casper WJ, DePaulo B. A new layer to inclusion: creating singles-friendly work environments. In: Reilly NP, Joseph Sirgy M, Allen

Gorman C, editors. Work and quality of life: ethical practices in organizations. Dordrecht: Springer; 2012. p. 217–34.

133. Kislev E. Happy singlehood: the rising acceptance and celebration of solo living. Oakland: University of California Press; 2019. p. 152.

134. Hamilton EA, Gordon JR, Whelan-Berry KS. Understanding the work-life conflict of never-married women without children. Women Manag Rev. 2006;21(5):393–415.

135. Keeney J, Boyd EM, Sinha R, Westring AF, Ryan AM. From 'work-family' to 'work-life': broadening our conceptualization and measurement. J Vocat Behav. 2013;82(3):221–37.

136. Kislev E. Happy singlehood: the rising acceptance and celebration of solo living. Oakland: University of California Press; 2019. p. 153–60.

137. Crowther MR, Parker MW, Achenbaum WA, Larimore WL, Koenig HG. Rowe and Kahn's model of successful aging revisited positive spirituality – the forgotten factor. Gerontologist. 2002;42(5):613–20.

138. Ghaderi D. The survey of relationship between religious orientation and happiness among the elderly man and woman in Tehran. Iran J Ageing. 2011;5(4):64–71.

139. Levin J. Religion and happiness among Israeli Jews: findings from the ISSP religion III survey. J Happiness Stud. 2014;15(3):593–611.

140. Tapanya S, Nicki R, Jarusawad O. Worry and intrinsic/extrinsic religious orientation among Buddhist (Thai) and Christian (Canadian) elderly persons). Int J Aging Hum Dev. 1997;44(1):73–83.

141. Di Benedetto M, Swadling M. Burnout in Australian psychologists: correlations with work-setting, mindfulness and self-care behaviours. Psychol Health Med. 2014;19(6):705–15.

142. Hulsheger UR, Alberts HJEM, Feinholdt A, Lang JWB. Benefits of mindfulness at work: the role of mindfulness in emotion regulation, emotional exhaustion, and job satisfaction. J Appl Psychol. 2013;98(2):310.

143. Ghasemian D, Kuzehkanan AZ, Hassanzadeh R. Effectiveness of MBCT on decreased anxiety and depression among divorced women living in Tehran, Iran. J Novel Appl Sci. 2014;3(3):256–9.

144. Teasdale JD, Segal ZB, Williams JMG, Ridgeway VA, Soulsby JM, Lau MA. Prevention of relapse/recurrence in major depression by mindfulness-based cognitive therapy. J Consult Clin Psychol. 2000;68(4):615–23.

145. Rahimi A, Anoosheh M, Ahmadi F, Foroughan M. Exploring spirituality in iranian healthy elderly people: a qualitative content analysis. Iran J Nurs Midwifery Res. 2013;18(2):163–70.

146. Udhayakumar P, Ilango P. Spirituality, stress and wellbeing among the elderly practicing spirituality. Samaja Karyada Hejjegalu. 2012;2(20):37–42.

147. Mood YS, Kim DH. Association between religiosity/spirituality and quality of life or depression among living-alone elderly in a South Korean City. Asia Pac Psychiatry. 2013;5(4):293–300.

148. Antonovics K, Town R. Are all the good men married? uncovering the sources of the marital wage premium. Am Econ Rev. 2004;94(2):317–21.

149. Liebenson D. Young married men make more money than single men do. Business Insider 16 Apr 2015.

150. De Paulo BM. Singled out: how singles are stereotyped, stigmatized, and ignored, and still live happily ever after. New York: St Martin's Griffin; 2007.

151. Martin SC, Arnold RM, Parker RM. Gender and medical socialisation. J Health Soc Behav. 1988;29:191–205.

152. Allen I. Doctors and their careers. a new generation. London: Policy Studies Institute; 1994.

153. Tracy EE, Wiler JL, Hoschen JC, Patel SS, Ligda KO. Topics to ponder: part-time practice and pay parity. Gend Med. 2010;7(4):350–6.

154. Lahad K. A table for one: a critical reading of singlehood, gender and time. Manchester: University of Manchester; 2017.

155. Morris WL, Sinclair S, DePaulo BM. No shelter for singles: the perceived legitimacy of marital status discrimination. Group Process Intergroup Relat. 2007;10(4):457–70.

156. Jordan AH, Zitek EM. Marital status bias in perceptions of employees. Basic Appl Soc Psychol. 2012;334:474–81.

157. Pisani MA. Women in medicine struggle with mentorship and sponsorship. Op-Med.doximity.com, 12 Oct 2018.

158. Matsui T, Sato M, Kato Y, Nishigori H. Professional identity formation of female doctors in japan – gap between the married and unmarried. BMC Med Educ. 2019;19(1):55.

159. Gjerber E. Women doctors in Norway: the challenging balance between career and family life. Soc Sci Med. 2003;57:1327–41.

160. Lorber J. Women physicians: careers, status and power. New York: Tavistock; 1984.

161. Keizer M. Gender and career in medicine. Neth J Soc Sci. 1997;33:94–112.

162. Desai S, Waite LJ. Women's employment during pregnancy and after the first birth: occupational characteristics and work commitment. Am Sociol Rev. 1991;56:551–6.

163. Berquist S, Duchac BW, Schalin VA, Zastrow JF, Barr VL, Borowiecki T. Perceptions of freshman medical students of gender differences in medical specialty choice. J Med Educ. 1985;60:379–83.

164. Chertoff JD, Bird CE, Amick BC III. Career paths in diagnostic radiology: scope and effect of part-time work. Radiology. 2001;221:485–94.

165. Arnold L, Campbell C. The high price of being single in america. The Atlantic. 14 Jan 2013.

166. DePaulo B. Discrimination against singles in the health care system. Psychology Today (website). 21 March 2018.

167. Fischer AR, Shaw CM. African Americans' mental health and perceptions of racist discrimination: the moderating effects of racial socialization experiences and self-esteem. J Couns Psychol. 1999;46(3):395.
168. Noh S, Beiser M, Kaspar V, Hou F, Rummens J. Perceived racial discrimination, depression and coping: a study of Southeast Asian refugees
in Canada. J Health Soc Behav. 1999;40(3):193–207.
169. Huntre HER, Williams DR. The association between perceived discrimination and obesity in a population-based multiracial and multiethnic
adult sample. Am J Public Health. 2009;99(7):1285–92.
170. Kriegar N, Sidney S. Racial discrimination and blood pressure: the car-
dia study of young black and white adults. Am J Public Health.
1996;86(10):1370–8.
171. Borrell LN, Diez Roux AV, Jacobs DR, Shea S, Jackson SA, Shrager S,
Blumenthal RS. Perceived racial/ethnic discrimination, smoking and
alcohol consumption in the multiethnic study of atherosclerosis
(MESA). Prev Med. 2010;51(3):307–12.
172. Gibbons FX, Gerrard M, Cleveland MJ, Wills TA, Brody G. Perceived
discrimination and substance use in african american parents and their
children: a panel study. J Pers Soc Psychol. 2004;86(4):517–29.
173. Noh S, Kasper V. Perceived discrimination and depression: moderating
effects of coping, acculturation, and ethnic support. Am J Public Health.
2003;93(2):232.
174. United Nations General Assembly. Sixty-fifth session, Agenda item 15,
Culture of peace, 27 Apr 2011.
175. Zuckerberg M. Celebrating friends day at Facebook HQ, Facebook. 4
Feb 2016. www.facebook.com/zuck/videos /vb.4/10102634961507811.
176. Bureau of Labor Statistics. Consumer Expenditures in 2014. In:
Consumer expenditure survey. Washington, DC: US Bureau of Labor
Statistics; 2016.
177. Klinenberg E, Solo G. The extraordinary rise and surprising appeal of
living alone. New York: Penguin; 2012.

Navigating a Traditionally Male-Dominated Specialty as a Woman

10

Pelagia Kouloumberis

It was just past midnight on a night in mid-2004. The paramedics were just about done giving me report on a critically ill gentleman in his mid-forties who was found unresponsive at home by his wife. This man had suffered a subarachnoid hemorrhage from rupture of an intracranial aneurysm. I was near the end of my first year as a neurosurgery resident and, at this point, was quite adept at taking care of these types of patients once they arrived in the intensive care unit of the Chicago hospital where I trained.

The dangers of intracranial aneurysm rupture are many. However, my first priority was to assess him and determine if he needed an emergent bedside procedure to help drain the cerebrospinal fluid that normally bathes the central nervous system which was no longer being absorbed normally by his stunned brain. Following my initial assessment, my next task involved discussing his condition with his family in a manner that addressed all of their concerns, while staying focused on the fact that this procedure needed to happen in an expedited fashion to provide the best possible clinical outcome for my patient. I reviewed the disease process with his wife and her sister; explained to them my role on

P. Kouloumberis (✉)
Department of Neurosurgery, Mayo Clinic, Phoenix, AZ, USA
e-mail: Kouloumberis.Pelagia@mayo.edu

© Springer Nature Switzerland AG 2020
C. M. Stonnington, J. A. Files (eds.), *Burnout in Women Physicians*,
https://doi.org/10.1007/978-3-030-44459-4_10

his team, clearly stating that I was a physician; and obtained informed consent for the procedure that would take place within the next few minutes.

I was very pleased when following the procedure, he showed promising signs of recovery within the first few hours. His family was also overcome with emotion and immediately declared that with what I had just accomplished, "they" should just allow me to become a doctor. This was one of the first times in my medical career that, I can very clearly recall, someone had very poignantly distinguished me from my colleagues based solely on my gender. Despite my introducing myself as Doctor, that declaration reinforced by the MD following my name on my hospital ID badge, and the embroidered indication of my station in life on my white coat, these family members instead chose to believe that I was not a physician. This was my conscious introduction to a life of being constantly underestimated. It is not lost on me that, in this particular case, I have chosen a certain interpretation of that statement that may not reflect the actual meaning intended by the family. However, I assure you, I have suffered through many other conversations during my professional life that lend themselves to much less ambiguity.

Throughout the years, I have lost track of the number of times patients, colleagues, and sometimes perfect strangers have ventured a guess on what my role within the health-care system is. On more than one occasion, I have entered a patient's room and have been asked to place a pillow behind his head, followed by the question "do you know when my doctor will be here?" I have listened to wives, mothers, husbands, and sons end calls with loved ones because their physical therapist has arrived. I have even been asked who will actually be performing the surgery at the end of a clinic consultation. On rare occasion, I have entertained the occasional request from patients who have requested that a male colleague assist me with their procedures at the begining of a consultation.

In 1995, Dr. Greenwald lay the groundwork that demonstrated our social behavior is not always necessarily under our conscious control [17]. In developing the Implicit Bias Test, he established that we are not in complete control of our reaction to every situation. As a female neurosurgeon, I have often had to remind myself of this throughout the years. Also as a result, I have become more aware of my own implicit biases.

The History of Women in Neurosurgery

I was asked many years ago, during an interview, what it felt like being a female neurosurgeon [15]. At that time, I only personally knew two other female neurosurgeons. My answer to that question was very calculated and safe. I responded that I did not see myself as a female or male neurosurgeon, but simply as a neurosurgeon. Despite my many experiences to the contrary, I wanted desperately to believe that neurosurgery saw no gender. We all take calls, we endure long hours, and we treat our patients to the best of our ability, regardless of our gender identity, ethnicity, or religious beliefs. Throughout my entire training, I had been the only female resident. I had a very strong female mentor who never made gender the focus of any discussion. If asked that question again today, I would answer it with a bit more grit and I would shed the idealism. Years of being in practice has made me acutely aware of the challenges that women face in traditionally male-dominated fields. Neurosurgery is no exception. As Dr. Stamp stated in a recent piece she wrote for *The Washington Post*, "When girls or women ask me if they can be a surgeon, I'll still say yes, they can. I'll still encourage them because despite the obstacles, I love my job and I want to see the ranks swell with more women. And I will still tell them that just because they are female, it has no bearing on whether they can or should do a job. But I will then tell them that it may not be an easy or fair road, and that I am going to keep fighting and holding accountable the people and the system who will make a liar out of me and a tough road ahead for the next generation. Despite my fears, I don't lie to the next generation, but I am determined to change the system, not the women who try to survive in it" [52].

In 1965, women represented only 9% of US medical school enrollment and only 7% of medical school graduates [41]. Since 2011, more women have graduated from medical school than men [13]. In 2017, for the first time in history, there were more females enrolled in medical school than males [20]. Despite this trend, following the 2018 Neurosurgery Match, only 17.5% of neurosurgery residents were women [13, 43]. This represents a slight improvement from 2015, when only 15.8% of neurosurgery residents were female, even though women represented 46% of all

US medical residents [41]. While there has been an increase in female representation in neurosurgery, these gains do not parallel those seen in the general population of residents, neurology, or even general surgery. We are bridging the gap, but at a significantly slower pace [5, 58, 10]. Retention of female neurosurgery residents is also lower than their male counterparts. Eighteen percent of women do not complete residency, while the male attrition rate is only 10% [1].

Mentorship

What drives the decision process when medical students are choosing what field to pursue after graduating? While there are many factors involved, mentorship is one of the most important. Mentorship has repeatedly been shown to be very important when deciding what field to pursue following medical school. Females lacking a female mentor were less likely to apply to surgical residency [26]. Females also reported greater interest in applying to programs with other female residents and faculty members [48]. I can personally attest to this influence. When I was rotating at my home institution as a medical student, a very outspoken female chief resident encouraged me to consider applying to neurosurgery. Up until that point, while I had a very strong interest in neuroscience, neurosurgery seemed like a pipe dream. However, not only do we need mentors to advise us, sponsorship from our mentors is critical for advancement. And yet, male neurosurgery mentors are more likely to advocate for their same-gender mentees on a professional level, whereas females are more likely to receive psychosocial guidance and personal advice from their male mentors [58].

Leadership

There is a paucity of female physicians in academic medicine and leadership roles. The ones that are there earn, on average, 10% less than their male colleagues [4]. The first female chairperson of a neurosurgery department was not appointed until 2005, when Dr. Karen Muraszko was appointed at the University of Michigan [4]. If we review the academic genealogy of neurosurgery, it quickly becomes very apparent why there has not, until recently, been a female chair of neurosurgery. Of the 377 chairs identified, none were women [59]. I can confirm from my personal experience that several female peers approached me after learning that I would be entering a neurosurgical training program and commented that they did not realize that neurosurgery was an option for them. Reflecting on these comments now makes me realize how rapidly one's perspective can change. I consider myself beyond lucky, as I was also fortunate enough to be taken under the wing of the then chief resident of the neurosurgical service during my medical school elective rotation. I am not sure if I would be where I am today were it not for the strong female role models I was fortunate enough to encounter along my journey. Even since my graduation from residency in 2010, there are now five female residents in the program in which I trained. Up until 2010, there were only two female graduates from my program. The only other female resident before me graduated in 1983 [4].

Jaclyn Janine Renfrow, MD, and her colleagues from the Wake Forest School of Medicine reviewed data from the American Association of Neurological Surgeons (AANS) and the American Board of Neurosurgery (ABNS) from 1964 through 2013 in an attempt to determine the number and trajectory of female neurosurgery graduates. During that time period, there were 379 female neurosurgery residency graduates. Only 70% became ABNS-certified and 27% pursued fellowship training. Between 1960 and 1969, only two women were board-certified in neurosurgery [43].

The ABNS was formed in 1940. As of March 2018, in its 78 years, the ABNS has certified 7142 neurosurgeons. Less than 8% of all neurosurgeons receiving board certification in the ABNS' 78-year history have been female. Board certification is an arduous process in all medical fields. In neurosurgery, you are first required to take written boards, which most programs require before being allowed to serve as chief resident, followed by the dreaded oral board examination that takes place anywhere from 2 to 5 years following graduation from residency. The first female diplomate of the ABNS was Ruth Kerr Jakoby, MD, JD [51]. She was board-certified in 1961. This was 21 years after the formation of the governing body. After developing an interest in medical-legal issues, she also received her JD from Northern Virginia Law School in 1936, becoming the first female neurosurgeon to also be a lawyer. She is still living and is 89 years old.

Another important milestone was reached this past year. In 2018, the AANS inducted its first female president, Dr. Shelly Timmons. It has taken 78 years for the field of neurosurgery to elect a female as the leader of one of its two main congresses: American Association of Neurological Surgeons (AANS) and Congress of Neurological Surgery (CNS).

It seems difficult to believe that as late as the 1990s, more than 30% of all US neurosurgical residency programs had never graduated a female neurosurgeon. As of 2007, there were still 4 programs that have never had a female resident [4]. Another milestone was reached in 2017, when Johns Hopkins Hospital accepted its first black female resident, Dr. Abu-Bonsrah [27].

I feel very fortunate to have been exposed to neurosurgery in medical school at a time when not many women received this opportunity. When reflecting on my journey, I feel a sense of pride at being a part of something so wonderful. I do not deny that many days are filled with unique challenges. Yet many of today's medical students are not afforded the early exposure to neurosurgery I had. For our current generation of students to flourish in a field that would benefit greatly from a greater presence of women, we must actively combat gender discrimination, lack of female role models, and abjuration of work-life conflicts [39].

The Impact of Gender Discrepancy in Certain Fields of Study

Since graduating in 2010 from residency, I have held two faculty positions. In both environments, I have been the only female attending. I have often wondered why there are so few women in my field and the impact this has on how neurosurgery has evolved and continues to evolve as a profession. Neurosurgery, like other fields in medicine and outside of medicine, has always suffered from a lack of gender diversity. These inequalities have been shown to become even greater as one ascends in the educational hierarchy [57].

Despite the fact that higher education is available to both men and women in our current society, it seems that the environment that awaits following graduation is not always the welcoming one we would hope for as women. In 1998, Benokraitis very aptly wrote in her book, *Career Strategies for Women in Academia: Arming Athena,* "Subtle sex discrimination refers to the unequal and harmful treatment of women that is typically less visible and less obvious than blatant sex discrimination is. It is often not noticed because most people have internalized subtle sexist behavior as normal, natural, or acceptable. It can be innocent or manipulative, intentional or unintentional, well-meaning or malicious" [9]. What makes this behavior difficult to label and, therefore, correct is that it lends itself to multiple interpretations. What may seem offensive to some may appear harmless to others. The example she gives is a classic one: a man and woman are having dinner. When it comes time to pay the bill, the woman hands the waiter the credit card and bill. The waiter returns with the receipt, handing it to the man. No atrocious crime has been committed. Yet the waiter's action implies a certain male authority. This authority is recognized in most settings. I have lost count of the number of times I have entered a patient's room with a male nurse or midlevel provider, only to have the patients and their family members address my male counterpart as their doctor and me as his assistant.

Examples similar to the one above exist in everyday life and color our world. Eventually, if allowed to fully evolve, they help form our self-identity. If left unchecked for too long, Imposter Syndrome imposter syndrome may result [8]. For a female in a male-dominated field, it may be something as simple as being less likely to be called on during a meeting to share an opinion, not having your male colleagues ask what you thought of last night's football game, having to endure sexist humor for fear of exclusion if you object, or co-workers assuming that you are always the right person with whom to discuss a difficult personal situation. Over time, as self-worth devolves, we are less likely to reach heights that a more supported individual may reach. Therefore, while subtle sexist behavior may be just that, it is important to recognize early the effect it may have on us, so that we may change our course. While we may not be able to eliminate these behaviors in others, we can at least become aware of them and alter the way we process them.

Over the years, I have used humor on many occasions to diffuse otherwise tense patient interactions involving my gender and being a surgeon. As it is not infrequent enough that patients ask who will actually be performing their surgery, I assure them that I am better at sewing than some of my male colleagues. While I find this type of humor necessary during those especially awkward times, it is also a form of self-deprecation that I do not condone. I am ashamed to admit that, on occasion, self-deprecating humor has been my escape, especially when my gender in relationship to my career choice has been called into question. However, as Hannah Gadsby so eloquently stated in her recent Netflix comedy special, *Nanette*, self-deprecating humor from an individual who already exists in the margins is not humility. Instead, it is a form of humiliation [34]. Using self-deprecating humor to speak is perhaps a way by which a minority seeks permission to speak – to be heard. This may perhaps be one manifestation of the commonly discussed *Imposter Syndrome*.

The impact on a field has to be considered from two different perspectives: First, we have to consider what it means to be a minority in your line of work. Second, we have to consider the evolution of a field. Does it follow a different trajectory when there is gender diversity? Stated in simple terms, what could a female colleague bring to the table that differs from her male counterpart?

As far as neurosurgery is concerned, women are given "less than minority" status. This is defined as a group with fewer than 15% representation [4]. A group that is assigned "less than minority" status does not meet the criteria for critical mass. Being part of such a small group does not allow that group to function as a minority, but rather as isolated individuals.

Being "the only" in any situation, a term used by David Goggins in his book *Can't Hurt* Me, changes your constitution [16]. As adolescent and teenage girls, we congregated in the halls to share secrets and discover the norms of society. In a workplace where you are the only female, the congregation changes. Friendship among colleagues is an important component of any work environment. We all have an inherent need to belong. Belonging has to be very clearly distinguished from just fitting in. *Fitting in requires changing who we are to be a part of a group. Belonging, on the other hand, does not require this change.* We are a part of a group because of who we are. Belonging feels natural and there is no need to hide or alter our fundamental values and beliefs. We enjoy the company and value the opinions of those in our circle. In an environment such as this, one can thrive. On the other hand, when we do not belong, we are emotionally exposed, which leads to an increase in stress and distress [6]. Eventually, these may manifest as physical symptoms. One study out of Sweden found that females in male-dominated fields take twice as much sick leave as their male colleagues [46]. This corresponds to the deterioration in the psychosocial work environment as the number of women decreases in the workplace. Furthermore, absences secondary to illness are multidimensional and did not only comprise biomedical complaints. One of the most convincing findings is that the amount of sick leave was also proportional to the employees' resources, demand of the work, and social factors. Much of the leave was related to burnout, depression, and other stress-related illnesses. A lack of mentorship was also mentioned during the interviews regarding the work environment. It has also been reported that emotional burnout may lead to changes in serum lipids [49].

Men and women have different styles of friendship formation. As a result of this, underrepresented genders are likely to have a more negative experience than those in gender-typical occupations. This includes increased psychological stress and a poorer self-assessment of overall health. This also manifests as a higher rate of sick leave in individuals working in gender-atypical occupations [42]. Women in male-dominated careers face many struggles when it comes to successful social assimilation in a gender-atypical environment. Many male-dominated work environments are described as agentic, where assertiveness, competitiveness, and a hierarchical approach to workplace dynamics are valued. This is contrary to the characteristics typically associated with women, which include collaboration, process, and equalizing behaviors [14]. This creates the dilemma of either trying to fit in or being true to one's nature.

I offer a different perspective for the reader to consider. In my personal experience, I do not believe that the work dynamic described above is quite so simple. I believe that women working in a male-dominated environment adapt and may, on the contrary, find it difficult to make friendships with other women outside of the workplace. Over the years, while I am still a mother with maternal tendencies, I have found it increasingly difficult to form friendships with other women in the conventional sense. I do not have a group of close girlfriends and rarely find myself attending "girls' night." Furthermore, when attending social functions with work colleagues, I find myself in the awkward position of figuring out where I belong. Do I socialize with the "work wives," or engage my colleagues in social banter? These types of situations defy the commonly held ideals of gender socialization. Gender socialization is a concept that describes how we are taught to socialize from a very young age. As the term implies, these norms are predominantly defined by society and are not solely rooted in biology.

When it comes time to secure a position, climb the academic ladder, or merely survive residency, negotiation is paramount. Women and men have, on average, very different approaches to negotiating. Women tend toward a "relational style." The relationship between the two, or more, parties involved is the focus when attempting to achieve a goal. Men, on the other hand, rely on a "competitive style" that focuses more on achieving the desired result [33]. In 2002, Sandra Ford Walston wrote a piece entitled "Women Integrating Workday Courage." In it, she describes that being more courageous in our place of employment allows us to design our lives rather than being told who we are and led down a path created *for* us, instead of *by* us. It is very common for a woman to thank an employer for a raise or an opportunity instead of understanding that it was her hard work that led to the recognition. My favorite quote from her writing should serve as a mantra to anyone and everyone who goes to work and wishes to rise above the daily chaos: "Remember, getting a promotion or some other accolade at work isn't a gift. It's something you've worked hard for and deserve. The action you take or don't take during such a situation reveals your true courage quotient. When you fail to insist on credit for your accomplishments, your spirit slowly shrinks" [56].

There is no canon that defines with unwavering certainty what comprise the expectations of a specific role and, therefore, no objective standards by which to judge oneself. In today's shifting society, we must all learn to wear multiple hats. Women who work and are also mothers experience a role conflict that can put them at risk for burnout. Mentoring and self-care are two techniques we can employ to prevent burnout before it happens. Recognizing that it is not easy, or maybe even impossible, to be everything to everyone is important. As such, women who work in male-dominated fields often describe feelings of social isolation and loneliness. Loneliness has been linked to almost all forms of mental illness [44]. Last year, loneliness was reported as a potentially bigger health risk than smoking or obesity [54].

As physicians, it is in our DNA to find solutions to problems. However, we cannot begin to solve the problem of gender inequality within certain fields until it has been clearly defined. Especially because women who work in traditionally male-dominated fields also defy the model of the nuclear family discussed by Talcott Parsons in 1955. In this model, there is clear role segregation, placing the female in charge of maintaining the household, while the male is expected to be in the workplace.

Current trends in the United States now tend more toward a social construct of role integration, as opposed to role segregation, e.g., work-life integration versus work-life balance, as a more realistic approach to the reality of multiple roles when managing work and home. The proportion of women comprising the total labor force participation has been steadily rising. Today, almost half of the workforce is female, which is a significant increase when compared to approximately 34% in 1950 and 43% in 1970 [53]. Despite this progress, many fields of medicine still lag behind. And regardless of the percentage of women in any given field of medicine, women still take on the majority of household responsibilities [30]. The conversation regarding gender parity in the workplace is an important one that cannot be disregarded. Until there is organizational citizenship that addresses the role conflict many women face today, we need to keep talking.

If one performs a Google search of *women in male-dominated* fields, it may come as no surprise that there are 27,900,000 results. You are then confronted with titles such as *Male-dominated fields should remain male-dominated*, as well as a piece from The Guardian published in February, 2019 entitled *Female surgeons frustrated by male dominated field – study*. There is no paucity of literature on this topic. I do not claim to have reviewed all these results for pertinence to this chapter, but what struck me with most everything I did read was the insistence that we are unable to look past the negative aspects of the gender discrepancy and, instead, make lemonade. It seems that it is time to move forward with embracing the inherent differences between men and women and extracting their best qualities to create a rich and diverse workplace. Gender equity in the workplace may enhance job satisfaction for women, as well as men. While a woman's job satisfaction is not as strongly correlated to pay as a man's, working in family-friendly work environments, and believing their place of business practices this, the perception of gender equality in the workplace has been shown to correlate with high self-reported levels of job satisfaction [22].

Navigating the Waters of Traditionally Male-Dominated Fields: How We Adapt to Our Environments

Women in male-dominated careers face unique challenges when compared to those working in gender-balanced positions. While some women integrate femininity into their work environment, it is not uncommon for women in predominantly male environments to adopt classically male behaviors in order to fit in [31]. The reality is that many female physicians experience burnout at some point in their career. One study found that female physicians were 1.6 times as likely to suffer burnout when compared to their male counterparts [32]. Some of this is due to the gendered expectations placed upon us by colleagues and patients. One theory is that patients have different expectations of care provided by females than of that provided by males. Females are expected to be more empathic and as such are often confronted with patients that offer more psychosocial complexity [28]. The result of this expectation differential may be reflected in the Press Ganey Patient Satisfaction Scores. In a 2017 study, the Press Ganey scores of female gynecologists were significantly lower than their male colleagues [45]. Please see Chap. 2 for further details regarding gender differences in patient satisfaction scores and outcomes.

Even after removing gender from the equation, some fields have a high risk of burnout. In a very poignant essay entitled "Physician Burnout: Is the Foundation of Your Life Crumbling?", Dr. Kraig Burgess, a hand surgeon, describes the insidious nature by which neglect of our personal lives may result in the dissolution of the family unit and offers personal insights as to how one might assuage the negative effects of a surgical career on one's family life [7].

There are many cautionary tales to be told. You can find them by the hundreds on social media sites. As that is the case, why is it taking so long for people to listen and act? How many times must history repeat itself before we remove the blinders? To some extent, we all believe that we are impervious to the ordinary. Our lives will somehow manage to defy reality. We are extraordinary. However, once you reach the summit of that hill, the fall can be steep. The abovementioned essay and many others like it are perfect illustrations that by the time you are rolling down the hill, momentum makes it difficult to reverse course.

The reality is, however, that although most physicians, both female and male, probably experience varying degrees of burnout throughout their careers, we are very likely to attribute those feelings to long hours and the emotionally demanding nature of our work and our current regulatory and electronic environment. That stress may be compounded by added sexism experienced outside the workplace. Many times, we may suffer at the hands of our own friends and family. I have been asked countless times why I decided to pursue neurosurgery as a career, given the demanding nature of the work and the impact it will have on my ability to take care of my family. I have come to the point now where I have pretty much worked out the following standard response: The fact that I work *is* the very reason I am able to take care of my family. Having a demanding and rewarding career like neurosurgery also fosters a desire in my daughters to seek independence and knowledge as they believe this to be the modus operandi of all individuals. While living in a dual-income household means that we rely on the help of substitute caregivers, we stress to ourselves and to our children that while our careers fulfill us, it is our family that completes us.

There is a common perception that women and men have different leadership styles. Most perceive women as having a leadership style that is more people-oriented, while men tend to be more task-oriented [24]. This misconception may be in part attributed to the social role theory in which women are viewed as nurturing and men "get things done." This characterization pervades our society as demonstrated by the adjectives *masculine* and *feminine*. The word masculine implies strength, while feminine brings to mind something delicate. Even when describing music, feminine refers to a final chord occurring on a weak beat, while masculine is a final chord occurring on a strong beat. It is a hybrid approach that I believe characterizes the strongest leaders.

Work-life balance is perhaps the most talked about conflict that affects working women. Drs. Toby Parcel and Elizabeth Menaghan have authored multiple research articles and books regarding the effect on a child's well-being when both parents are employed. They have written extensively about the detriment to both cognitive and social development in children who are raised by substitute providers and the resulting attachment insecurity [38].

The term work-life balance itself implies two opposing forces. Instead, they should be experienced on a continuum. While I do work longer hours than the average gainfully employed individual [3], I strive to involve my family in decisions regarding my work life. I am clear with my children regarding my work responsibilities and the importance of the work I do, all the while emphasizing that they will always be my top priority. I also involve them, when appropriate, by taking them to work functions with me, as well as visiting my office on off-hours occasionally so they can see where I am when I am away from them. Conversely, my colleagues and I speak often about our families and lives outside of medicine. Of course, in a field like neurosurgery, social capital is not viewed as important as professional capital. Despite this, even though the care of my patients is wildly important to me, I have not been able to think of myself as a neurosurgeon first since becoming a mother. While some may define this as a weakness, I believe this has helped shape me into a more present and compassionate doctor. While empathy has been shown to decline through the course of medical school and residency [35], it is through interaction with society's most innocent citizens, our children, that we can reawaken our emotional understanding of another individual's experience and needs [40].

As I mentioned above, while I do not miss an opportunity to tell my family they remain my top priority, that does not translate to my presence at every school function or extracurricular activity. Also, the fact that I occasionally sacrifice professional opportunities to be present at times when most of my contemporaries are not has taught me an important lesson in the last decade. We place too much pressure on ourselves to have it all. Instead of having it all, I have found a new equilibrium that has worked very well for me. I no longer strive to *have it all*. I strive to *have enough*.

Bridging the Gap and Moving Forward

We all strive to create a workplace with gender parity, so much so that we do not want to treat individuals differently. What we fail to realize is that women and men *are* quite different. Years of misinformation has created the belief that those difference lie in their intellectual abilities. In our pediatric rotations during medical school, we are repeatedly reminded that kids are not just small adults. I think a similar statement may be made regarding females and males: women are not just men with less bodily hair. We do not want to be treated exactly the same. We want our unique qualities and skills to be recognized, accommodated, and celebrated so that we can thrive in the professional world just as men have for hundreds of years.

Creating Awareness and Comfort

First, and foremost, we need to create awareness of the gender discrepancy that exists in some fields. Whenever there is any imbalance in nature, scientists have jumped into the field to determine the cause in order to begin work on solutions. Gender discrepancy is no exception. There is a growing body of literature regarding this topic. When performing a literature search for "females in male-dominated careers," there are almost 28 million results. However, when researching "burnout of females in male dominated careers," there are 4.5 million results. We have spent a lot of time observing, and now we need to systematically begin working on actionable solutions. By clearly defining an issue and assigning vocabulary to it, only then can it be tackled.

When one is a minority in his or her environment, the risk of isolation and attrition increases. Small work groups, referred to as "microenvironments," have been shown to be beneficial in increasing confidence and comfort with speaking up and contributing to assignments [11].

Professional women need to be more visible and available to medical students throughout their training. We need to be seen. In my field, the image that most people conjure in their mind when they hear the word neurosurgeon is someone sitting under a microscope for 12–24 h. The question I am still most frequently asked when people find out that I am a neurosurgeon is how I can operate for so long without going to the bathroom. Never mind that the majority of the procedures I perform require less than 3–4 h. Also, I believe one of my patients said it best when she declared, "I expected someone much older and more male."

Eliminating Negative Stereotypes Through Mentorship

All individuals are biased to a certain degree. Cognitive biases are shortcuts that have evolved during our socialization that allow our brain to decipher what it sees without wasting time. The most automatic calculations our brains make revolve around age, race, and gender. A person's gender allows us to socially categorize every individual we meet [25]. In order to eliminate negative stereotypes, we need to reprogram the way we think. Implicit biases exist in most of us, despite our best intentions and conscious declarations. The Implicit Association Test (IAT) has become one of the most commonly used tools in the workplace to evaluate our implicit biases.

Research in child development indicates that the performance and interest in STEM topics is equal during early childhood between girls and boys. It is only later, due to societal standards, that participation in these fields changes [18]. The factors involved are multiple and complex. They are beyond the scope of this chapter. However, awareness of this fact and early intervention may foster interest in females and males alike, which may change societal nuances to pave a drastically different road for future generations.

I often feel like I live somewhere in the gulf between surgeon and mother. After all, the two are not typically assigned to the same individual. The old riddle about the boy involved in a car accident continues to stump many people to this day. If you have not heard it, it goes something like this:

A young boy and his father are on their way home from a soccer game when they are involved in a motor vehicle collision. The father dies instantly, but the boy survives and is taken to the nearest emergency department. Upon arrival, it is determined that the boy requires immediate surgery.

However, the surgeon assigned to the case appears and states, "Call my partner STAT to the operating room. I cannot operate on this patient. He is my son!"

This riddle has stumped many well-intentioned adults. *Good Morning America* approached random people on the streets of New York. Surprisingly, the majority were unable to solve this riddle. Instead, it was a group of fifth-graders in Manhattan that were almost all able to answer without hesitation [55].

It has been clearly demonstrated that there is a positive correlation between the proportion of women surgeons on a faculty and the choice to pursue a surgical career in female medical students

[36]. It is often said the best way to lead is by example. It follows suit that we will only be able to shatter stereotypes through mentorship. As I mentioned earlier in the chapter, I truly believe that I am here today as a result of having positive experiences during my medical school and residency training supplied by strong, female role models.

There have been a lot of efforts made throughout the past few decades to integrate females into the STEM fields. One challenge, however, has been retention. The current environment has proven to be hostile and wrought with workplace incivility, resulting in female attrition. This can be as subtle as gendered language to interrupting someone while speaking, or addressing a colleague inappropriately [47]. By working to increase the number of female mentors in all fields, gender equity is sure to follow. In order to accomplish this task, we must continue to not only mentor, but sponsor, future generations [21].

Recognizing Gender Difference in Burnout

Burnout in medicine is an important area of study for multiple reasons. From a financial perspective, it results in a $4.6 billion burden to the US health-care system per year [19]. This is, in part, due to higher than expected physician turnover and decreased clinical hours. Burnout comprises two main components: emotional exhaustion and depersonalization. It may come as no surprise that women and men experience burnout differently. While many confounding factors prohibit any truly declarative statements from being made, it appears that women are more likely to experience emotional exhaustion, whereas men more commonly experience depersonalization. There is an inherent bias that burnout is more commonly experienced by women than men. This presents two very clear dangers: women may be less likely to be assigned more challenging tasks or receive promotions, while men experiencing burnout may go unrecognized and fail to receive much needed care [42]. As a surgeon, I am especially interested in correcting the course we are all on, as burnout affects the care I deliver to my patients, my patient satisfaction scores, and my personal risk for being involved in a malpractice suit [50].

Is "Self-Care" the Answer?

As a health-care provider, it is very easy to hide behind the work. I spend most days taking care of other people. I listen attentively to their problems. I offer advice. On the best days, I am in the operating room, surgically correcting what ails them. When we spend our days tending to the needs of others, it is not uncommon to forget our own. Over time, we become better at caring for others than of ourselves. In their book, "Leaving it at the Office," John Norcross and Gary VanderBos pose the following conversation opener, "You are fine. How am I?" [37]. It is not very often that we ask ourselves that question. The suggestions offered in this book are both realistic and do not require finding extra time in our schedules to implement. They include things such as setting boundaries and refocusing the rewards. During our fast-paced days, we rarely take time to receive the rewards our patients unknowingly offer us. They offer the following old Chinese proverb:

- If you want happiness for an hour – take a nap;
- If you want happiness for a day – go fishing;
- If you want happiness for a month – get married;
- If you want happiness for a year – inherit a fortune; but
- If you want happiness for a lifetime – help someone else.

We are given a gift that rare other professionals ever experience. We are entrusted with our patients' most vulnerable moments. It is not uncommon for patients to share with us information that does not fall on any other ears. They look to us for guidance and answers. Even though we are not always able to provide solutions to all problems, the reward is immeasurable when we do.

The focus on self-care these days has shifted to tangible activities, things like manicures, massages, and yoga; the list goes on and on. I think it was said best by Catherine Dietrich when she likened today's self-care as one more thing to add to our to-do list [12]. Self-care does not need to be complicated, but it is necessary. It can be as simple as sitting in a room alone with your thoughts for a few minutes meditating, or not.

Reproductive Life Planning

In examining the literature on reproductive planning, there are thousands of articles about how to discuss this with our patients. However, there is virtually no information specifically geared toward health-care providers and how this may contribute to burnout. Childcare in certain fields is regarded as an impediment to climbing the professional ladder. There have not been any studies that look at the importance of this for medical students, residents, or attending physicians.

I hope that a new world will be waiting for the trainees and students of the future. It was not too long ago when I found out that I was pregnant just before my chief year of residency. Although, alone in my bathroom staring at that little stick that notified me of the happiest news of my life, I was absolutely elated, the realization of what this might mean for my professional life was a different reality all together. I immediately felt complete and utter fear that I might be fired with only 1 year left in residency training. While I admit this was a rather intense reaction, the fact that the thought even entered my mind speaks to the culture at that time. Being the only female in my residency program did not offer any rational comparisons by which I could accurately calculate my fate. That, coupled with my first trimester routine of vomiting on the way in to the hospital at what I affectionately began referring to as "my" trashcan every morning, definitely made for an interesting experience.

Social Networking

It is estimated that by the year 2020, there will be almost 3 billion social network users (Statistica). Social media is how we connect on a social and professional level. This platform will continue to grow and gives us instantaneous, worldwide access to similar professionals. The role of social media in healthcare is multifaceted. It can be used to educate as well as network. It has been shown to assist with mentoring for women in male-dominated specialties by connecting them with mentors across the world [29].

Conclusion

In a recent book written by Siri Hustvedt, she states that "gulfs of mutual incomprehension among people in various disciplines may be unavoidable" [23]. Although her text does not specifically address the topics covered in this chapter, I feel that this gulf exists in any situation where all the moving parts are not necessarily the same. A multidisciplinary approach will be required to bridge the gap.

The most potent motivator for change is having a personal stake in the outcome. If society is headed for change, we will only be successful in a system where there is a culture of personal responsibility and accountability. The reason most diversity and inclusion programs fail is due to the fact that the parties involved feel as though they are being talked "at" and not an agent of change. Mutual respect is a prerequisite for any dialogue that will lead to meaningful, positive change.

At the end of the day, when I look back at my 16 years spent as a neurosurgeon, I have always been "a woman looking at men looking at women" [23]. This has offered me unique perspective. While I would seem to wax poetic if I refer myself as a perpetual outsider, my gender, ironically, has offered me an atypical advantage.

In order to transform our current society, we must draw on the collective knowledge of all its citizens. Even those considered to be "less than a minority." No one should be underestimated, as the input of the novice may, in some cases, be more flexible and brimming with infinite potential and possibility than that of an expert in the field. It should seem unacceptable to all parties that 88% of respondents to a recent survey in the UK reported that they felt surgical subspecialties remain male-dominated and that 59% have witnessed discrimination against females in their workplace [2].

Nowhere in the literature is it stated that women lack the intelligence required to enter specific fields. To the contrary, girls score at higher levels in some areas of STEM than boys during childhood [18]. Despite this, and the abundance of literature on the topic, no significant cultural shift has occurred even though the number of women in the workplace has been steadily increasing for decades. Instead, highly educated women find themselves falling prey to Imposter Syndrome and having to endure gendered language and adopting male personality characteristics to survive the daily grind.

In a quote commonly attributed to both Anais Nin and the Babylonian Talmud, "we don't see things as they are, we see things as we are," we get a glimpse at how our perception affects our reaction to everyday events. It seems that it may be time we reshape our preconceptions in order to alter our perception of previously fixed roles that, thus far, have not be fully available to women. Acceptance is an essential element to feeling whole. As mentioned earlier in the chapter, Brene Brown spoke very concretely about the distinct difference between belonging and fitting in [6]. Once we all stop trying to fit in and, instead, belong, we will be able to move forward as a cohesive community in a more constructive way.

Perhaps all of our current attempts at creating gender parity have been a bit short-sighted. As sociologists attribute gender socialization to predominate during the early childhood years, perhaps it is time to consider a paradigm shift in the types of gendered language, activities, toys, and expectations to which we expose our children. While the inherent biological differences between men and women cannot be denied, we should consider allowing our children to grow into themselves as opposed to molds we prepare for them, as a society.

In the meantime, until gender roles are redefined, I suppose we can continue going it alone, together.

References

1. Agarwal N, White MD, Pannullo SC, Chambless LB. Analysis of national trends in neurosurgical resident attrition. J Neurosurg. 2018;1 (aop):1–6.
2. Bellini MI, Graham Y, Hayes C, Zakeri R, Parks R, Papalois V. A woman's place is in theatre: women's perceptions and experiences of working in surgery from the Association of Surgeons of Great Britain and Ireland women in surgery working group. BMJ Open. 2019;9(1):e024349.
3. Bureau of Labor Statistics. 6 Sept 2019. https://www.bls.gov/news. release/empsit.nr0.htm. Accessed 10 Sept 2019.

4. Benzil DL, Abosch A, Germano I, Gilmer H, Maraire JN, Muraszko K, Pannullo S, Rosseau G, Schwartz L, Todor R, Ullman J. The future of neurosurgery: a white paper on the recruitment and retention of women in neurosurgery. J Neurosurg. 2008;109(3):378–86.

5. Blakemore LC, Hall JM, Biermann JS. Women in surgical residency training programs. JBJS. 2003;85(12):2477–80.

6. Brown B. The gifts of imperfection: let go of who you think you are supposed to be and embrace who you are. Center City: Hazeldon Publishing; 2010.

7. Burgess KM. Physician burnout: is the foundation of your life crumbling? ASSH perspectives. January 2019. http://asshperspectives.org/2019/01/physician-burnout-is-the-foundation-of-your-life-crumbling/. Accessed July 2019.

8. Clance PR, Imes SA. The imposter phenomenon in high achieving women: dynamics and therapeutic intervention. Psychother Theory Res Pract. 1978;15(3):241.

9. Collins LH, Chrisler JC, Quina K. Career strategies for women in academia: arming Athena. Thousand Oaks: Sage; 1998.

10. Corley J, Williamson T. Women in neurosurgery: final frontier of career women's movement. World Neurosurg. 2018;111:130–1.

11. Dasgupta N, Scircle MM, Hunsinger M. Female peers in small work groups enhance women's motivation, verbal participation, and career aspirations in engineering. Proc Natl Acad Sci. 2015;112(16):4988–93.

12. Dietrich C. When self-care is just one more thing on your to-do list. Motherly. 2017. https://www.printfriendly.com/p/g/WfCXRM. Accessed July 2019.

13. Dixon A, Silva NA, Sotayo A, Mazzola CA. Female medical student retention in neurosurgery: a multifaceted approach. World Neurosurg. 2019;122:245–51.

14. Eagly AH, Wood W. Explaining sex differences in social behavior: a meta-analytic perspective. 1988. https://files.eric.ed.gov/fulltext/ED303721.pdf. Accessed 12 July 2019.

15. Fabbre A. St. Joseph's female neurosurgeon would like to change minds. Chicago Tribune (Chicagoland Extra). 2010 May 7: Section 4: page 2.

16. Goggins D. Can't hurt me. Lioncrest Publishing; 2018.

17. Greenwald AG, Banaji MR. Implicit social cognition: attitudes, self-esteem, and stereotypes. Psychol Rev. 1995;102(1):4.

18. Halpern DF, Benbow CP, Geary DC, Gur RC, Hyde JS, Gernsbacher MA. The science of sex differences in science and mathematics. Psychol Sci Public Interest. 2007;8(1):1–51.

19. Han S, Shanafelt TD, Sinsky CA, Awad KM, Dyrbye LN, Fiscus LC, Trockel M, Goh J. Estimating the attributable cost of physician burnout in the United States. Ann Intern Med. 2019;170(11):784–90.

20. Heiser S. More women than men enrolled in US medical schools in 2017. AAMC News. 18 Dec 2017.

21. Helms MM, Arfken DE, Bellar S. The importance of mentoring and sponsorship in women's career development. SAM Adv Manag J. 2016;81(3):4.

22. Huang G. Employee satisfaction: the female perspective. Forbes. 18 July 2016. https://www.forbes.com/sites/georgenehuang/2016/07/18/employee-satisfaction-the-female-perspective/#79c128945a76. Accessed January 2019.

23. Hustvedt S. A woman looking at men looking at women: essays on art, sex, and the mind. New York: Simon and Schuster; 2016.

24. Jacobs P, Schain L. Professional women: the continuing struggle for acceptance and equality. Sacred Heart University. 2009. https://digitalcommons.sacredheart.edu/cj_fac/1/. Accessed May 2020.

25. Kang SK, Kaplan S. Working toward gender diversity and inclusion in medicine: myths and solutions. Lancet. 2019;393(10171):579–86.

26. Kerr HL, Armstrong LA, Cade JE. Barriers to becoming a female surgeon and the influence of female surgical role models. Postgrad Med J. 2016;92(1092):576–80.

27. Larkin A. Johns Hopkins has first black female neurosurgeon resident. CNN. 22 March 2017. https://www.cnn.com/2017/03/21/health/hopkins-black-woman-neurosurgeon-trnd/index.html. Accessed April 2019.

28. Linzer M, Harwood E. Gendered expectations: do they contribute to high burnout among female physicians? J Gen Intern Med. 2018;33(6):963–5.

29. Luc JG, Stamp NL, Antonoff MB. Social media in the mentorship and networking of physicians: important role for women in surgical specialties. Am J Surg. 2018;215(4):752–60.

30. Ly D, Jena AB. Sex differences in time spent on household activities and care of children among US physicians, 2003–2016. Mayo Clin Proc. 2018;93(10):1484–7.

31. Martin P, Barnard A. The experience of women in male-dominated occupations: a constructivist grounded theory inquiry. sa J Ind Psychol. 2013;39(2):01–12.

32. McMurray Julia E, Linzer M, Konrad TR, Douglas J, Shugerman R, Nelson K. The work lives of women physicians: results from the physician worklife study. J Gen Intern Med. 2000;15:372–80.

33. Miller LE, Miller J. A woman's guide to successful negotiating. New York: McGraw Hill Professional; 2010.

34. Nanette. Directed by Madeleine Parry and Jon Olb. Written and Performed by Hannah Gadsby. 2018. Retrieved from Netflix.

35. Neumann M, Edelhäuser F, Tauschel D, Fischer MR, Wirtz M, Woopen C, Haramati A, Scheffer C. Empathy decline and its reasons: a systematic review of studies with medical students and residents. Acad Med. 2011;86(8):996–1009.

36. Neumayer L, Kaiser S, Anderson K, Barney L, Curet M, Jacobs D, Lynch T, Gazak C. Perceptions of women medical students and their influence on career choice. Am J Surg. 2002;183(2):146–50.

37. Norcross JC, VandenBos GR. Leaving it at the office: a guide to psychotherapist self-care. New York: Guilford Publications; 2018.
38. Parcel TL, Menaghan EG. Parents' jobs and children's lives. New York: Transaction Publishers; 1994.
39. Peel JK, Schlachta CM, Alkhamesi NA. A systematic review of the factors affecting choice of surgery as a career. Can J Surg. 2018;61(1):58.
40. Pieris D. Empathy in medicine: what we can learn from children. Stanford Medicine. https://scopeblog.stanford.edu/2018/07/09/empathy-in-medicine-what-we-can-learn-from-children/. Accessed 29 Aug 2019.
41. Pilitsis J, Ben-Haim S. Women in neurosurgery: past, present and future. Congress of Neurological Surgeons. 2015. https://www.cns.org/publications/congress-quarterly/congress-quarterly-spring-2015/women-neurosurgery-past-present. Accessed March 2019.
42. Purvanova RK, Muros JP. Gender differences in burnout: a meta-analysis. J Vocat Behav. 2010;77:168–85.
43. Renfrow JJ, Rodriguez A, Wilson TA, Germano IM, Abosch A, Wolfe SQ. Tracking career paths of women in neurosurgery. Neurosurgery. 2017;82(4):576–82.
44. Reichmann FF. Loneliness. Psychiatry. 1959;22(1):1–5.
45. Rogo-Gupta LJ, Haunschild C, Altamirano J, Maldonado YA, Fassiotto M. Physician gender is associated with Press Ganey patient satisfaction scores in outpatient gynecology. Womens Health Issues. 2018;28(3):281–5.
46. Sandmark H, Renstig M. Understanding long-term sick leave in female white-collar workers with burnout and stress-related diagnoses: a qualitative study. BMC Public Health. 2010;10(1):210.
47. Saxena M, Geiselman TA, Zhang S. Workplace incivility against women in STEM: insights and best practices. Bus Horiz. 2019;62:589–94.
48. Schmidt LE, Cooper CA, Guo WA. Factors influencing US medical students' decision to pursue surgery. J Surg Res. 2016;203(1):64–74.
49. Shirom A, Westman M, Shamai O, Carel RS. Effects of work overload and burnout on cholesterol and triglycerides levels: the moderating effects of emotional reactivity among male and female employees. J Occup Health Psychol. 1997;2(4):275.
50. Sinsky CA, Cipriano PF, Bhatt J. Burnout among health care professionals. American Medical Association. 2017. https://www.ama-assn.org/sites/amaassn.org/files/corp/media-browser/public/ipp/i17-ipps-lotte-dyrbye-burnout-among-health-care-professionals.pdf. Accessed May 2020.
51. Spetzler RF. Progress of women in neurosurgery. Asian J Neurosurg. 2011;6(1):6.
52. Stamp N. I'm a female surgeon. I feel uncomfortable telling girls they can be one, too. The Washington Post. 2019. https://beta.washingtonpost.com/opinions/2019/07/29/im-female-surgeon-i-feeluncomfortable-telling-girls-they-can-be-one-too/?noredirect=on. August 2019. Statistica. https://www.statista.com/statistics/278414/number-of-worldwide-social-network-users/. Accessed 5 Sept 2019.

53. Status of Women in the States. Women's labor force participation. https://statusofwomendata.org/earnings-and-the-gender-wage-gap/womens-labor-force-participation/. Accessed March 2019.

54. Tate N. Loneliness rivals obesity, smoking as health risk. WebMD Health News. 4 May 2018. https://www.webmd.com/balance/news/20180504/loneliness-rivals-obesity-smoking-as-health-risk. Accessed 5 March 2019.

55. Torrey T. The importance of the surgeon riddle. 19 Aug 2019. https://www.verywellhealth.com/riddleme-this-who-is-the-surgeon-3969767. Accessed 1 Sept 2019.

56. Walston SF. Women integrating workday courage. Women Bus. 2002;54(2):28–9.

57. Ward L. Female faculty in male-dominated fields: law, medicine, and engineering. N Dir High Educ. 2008;143(Fall):63–72.

58. Woodrow SI, Gilmer-Hill H, Rutka JT. The neurosurgical workforce in North America: a critical review of gender issues. Neurosurgery. 2006;59(4):749–58.

59. Ziechmann R, Hoffman H, Chin LS. Academic genealogy of neurosurgery via department chair. World Neurosurg. 2019;121:e113–8.

Mind the Gap: Career and Financial Success for Women in Medicine

11

Kristine D. Olson and Jamie R. Litvack

> *Exemplary of a champion, NIH director Dr. Collins wrote...*
>
> "I want to send a clear message of concern: It is time to end the tradition in science of all-male speaking panels,".... "Starting now," he added, "when I consider speaking invitations, I will expect a level playing field, where scientists of all backgrounds are evaluated fairly for speaking opportunities. If that attention to inclusiveness is not evident in the agenda, I will decline to take part. I challenge other scientific leaders across the biomedical enterprise to do the same." [1]
>
> New York Times June 12, 2019

In 2019, the World Health Organization published "Delivered by Women, Led by Men: A Gender and Equity Analysis of the Global Health and Social Workforce." The authors reported that 70% of the global health-care workforce is female. Labor was segregated by gender norms, horizontally (across specialties) and vertically (through leadership). The gender pay gap in healthcare

K. D. Olson (✉)
Internal Medicine, Yale School of Medicine, Yale New Haven Hospital, New Haven, CT, USA
e-mail: kristine.olson@yale.edu

J. R. Litvack
Surgery, Washington State University, Pullman, WA, USA
e-mail: jamie.litvack@wsu.edu

© Springer Nature Switzerland AG 2020
C. M. Stonnington, J. A. Files (eds.), *Burnout in Women Physicians*,
https://doi.org/10.1007/978-3-030-44459-4_11

303

was higher than in any other sector of the economy. Female professionals were clustered into "low-status/less paid" roles. There was a lack of gender parity in leadership driven by "stereotypes, discrimination, power imbalance, and privilege," and that this disadvantage can be multiplied by other factors such as race, class, etc. The authors reported that bias, discrimination, and harassment were associated with attrition, low morale, and ill health. Whereas empowering women with education, financial well-being, and autonomy generally improves the well-being of her family, community, and society at large, and female leaders commonly improve health for all [2].

Men and women in medicine are held accountable to the same rigorous strictly enforced standards for entering and graduating from an accredited medical school, passing national licensing exams, completing approved residency training, achieving board certification, maintenance of certification, and credentialing and complying with the oversight of medical staff. Women pay the same tuition, make the expected personal sacrifices, and are as capable as their male colleagues. Since half of the medical graduates are female, it follows that we would want female physicians working at full capacity. Yet currently female physicians do not achieve the same level of success (professional rank or reward).

In 2017, the number of women entering medical school surpassed men (50.7%) [3]. However, in this chapter we will demonstrate that without a substantive change in the culture of medicine, the likelihood a woman entering medical school in 2017 will become chief medical officer, dean, department chair, full professor, editor in chief, RO1 grant recipient, first or last author on a manuscript, invited editorialist, or a specialist in the most lucrative specialties is significantly less than that of her male counterparts. It is less likely that she will marry or have children, and if she does, it is more likely she will carry more domestic responsibilities related to the care of the household and children. These discrepancies in her success, defined as personal and professional rank and rewards, cannot be completely explained by specialty, practice setting, work hours, productivity, race, ethnicity, year in academia, marital status, and parental status.

In this chapter we explore the gender gap in career success, explore some of the theories offered in the literature that underlie the gap and may explain a proportion of the phenomenon, and finally seek potential strategies and tactics to close the gap.

The Success Gap

Pay Gap

Female physicians have been reported to earn less than their male colleagues. Female physicians are reported to earn from 64% to 90% that of male physicians [4–8]. Women in other fields generally earn 80–82% of what men are paid for similar work [9]. These pay gaps start with the first job after training and persist over a women's career [10, 11] and can be especially problematic at the intersection of gender and race with Black, Native American, and Latino women making 52–58% of their male colleagues [9]. From the start of her career, at the time of this writing, female physicians earn an unadjusted average of $20,000 less in annual compensation than male counterparts [7, 8, 10, 12, 13]. Per these authors, this pay gap was not attributable to her specialty, practice setting, work hours, productivity, race, ethnicity, year in academia, marital status, or parental status. However, after adjusting for working part-time and taking leave, the pay gap shrunk to approximately $17,000 and did not reach statistical significance [7]. Part-time physicians reported lower compensation and fewer opportunities to advance, which in turn lowered career satisfaction [7, 14]. Women are more likely to work part-time.

Female physicians seem to be segregated into specialties with lower status and compensation. The gender pay gap was seen across 446 major US occupations examined by the Wall Street Journal; they found women earned less than men in 439 of these occupations, and this gap was magnified in some of the highest-paying occupations, specifically doctors and surgeons, financial specialists, and lawyers and judges [4]. In medicine, Desai et al. examined 13 medical specialties and found that the more lucrative the specialty, the more likely it was dominated by male physicians even after adjusting for hours, productivity, and years of experience [12]. Specialists stand to earn two to three times the salary of general medical doctors [15]. In 2012, cardiology was the medical specialty with the lowest percentage of women at 10.7% [12]. Whereas, general primary care was 49% female in 1999 and dropped to 33% by 2008 [10], which suggests evidence of diversification. Perhaps more importantly, female patients may benefit from having more female specialists. For example, cardiologist Dr. Donna Arnett advocates for more female cardiologists since heart attacks are the leading cause of death in women, and their presenting symptoms are currently described as "atypical" compared to those seen in men [16].

Leadership Gap

Women are less likely to be recognized as leaders. It has been reported that in the United States, approximately 95–98% of chief executive officers of Fortune 500 and S&P companies are men [17]. Both men and women have an implicit bias that leaders are men; perhaps the fact that men are in leadership positions serves as a confirmation bias to reinforce that perception [18]. In healthcare, approximately 3–18% of chief executive officers and chief medical officers, 6–16% of deans, 13–15% of department chairs, 9% of division chiefs, and 19% of full professors are female [19–22]. This is in spite of the fact that 70–80% of the health-care workforce, 50% of medical school classes, and 34–40% of the practicing physicians are female [21–23].

Women can be exceptional leaders, but face confirmation bias Women can be exceptional leaders, but seem to face some bias. Zenger et al., in one study published in Harvard Business Review, found that women were perceived as or more effective than men in 17 of 19 leadership competencies and were exceptional at taking initiative, practicing self-development, and driving for results and displaying honesty and integrity (men scored higher on strategic perspective and technical/professional expertise) [17].

In a different study, it was found that strategic roles are more often assigned to men, whereas operational roles are more often assigned to women, which can convey a bias that women have less aptitude for strategy and their absence in these roles serving as a confirmation bias [24]. Zenger et al. also evaluated how 40,184 men and 22,600 women assessed their own leadership effectiveness and found that women underestimated their abilities and men overestimated them [17]. Perception is not always reality, which suggests that men and women would both make better decisions if more aware of inherent bias in themselves and others.

Gender diversity in leadership improves organizational performanc *Gender diversity in leadership improves organizational performance.* Valerio et al. reported that after they sorted companies into quartiles based on their proportion of women on the board, the companies in the top quartile of female inclusion outperformed those in the bottom quartile by 15% for sales, customers, and profits [25]. Turban et al. examined 1069 companies in 35 countries over 24 industries and found that a 10% increase in Blau's index (a diversity index taking into account the ratio of men to women) increased the market value to 7% when coupled with the belief that gender diversity was important and "normatively" accepted (publicly declared and actively pursued in earnest) [26]. Furthermore, 67% job seekers look for diversity in the workforce, and 61% of female candidates look for gender diversity in the leadership team and opt to join a firm with diversity in the leadership team [26].

Clinical Care Recognition Gap

Female physicians were less likely than male physicians to be recognized as physicians by patients (78.5% vs. 93.3%, in one study of ER physicians) [27]. Yet female physicians perform as well as their male counterparts. In an analysis of 1.5 million Medicare patients treated by female versus male physicians, the patients treated by female physicians had a statistically significant lower 30-day mortality rate (15.02% versus 15.57%) and a lower hospital readmission rate (11.07% versus 11.49%) [28]. Female physicians have been shown to be more likely to spend more time with patients and engage in shared decision-making, counsel patients, tend to their psychological needs, attend to preventative services, and achieve better outcomes with less litigation [29, 30].

Academic Success Gap

Female physicians are less likely to be introduced by professional title when presenting at major meetings and are less likely to be invited to give these important presentations [31, 32]. In spite of being as equally committed to academic medicine as male counterparts and comprising 40% of the academic faculty at the time of this writing, female faculty make up only a quarter of tenured faculty [7]. Women advance to full professor more slowly and are less likely to make full professor with a ratio of female to male full professors of 1:4 [16, 21, 23, 33, 34]. Furthermore, a 2016 study of 10,241 academic physicians from 24 public medical schools reported that female full professor salaries were comparable to male associate professors and female associate professors salaries were comparable to male assistant professors [35]. Despite adjustments for potential confounders including age, years of experience, faculty rank, specialty, scientific authorship, NIH funding, clinical trial participation, and Medicare reimbursement, nearly 40% of the differences in salaries between men and women remained unexplained. In academia, if one does not advance to full professor, it can account for a $60,000 annual pay gap [7]. These financial inequities compound over decades.

Academic institutions have been reported to give less generous start-up packages to women than men, reporting a difference of $585K versus $980K, respectively [36]. In another study, Bates et al. reported a similar disparity of $400 K for junior facility doing basic research [36]. Compared to men, the women are less likely to transition from a K Award to an established RO1 within 5 years, 19% versus 25% [34]. Women seem less likely to apply for RO1 grants, compared to men, 27% to 73%, respectively. In published work in the medical journals, women account for a third of the first authors, 4–19% of senior authors, 11–19% of invited guest editorials in the prestigious journals NEJM and

JAMA, and account for 7% of the editors in chief [34]. The slow-down during the critical early years in a woman's career has been often been referred to as "the motherhood tax," "the maternal wall", which will be discussed below.

Family and Citizenship Gap

Female physicians are less likely to marry (79% versus 89%) or have children (81% versus 92%) [7]. Half of female physicians are married to another physician (42–50%), whereas, a less than a third of male physicians are married to another physician (15–30%) [37]. Compared to their male colleagues, women are less likely to have a partner who works less than full-time outside of the home (85.6% versus 44.9%) [38], and it is not clear what proportion of these female physicians are the primary bread winner for their families. Women are more likely than men to work part-time or to take an extended leave (22% versus 15%). Female physicians are more likely to be the one who is primarily responsible for domestic duties, including care of the children and elderly. On average, female physicians with children were found to perform 10 hours less professional work per week than those without children, and female physicians perform 100 more minutes per day or 8.5 more hours per week on domestic work (caring for children and running the household) than male physicians [38, 39]. In addition to a disproportionate share of household and family responsibilities at home, many women also report discrimination at work for having these responsibilities. In one survey of 5782 female physicians, 66.3% reported gender discrimination at work, and 35.8% felt discriminated against for issues related to motherhood. Of those who experienced maternal discrimination, 89.6% reported discrimination against pregnancy and taking maternity leave [40]. Female physicians felt judged as "lazy" professionals if working part-time and judged as a bad mother if working full-time [22, 40]. For men, the family is considered a support system. For the women, the family is considered an additional responsibility. This shift for women to cut down on professional work to take on more domestic work is coined the "motherhood penalty" and the "fatherhood bonus" [8]. This is not to say that men would not also prefer to have equal time bonding with and raising their children.

Exploring the Gap

The segregation of women in medicine into low-status, low-earning areas horizontally (across specialties) and vertically (in the hierarchy) raises the question of whether women self-sort as a reflection of women's preferences toward "caregiving" traits, or whether they are marginalized by a male-dominated profession [41]. Riska et al. offer several models to consider. Perhaps women are socialized into gender norms based on a "deficient focus" (lacking traits as a gender needed to advance within the profession), or "asset focus" (possessing traits, for example, suited to compassionate care for children and the elderly). Or, perhaps the status of the male-dominated profession must be defended by subjugating or excluding women. Another possibility is viewing the medical profession as what Riska calls "discourse and relational," and thus discursive strategies are used by the male-dominant in-group to create cultural practices that define women's roles (e.g., women's health specialty) [41]. The dominant group might also claim a lack of qualified candidates to explain the underrepresentation of women – the "meritocracy myth" [42–44]. However, the female may not be deemed as qualified because she has not had the opportunity, through position and promotion, to demonstrate her qualifications; this privilege might be considered an "asset" that the nondominant group members do not possess [45, 46]. Compared to a member of the dominant in-group, the nondominant group member may have to work much harder to "merit" the opportunity. For example, as reported in the review by Kang et al., women had to be 2–5 times more productive than men to be hired for similar postdoctoral positions [47]. Those that succeed lead in shaping the future of medicine.

Perhaps, men and women have a different notion of success. One hypothesis for the gender gap is that men and women define success differently and pursue it accordingly. One study of physicians asserted that men define success as achieving goals and social recognition through income and promotion, whereas, many women define success by their social relationships, "personal challenges," and the desire to be more "autonomous and less dependent on external recognition." These authors defined *objective career success* as titles, publications, and organizational metrics and *subjective career success* as satisfaction and self-efficacy in teaching, research, and clinical work. The authors found a gender gap in objective career success, but not in subjective career success. These findings seem to conform to gender norms, and the conclusion drew criticism for not accounting for the social constructs that could have produced the results such that they may not be reflective of women's preferences [48]. Others have speculated that due to estrogen women may be more emotionally attuned, nurturing, and relational, whereas men, due to testosterone, may be more competitive, risk-takers, aggressive, and more independent-minded. It remains unknown to what extent female and male physicians self-sort into their preferred roles versus are expected to maintain the norms of the dominant culture.

Women will self-silience themselves for fear of losing critical relationships. A 2019 review on "self-silencing and women's health" explains the phenomenon [49]. More than men, perhaps due to a combination of gender norms, lower social status, and biologic sex, women have been more dependent on and gain power through relationships and communication. As such, the authors explain, many women develop "rejection sensitivity" through which she knows when to silence herself in order to survive, feel protected, or accepted. Women may silence themselves to avoid conflict and loss. Women may also self-silence if they believe self-sacrifice is a form of love and care, making them more valuable, as a way to raise their status in society. Some will conceal their true self to present the external false self that is expected by others and to conform to the social norms of feminine "goodness." Those who have an "externalized self-perception" dependent on what others think of them lack confidence or suffer from perfectionism and are even more prone to strictly conform to perceived gender norms in order to fit in. The authors explain, she may hide her anger and sense of unfairness, as these displays are socially unacceptable for women. However, as Maji et al. describe, concealing one's authentic self can lead to internalized anger, frustration, unmet needs, and risk becoming disconnected from others. Self-silencing is also considered a form of abandonment of one's true self, perpetuates self-doubt, and has been linked to depression [49].

The confidence gap between men and women has gained attention through investigative journalists Claire Shipman of ABC News and Katy Kay of the BBC World News [50]. They report, women exhibit more perfectionism and are more likely to experience the "imposter syndrome," in which they feel inadequate and fraudulent in their success, despite the evidence they are performing as well as men. The authors reported that the sense of mastery and confidence comes from learning from trial and error, but women miss out on opportunities to grow from mistakes when they are worried about being perfect, being liked, and fear failure. This may explain why women consistently underestimated their abilities and men consistently overestimate their abilities, though both perform equally well. Women are more likely to blame themselves (internal forces) for shortcomings, whereas men are more likely to blame external circumstances. These journalists go on to report that women are less likely to speak up or apply for a job unless they are absolutely certain they are correct in their statements or that they meet all of the stated job qualifications. Whereas, men will apply if they meet 60% of the qualifications and expect they will learn what they do not know on the job [50].

Zenger et al. found that the confidence gap between the genders starts at an early age. Between the ages of 8 and 14 years, a girl's confidence drops 30%, and their fear of failure increases 150%. The perception of being "liked" drops from 71% to 38% in the early teen years. Perhaps this is due to the fact that adolescent girls get the message to value perfection and avoid risk, therefore, they may miss out on the opportunity to grow confident through learning from mistakes. At age 25, women will start to gain confidence and finally close the gap by age 60. During this period, from 25 to 60 years old, women gain 29 points on the confidence scale, compared to the men who gain 8.5 points during the same period of time. Because women lack confidence during the early stages of a career, she may not assert her competence and capabilities thus losing out on opportunities [17, 50].

Double standards and "the double bind" can be particularly challenging for successful women. Unlike men, in the current climate women are not perceived to be both assertive and warm, competent and "likeable," simultaneously. The presence or absence of one infers the presence or absence of the other, called the "innuendo effect." To say that a woman is "not likable" or "not a good fit" may sometimes be a euphemism for discrimination by gender norms against her ambition, even if unintentional. This can be confusing for women in leadership who get high marks and often exceed expectations on tasks but are held to "double standards" in managing work relationships. For example, researchers found that in the same performance reviews women may be told to "say no more often" and "not be afraid to make decisions that are unpopular," while at the same time needing to "take others viewpoint into account" and "be more collaborative." An aspiring female physician leader may try to be everything to everybody simultaneously. Or she may feel the need to conceal parts of herself (such as her strengths), unable to be fully authentic, expressive, or efficacious. This can be likened to the feeling of "walking a tight rope" or "walking on eggshells," which feels isolating, stressful, and exhausting. The energy needed to conform to gender norms and be "liked" by everyone can detract from the primary work. Furthermore, the pressure to conform to the gender norms along with the biased double standards and double binds perpetuates the "hidden curriculum," in which one generation of women teaches the next generation of women to conform to gender norms and conveys the message that her authentic self is unacceptable [42, 51–53].

Women are expected to put others first. Compared to men, women have been shown to generally behave more collaboratively and look after the greater good, which has also been demonstrated in research and education [22]. Still women are often chastised for too much ambition and self-sacrifice to attain success, even if her ambition is to serve others. Per gender norms, she may be shamed for expecting credit for her own work. Some say, "nice girls don't get the corner office" [54]. However, she may need to be "liked" and to "fit in" with the male-dominant "in-group" to get an opportunity. She may even be expected to downplay her achievements to be deemed more "likable." To be "liked", she may be relegated to the "helper role" by the dominant group, and vulnerable to others taking credit for her labor, such that being a "teamplayer" does not necessarily translate into advancement. This is a "double bind". And if she were to express anger about the situation, her anger is more likely to be perceived as irrational and evidence of her lack of competence, whereas a man's anger is more often attributed to external conditions and deemed reasonable, rational, and persuasive [51], which is a "double standard".

The "token" status of women in certain aspects of medicine does not fully explain the challenges they face to be accepted, fully participate, and advance in her field. By "token", we mean being less than 15% of a group. By raising the proportion of women in the group, it does not necesssarily resolve the obstacles women's face for upward mobility. In the comprehensive review on the subject of "tokenism" by Zimmer [55], the author provides some examples. For example, a decision-maker may purposefully promote a "token" outsider from the nondominant group as proof that he or she, the decision-maker, is not discriminatory and as evidence that they are compliant with expectations for desegregation, diversity, equity, and inclusion. However, these motivations do not guaruntee that those selected from the token group are most likely to succeed. Furthermore, it also suggests that a smaller proportion than than those qualified will be advanced. And furthermore, those token women that are hired into male-dominated fields such as medicine, police work, or the military are often segregated into positions with less power and less opportunity to advance. In contrast, men in female-dominated fields such as teaching and nursing are often disproportionately upwardly mobile and powerful. Moreover, as women rise in proportion in male-dominated fields, there was found to be a proportionate backlash of harassment to prevent them from advancing [55].

Women may fear rejection and retribution from the "in-group" that holds authority over her success. In a 2019 study of 7409 resident surgeons, 30% of women and 4% of men who felt sexually harassed feared the negative consequences if they complained about it. Hu et al. found that 65% of female surgery residents reported experiencing gender discrimination and 20% experienced sexual harassment, compared to 10% and 4% of males, respectively. Their supervising attending physicians were the most frequent source of sexual harassment (27%) and abuse (52%). This study also reported these experiences were associated with symptoms of burnout and suicidal thoughts, and these consequences were no longer present after adjusting for such mistreatment [56]. Women face hostility in the workplace and for reporting it [57]. A sexualized workplace can make women and men fearful of one another and therefore less likely to hire women in order to avoid risk, especially if it is believed that there is little to gain [58]. Perhaps this will resolve by normalizing gender diversity in the workplace.

Unconscious, implicit, second-generation bias is unintentional, yet omnipresent and detrimental to the advancement of women. Thus, it is imperative to deconstruct gender stereotypes that impose "double standards," put women in the "double bind," impose "self-silencing," and undermine women's confidence, forbid their ambition, and perpetuate the expectation that they behave according to gender norms to "self-sacrifice" and help others without the expectation of credit or reward. Making the necessary corrections role model for young girls and the next generation of female physician that their hope to be successful is acceptable and attractive, to be celebrated and not concealed. She should have permission to be simultaneously strong and warm, competent and likable, ambitious and collaborative, and authentic. This should strengthen her relationships and not detract from them. Like men, she should be able to be a parent and a professional. In achieving all of this, women should not be penalized with the "minority tax" in which she is tasked to resolve her own marginalization and devaluation, which further detracts focus from the primary work. It is a societal problem that requires a societal solution.

Closing the Gap

Negotiation training can help women navigate gender stereotypes. In "Negotiation Strategies for Women, Secrets to Success" by the Program on Negotiation at Harvard Law School [24], the authors refute the claim that women are less skilled or assertive in negotiation; however, they negotiate less frequently and they often ask for less in order to protect against the backlash they face for breeching gender norms. The authors write that women are expected to be "accommodating and cooperative," "nice and empathetic," and "warm not assertive," and to put others needs ahead of their own. The authors report that women may advocate forcefully for others, but not themselves, and ought to avoid negative masculine traits such as "dominance, arrogance, and entitlement" [24]. Their goal is to get their request granted while remaining likable, lest an "unlikability" judgement taint their career long term. Therefore, Professor Bohnet refers to Sheryl Sandberg's advice to "combine niceness with insistence" to be "relentlessly pleasant" and "adhere to biased rules and expectations." To avoid backlash, Professor Bowles recommends to "link aggressive demands to the needs of others, such as the organization," and men and women ought to "audit their judgements for the subconscious tendency to view assertive women negotiators as unlikeable and overly demanding" and otherwise "reference relevant [objective] standards that would be difficult for the other side to ignore." Bowles suggests communicating that she cares about the relationships and "legitimize" her negotiation behavior (e.g., such as by referencing that a "team leader suggested asking about compensation").

Protecting against the backlash of breeching gender norms may be possible under some circumstances. For example, women perceived as "high status" may not experience as much backlash. Professor Bowles referred to the work by Professor Amy Cuddy and Professors Amanatallah and Tinsley in stating that even striking a pose or anything that generates a psychological sense of power can improve negotiations for women. Professor Bohnet relays how habitually facing your fears to "overcome stereotypical expectations through positive experiences" can increase your mastery and confidence in future negotiations [59]. Martin et al. found that women with "gender blindness" are more likely to feel confident, take initiatives, and take risks, than those who were "gender aware"; there may be some advantages to downplaying gender [60].

Women in male-dominated fields may benefit from being self-aware of their implicit tendencies to compensate for social constructs of gender norms, thus be more intentional in choosing a particular non-gendered response. For example, in "Tokenism and Women in the Workplace: The Limits of the Gender Neutral Theory" [55], Zimmer reports how women respond to being in positions that lack power or opportunities to advance. The author describes that those who lack power may exercise *"authoritarianism and use of coercion over subordinates."* Those who lack opportunities for advancement may *"respond with lower aspirations, parochialism and heightened commitment to nonwork rather than work activities."* If working alongside men in leadership, the "token" women may be *"highly visible and intensely scrutinized"* and respond by *"overachievement or underachievement."* The dominant group may differentiate from the "outsider" by grossly exaggerating stereotypes, thus *"boundary heightening"— increasing the obstacles for the "token" women to advance.* The minority may experience a sense of isolation. Zimmer, citing Kanter, explains how some women may assimilate via *"role encapsulation,"* by acting within a female caricature – *"the mother, the pet, the seductress, the iron maiden"* – which influences the responses and evaluations from the dominant group but limits one's ability to be a successful authentic leader. As Kanter wrote, *"Tokenism is stressful: the burdens carried by tokens in the management of social relationships take a toll in psychologic stress, even if the token succeeds in work performance. Unsatisfactory social relationships, miserable self-imagery, frustrations from contradictory demands, inhibition of self-expression, feelings of inadequacy and self-hatred all have been suggested consequences of tokenism"* [55, 61, 62].

Male sponsors and mentors are critical in the advancement of women [20, 25, 47]. After interviewing 500 company executives, Valerio et al. found that effective male "champions" considered gender equity integral to talent management, ensured equal opportunities for women, and involved both men and women in working toward gender equity. As "sponsors," those in the dominant group often transfer some of their own social privilege and power in support of those they sponsor, to raise the visibility and credibility of the individual they sponsor. As "mentors," the male senior executive integrated the mentee into their work to role-model and teach the leadership process. Ibarra et al. found that men were more likely to have been mentored by the CEO or another senior executive, 78% versus 69%. Within 2 years the men had received 15% more promotions. Furthermore, women in top positions were nearly twice as likely to be hired from outside their firm [63], meaning they were less likely to be hired into top positions at their home institution. It is also worthy to note, that in calling out gender bias, male champions often risk resistance from their own dominant in-group [25].

Engaging male allies can triple the chance that organizations will improve gender inclusion (96% versus 30%), say Johnson and Smith [64]. Smith et al. reported on reasons why male allies may remain on the sidelines and how they might be more willing to show more public support for gender equity [64, 65]. To overcome the "bystander effect," in which a potential ally thinks someone else will do something about gender bias, the would-be bystanders might benefit from learning well established techniques that they can easily do to help in reduce unconcious bias [65]. For example, they might call out"microaggressions" by unwitting transgressors, in order to increase our collective awareness of bias. In the case of inactivity due to "psychological standing," in which he may think it is not his place to speak on this issue in which he does not have a stake, the potential male ally may be more willing to engage if they knew their role was important and dignified [64, 65]. It is also important for women to appreciate that male allies sometimes give up their comfort in choosing to confront the dominant norms upheld by their own dominant in-group and sometimes risk "stigma by association" or the "wimp penalty" or may be considered less masculine for "power-sharing" and working collaboratively with women [64]. At the same time, men and women might wish to avoid the "pedestal effect" in which the appreciation of these male allies overshadow the long-sustained work done by women over the years, thus reinforcing the hierarchy. Similarly, the authors make note of the possibility of "fake male feminists" who may use the title for praise or to wield influence over women [64]. Overall, men and women will be more successful teaming up together to improve gender diversity, equity, and inclusion for the good of all. Both men and women would benefit from developing more self awareness and situational awareness for bias that mascarade as "the norm".

Role modeling, peer mentoring, and coaching can help reduce the sense of "otherness" that women may feel as the minority group at the top, especially if caught in one of the seemingly impossible "double binds" as described above. The Physicians Mom's Group started online through Facebook in 2014 and now has over 70,000 members [66]. Here, female physicians share common experiences and find peer support. These peer groups provide role models, mentors, and coaches to help women reframe their experience and gain confidence in navigating the road to success [22]. President of Barnard College and cognitive scientist, Professor Bellock emphasized how important it is to practice cognitive reframing to combat the self-doubt, "learned helplessness," and "imposter syndrome" that can sometimes result from environments with pervasive though subtle bias against women. She advocates that journaling is one method that can help to work through emotions, maintain confidence, and focus inner voice [67].

Affirmation will be needed to keep female talent engaged. Women in leadership may be given resources to learn the skills needed for the job. She may be offered resources on how to have an "executive presence" in how she looks, speaks, and behaves. However, as Ibarra et al. advise, it is also important to be aware of the mismatch between how these traits are portrayed and perceived within current gender norms. Ibarra et al. describe that people will recognize the emerging female leader to not be what they expected (as they are accustomed to the current culture in that white males define executive leadership) and may accept or reject her or affirm or deflate her self-perception as an able leader. Thus, it is important to have opportunities for substantial achievements and to gain organizational endorsements. Ibarra et al. explain that through positive experiences, facing fear, and moving out of the comfort zone, the emerging leader will internalize her leadership identity. Ibarra et al. recommend facing the likability conundrum by neither being too feminine nor too hard charging, but to anchor in a sense of purpose that is value-aligned and serves the collective good. As the authors note, such an approach provides a compelling clear reason for action, conveys authenticity and trustworthiness, lends authority, and builds relationships [24].

How leaders might manage the "double bind" to be simultaneously tough and nice was investigated by Zheng et al. who interviewed 64 women in leadership (VP level or higher). They identified four "double bind" scenarios and five strategies to manage them. The four scenarios included 1) the need to be highly demanding of others while demonstrating warmth and care and 2) assert competence and decisiveness (strength) while showing vulnerability (weakness) and asking for collaboration (help), 3) advocating for oneself (so as not to feel taken advantage of) while focused on serving others (not being too aggressive with stakeholders to advance goals), and 4) maintaining distance (to generate leadership presence and maintain respect) while being approachable and accessible (without being perceived as informal, not serious, playing favorites). The strategy offered by the authors is to choose appropriate times when to use and signal niceness or toughness, distance or approachability, caring-collaborative or tough-directive traits for a particular situation and when it will first and foremost build relationships and trust and engage people. The authors suggest seeing assertiveness as a form of genuine care. They quote, "be tough on tasks and soft on people" [68]. Perhaps, this is not unlike parenting.

Implicit bias training can reduce bias. Implicit, unconscious, or second-generation bias is that which is inherent to existing organizational structures and practices and go unnoticed but harbor unintentional prejudices with adverse effects on women's access to opportunities and rewards. Unlike first-generation bias which has been made illegal in the workplace, second-generation bias goes unchecked (e.g., judging men and women differently for being assertive and advocating for themselves) [24, 69, 70]. Decision-makers who scored high on the implicit association tests (assessing one's unconscious associations with stereotypes) are more likely to hire the status quo; they are more likely to perceive those who are different from themselves or the dominant in-group as a risky choice. If the individual's difference is overt, i.e., cannot be concealed, it is even more likely that the decision-maker will infer competence based on the difference (e.g., gender, weight, race, etc.), making it more likely that the individual who is not in the "in-group" will be ostracized [71]. The implicit bias scores amongst health-care professionals are similar to those found in the general public, which is especially concerning given healthcare's pressured fast-paced environment, and thus prone to overly rely on cognitive shortcuts, fraught with bias to make quick decisions [42, 52, 53, 72].

An implicit bias course may make individuals more self-aware of their inherent bias, making them less likely to inadvertently perpetuate it. Gonzalez et al. describe one such method in which a course might provide the psychological safety necessary for a "transformational learning experience", in which the learner is faced with a profound example of a biased-based experience, followed by critical reflection and a "deeply moving" guided discourse, resulting in growth-enhancing behavior change in which the learner is made more aware of bias and the adverse effects such that they are less likely to inadvertently prejudice their judgements in the future [73]. Also, Kang et al. bring our attention to the resources available from the Center for Worklife Law at the University of California Hastings College of Law and those created by the Engendering Success in the STEM consortium, namely, the "Bias Interpreters" and the "Bias Busting Strategies," respectively [47].

A gender-diverse "promotion-focused" C-suite and board improve the financial success of the organization (as described above). Johnson et al. explained how the CEO and existing board members may inadvertently employ a "regulatory focus" in selecting individuals to steer the organization. Based on "regulatory focus theory", decision-makers may unconsciously employ a "promotion focus" or a "prevention focus" in considering what they have to gain versus what they have to lose, respectively. Those that adopted a "promotion focus" are less likely to engage in "group think" and achieve greater financial success. However, 84% of existing board members reported they are less likely to endorse an independent thinker. Existing board members may feel beholden to the CEO and the fellow board members who recruited them and wish to avoid dissenting views or see change as risk to be feared. The CEOs may prefer to appoint a known entity, such as other active CEOs. New members are likely to come from the same networks as the existing individuals and therefore likely to be of a similar race, sex, sociodemographic, behavioral, and interpersonal characteristics – predominantly white men (6% female). However, those with "promotion focus" were more likely to have diverse members that would challenge the CEO's position. They also reported more enjoyable dynamics, avoided group think, and had better financial performance. Disruptions in the organization or board are a good time to integrate new members, say Johnson et al. [74].

The ability to report harassment without fear of retaliation or stigmatization improved reporting and increased satisfaction for medical students, reported Mangurian et al. [22]. In "Organizational best practices toward gender equity in science and medicine" published in the Lancet by Coe et al., it was noted that women are at risk of a "double dose of hostility," given the prevalence of bias and risk of backlash for confronting it. Therefore, Coe et al. recommend that, as a starting point, those in power "listen to women, without comment, and believe them as they share their stories and experiences" [42].

Organizational accountability can improve diversity. Given the prevalence of unconscious bias by gender and the fast-paced nature of healthcare prone to cognitive shortcuts reliant on pattern recognition, which reinforces the status quo, health-care organizations might set a goal for gender equity as a proportion of women in all facets of healthcare vertically and horizontally and create a plan to achieve it and check the progress regularly [23, 42].

Add more women to the pool of candidates. Johnson et al. had 200 undergraduate students determine who to hire as the researchers changed the proportion of female candidates by changing the names on the applications for a fictitious nurse manager job. When two of three candidates were men, the participants were statistically more likely to hire a man for nursing leadership. In a follow-up study of university hiring patterns, Johnson et al. aggregated the finalists for jobs (an average of 4 individuals per finalist group for a total of 598) and examined those 174 who were extended a job offer. They found that the woman had zero chance of being hired if there was only one woman in the finalist pool, and she was 79 times more likely to be hired if there were two women in the finalist pool; however, the chances did not improve for each additional woman added to the pool [71]. To avoid anchoring expectations based on a male in the role, Johnson et al. suggested that the decision-makers interview the women first. Beware that when there is only one female candidate, her candidacy may be seen as a token of attempted gender diversity and undermine her chances [74].

Blinded assessments can reduce bias. Bates et al. reported on ways that blinding applications can improve gender parity, just as orchestras had increased the hiring of females by 25% when they blinded the audition. Similarly, the authors' commentary suggests that masking the gender of the principal investigator for grant applications to the National Institute of Health may reduce the bias against women's grant applications [36].

Structured interviews have been shown to be less biased than unstructured interviews. Bohnet et al. found that unstructured interviews are more prone to bias and less likely to determine job performance. For example, the authors found that three-quarters of the ratings that determined whether medical students were initially accepted to or rejected from medical school were based on perceptions and not objective facts, and it was not predictive of their future success. The authors explain that decision-makers can be overconfident in their own judgments and impressions, favoring those who "look the part" or "best person for the job," often hiring someone like themselves, thus reenforcing the status quo and gender-based segregation of roles. Bohnet suggests keeping interviewers as independent as possible, compiling objective data, establishing a question set to which interviewers can compare answers, having a scoring system, scoring and submitting the interview immediately, and aggregating the assessment before the meeting to discuss the candidates. The authors suggest eliminating group interviews in order to reduce "group think" [23, 75].

A *6-point rating scale may be less biased than a 10-point rating scale* when making assessments of men and women. Rivera et al. explain that when qualifications and behaviors are equal, women are less likely to be given a "perfect 10." Men are more likely to receive praise and the women are more likely to receive scrutiny. The authors examined 105,034 college student ratings made by 369 instructors in 235 courses after switching from a 10-point to a 6-point rating scale and found this eliminated the gender gap in the assessment of these otherwise equally qualified individuals. In a follow-up study in which they had a male and female deliver the exact same lecture, the female was scored 10–20% lower on a 10-point scale by 400 students, but had equivalent marks on a 6-point scale. This is important because these assessments determine wages and who will be given opportunities to advance to the top level of the organization. Over time, these discrepancies add up, determining one's level of success [76].

Wage transparency and an accurate accounting of work have been shown to shrink the wage gap between male and female physicians and slow the wage inflation for men [77]. As case in point, there was no pay gap for male and female otolaryngologists working in level I Veterans Affairs Medical Centers [78]. The authors attribute this in part to several decades of government-mandated initiatives starting with the 1963 Equal Pay Act. Salary data is transparent and publicly available. Stepwise increases are provided for years of service. Every 2 years, an objective review including an updated market evaluation is available. When oversights occur, adjustments can be made at later dates and retroactively applied. These researchers expanded the work to examine whether this phenomenon held true for other surgeon specialists. On univariate analysis, there was no difference in pay across 13 surgical subspecialties. On multivariable linear regression analysis, gender was a significant predictor of pay ($p < 0.001$), but the absolute differences were substantially reduced when compared to other work environments and absent in some specialties [79]. Other models of gender-blind value-based payments exist including the Mayo Clinic and Kaiser Permanente. Common themes emerge: similar starting salaries, stepwise increases, objective market review, and pay transparency.

Annual salary review can correct course. For example, as Warner et al. reported, Johns Hopkins found they were paying female physicians 3.4% less per FTE salary and 8.6% less in total salary. The University of California San Francisco Medical School could not justify the wage gaps between male and female physicians under the California Fair Pay Act and made $1.58M in salary adjustments [8]. Other prestigious medical schools followed suit.

Institutional funding, bridge grants, and skill building can help retain and promote junior faculty [23]. Female junior faculty are eager for professional development programs. Valantine et al. reported that of the 657 who participated in workshops, 64% were women. The topics covered included how to negotiate and delegate, write grants and manuscripts, communicate and present, time management, navigate work-life balance and implicit bias, and get reappointed and promoted.

Recognize the value of clinical work and clinical educators, which has a predominance of women. For example, Duke University, Dana Farber Cancer Institute, and Brigham and Women's Hospital have created ways to recognize clinical prowess and some have created a tenure track for these positions [21].

A *more flexible "academic clock"* may allow more women in academia to achieve full potential [23, 36, 80]. Advancement in academic medicine is often dependent on the rate at which a faculty member procures grants, publishes papers, and becomes engaged and renowned in their field. Often, eligibility for key grants and promotion is time limited, within the first 10 years of one's career. This may be when women, who have already delayed childbearing during training, now plan to have their children. An updated, flexible academic "clock" supported by academic promotion policies may be more effective in retaining and engaging top talent and promoting diversity, as top talent is a precious resource. Valantine et al. describe "Academic Biomedical Career Customization" with flexible policies that allow women to be available at home at critical times, such as tenure track extensions and parental leave, individualized career plans, flex up and down in research, patient care, administration and teaching, and facilitating physician engagement and satisfaction [20].

Support for work-life integration eliminates obstacles for women, especially mothers. Per the review by Mangurian et al., currently family leave policies at US medical schools are not compliant with the advice physicians give patients and society. For example, the Academy of Pediatrics is recommending

6 months of paid leave after childbirth, and most US medical schools only allow 8 weeks. Furthermore, family leave is often restricted to the "primary caregiver," which often defaults to the women to care for the children and elderly while limiting the option of "cooperative parenting" or shared caregiving, especially as half of physician mothers are married to a physician father. Mangurian et al. recommends a universal standard of at least 12 weeks paid childbearing leave, additional 4–12 weeks for childrearing for all new parents, lactation rooms and time to pump breast milk, on-site childcare, paid catastrophic leave for life-threatening illness or injury, flexible schedules and promotion policies, and legislative protection against employment discrimination against those with family caregiving responsibilities [22]. In Scandinavia where there is maternity-paternity leave for children under 1 year and accessible and affordable childcare for children under 6 years old, work and children were not considered an obstacle, and it has improved women's position in the workplace [41]. Warner et al. cite that companies such as Home Depot, Clif Bar, and Patagonia argue there is a strong business case for offering on-site child care, especially in improving engagement and reducing turnover; furthermore, 91% of the cost could be recouped in tax credits. The business case is likely to be more true for physicians, with replacement costs ranging from $250,000 to $1M per physician [8, 81]. Valantine et al. argue now that 50% of the American physician workforce comprises women, and work policies should not remain predicated on the idea that one spouse stay at home full-time [20].

Financial Freedom

Women need to achieve financial independence, perhaps more than men. On average, women live longer, are paid less, and are more likely to have work gaps. These gaps affect early, middle and late career. Childbearing and child rearing may affect early and early-middle career, and acute and/or chronic illness and care of elderly and aging family members may be more likely to affect middle and/or late career. Divorce and job prospects dependent on her partner's professional obligations can also affect a woman's career. Since women live longer than men and her wages peak earlier, and she is less likely to have as much invested for retirement; she is more likely to be widowed and at risk of financial "illness." Financial self-care reduces stress, increases confidence, and allows one to have more control over life choices. Strategies for achieving financial health and financial independence depend on managing debt, behavior (i.e., living below one's means), investing, and asset protection [82].

Manage debt by paying off high interest loans first. Alternatively, choose to pay off a smaller debt first and use the momentum from that success to inspire the next round of debt reduction. What about paying off medical school debt? Generally, if the interest rate is low, your money may be better spent investing in another investment vehicle with higher returns and paying down the difference. If the interest rate is high, it is better to pay off the student loan directly.

Set goals, budget, and save. In addition to traditional forms of information, such as books and brokers, there are a number of online resources such as The White Coat Investor [83], Physician on FIRE (Financial Independence and Retire Early) [84], and Wealthy Mom MD [85]. These resources are geared toward physicians and women physicians, respectively. In addition to saving and investing, factors such as specialty choice, practice type, and geography can substantially influence one's ability to build financial independence [6]. The highest paid specialties are typically procedural and/or surgical in nature. On average, owners/partners make more than independent contractors, who make more than employees. While compensation in the highest paying metro areas may be 37% higher, the cost of housing can vary tenfold, so living in a less expensive city with a slightly lower pay check may make more sense in the long-term. National cost indexes can be used to compare cost of living in metro areas to make sound decisions based on professional opportunities, family needs and quality of life.

Minimize medical school debt. For those of you reading this before or during medical school, minimizing school debt can help reduce stress and achieve financial freedom. In 2018, the median debt for medical student graduates who borrowed money was $200,000; this debt may increase by 20–50% by the completion of training [82]. Unfortunately, increased medical student debt has been associated with delays in making major life decisions such as marriage, children, and/or purchase of a home [86]. Several studies have associated medical school debt with choosing higher paying specialties [87]. In addition, medical student debt may be negatively associated with mental health, well-being and academic outcomes [87]. Some strategies to minimize school debt include choosing a state school over a private institution, sharing housing with a roommate, and selecting a less expensive city or one with good housing subsidies.

Investing is a critical part of growing wealth. Compared to men, women tend to be more likely to save and less likely to invest, which can hurt long-term growth. While some prefer traditional financial advisors, there are now online robo investing tools such Ellevest (ellevest.com), Betterment (betterment.com) and Wealthfront (wealthfront.com) to consider as part of your investment strategy. Ellevest is one of the few designed specifically for women and takes into account that women have a higher risk of gaps in work and a longer life span on average. Additionally, Ellevest provides resources to help educate oneself on financial decision making. Readers are advised to do their own research and vetting prior to making any investment decisions.

Anticipate life events, learn and plan accordingly. Many of the tools available are beyond the scope of this chapter, but they may be found in some of the online resources listed above. It is useful to educate yourself on topics such as the financial benefits of marriage and the cost of divorce, managing a dual physician household, delayed child-bearing and the cost and logistics of fertility treatments, the cost of childcare and education, the state variations in child education pre-tax investment devices, the rules for calculating and claiming social security benefits, retirement accounts, disability insurance, health insurance, life insurance, malpractice insurance, umbrella insurance, and state to state variations on what aspects of your personal financial portfolio would be at risk in case of a malpractice suit. While you build your financial security, you will also have to defend it.

Financial independence is defined by some as the ability to live on 4% of the overall value of one's investment portfolio annually [82]. For example, a $1,000,000 portfolio should generate $40,000 of income per year on average, a $2,000,000 portfolio should generate $80,0000 per year on average, and a $3,000,000 portfolio should generate $120,000 per year on average. Keep in mind that investing for a steady and reliable source of income is different than investing for long-term growth; the expected return on investment will be lower on average, but less volatile. Another simple way to calculate the amount needed to reach financial independence is to multiply one's annual cost of living by 25. For example, if your family lives on $200,000 per year, you will need a portfolio worth $5,000,000 to be financially independent.

Invest in yourself. You must invest in your most important asset: yourself. Disability insurance, particularly specialty-specific insurance and one that is portable, can help insure you against loss of income. Life insurance may be important if you have others that depend on you. Liability coverage can help protect you and your assets from other types of risk. Most importantly invest in your physical and mental health, carving out time to invest in your rest and rejuvenation for a long life of personal and professional success.

Conclusion

Now that women have achieved parity in medical school, it is essential to be sure that women physicians have equal opportunity to achieve career success. The reasons for the gaps in pay and promotion are multifactorial and will require a multifaceted approach involving both men and women, individuals, and institutions. Personal and professional freedom to participate and achieve rank and reward is a key component to women physicians' professional success, financial independence, and mental well-being.

References

1. Bulluck P. N.I.H. head calls for end to all-male panels of scientists. New York Times. 12 June 2019.
2. Manzoor M, Thompson K. Delivered by women, led by men: a gender and equity analysis of the Global Health and Social Workforce: World Health Organization; 3 Mar 2019. 60 p.
3. Heiser S. More women than men enrolled in U.S. medical schools in 2017: Association of American Medical Colleges; 2018 [updated December 18, 2017]. Available from: https://www.aamc.org/news-insights/press-releases/more-women-men-enrolled-us-medical-schools-2017.
4. Overberg P, Adamy J, Thuy L, Ma J. What's your pay gap? wsj.com: Wall Street Journal; 2016 [cited 2016 May 17]. Available from: http://graphics.wsj.com/gender-pay-gap/.
5. Miller C. Pay gap is because of gender, not jobs. New York Times. 23 Apr 2014.
6. Doximity 2019 physician compensation report: doximity. 2019. Available from: https://blog.doximity.com/articles/doximity-2019-physician-compensation-report-d0ca91d1-3cf1-4cbb-b403-a49b9ffa849f.
7. Freund KM, Raj A, Kaplan SE, Terrin N, Breeze JL, Urech TH, et al. Inequities in academic compensation by gender: a follow-up to the National Faculty Survey Cohort Study. Acad Med. 2016;91(8):1068–73.
8. Warner AS, Lehmann LS. Gender wage disparities in medicine: time to close the gap. J Gen Intern Med. 2019;34(7):1334–6.
9. Newcomb A. Women's earnings lower in most occupations 2018 [May 22]. Available from: https://www.census.gov/library/stories/2018/05/gender-pay-gap-in-finance-sales.html.
10. Lo Sasso AT, Richards MR, Chou CF, Gerber SE. The $16,819 pay gap for newly trained physicians: the unexplained trend of men earning more than women. Health Aff. 2011;30(2):193–201.
11. Carr PL, Raj A, Kaplan SE, Terrin N, Breeze JL, Freund KM. Gender differences in academic medicine: retention, rank, and leadership comparisons from the National Faculty Survey. Acad Med. 2018;93(11):1694–9.
12. Desai T, Ali S, Fang X, Thompson W, Jawa P, Vachharajani T. Equal work for unequal pay: the gender reimbursement gap for healthcare providers in the United States. Postgrad Med J. 2016;92(1092):571–5.
13. Baker LC. Differences in earnings between male and female physicians. N Engl J Med. 1996;334(15):960–4.
14. Pollart SM, Dandar V, Brubaker L, Chaudron L, Morrison LA, Fox S, et al. Characteristics, satisfaction, and engagement of part-time faculty at U.S. medical schools. Acad Med. 2015;90(3):355–64.

15. Foundation TP. Health Reform and the Decline of Physician Private Practice. A White Pater Examining the Effects of the Patient Protection and Affordable Care Act on Physicians Practices in the United States: Merrit Hawkins; 2010. p. pp 116.
16. Arnett DK. Plugging the leaking pipeline: why men have a stake in the recruitment and retention of women in cardiovascular medicine and research. Circ Cardiovasc Qual Outcomes. 2015;8(2 Suppl 1):S63–4.
17. Zenger J, Folkman J. Research: women score higher than men in most leadership skills. Harvard Business Review. 2019.
18. Murphy H. Picture a leader. Is she a woman? New York Times. 16 Mar 2018.
19. Rosenstein AH. Strategies to enhance physician engagement. J Med Pract Manage. 2015;31(2):113–6.
20. Valantine H, Sandborg CI. Changing the culture of academic medicine to eliminate the gender leadership gap: 50/50 by 2020. Acad Med. 2013;88(10):1411–3.
21. Rotenstein L. Fixing the gender imbalance in healthcare leadership. Harvard Business Review. 2018.
22. Mangurian C, Linos E, Urminala S, Rodrigez C, Jagsi R. What is holding women in medicine back from leadership. Harvard Business Review. 2018.
23. Valantine HA, Grewal D, Ku MC, Moseley J, Shih MC, Stevenson D, et al. The gender gap in academic medicine: comparing results from a multifaceted intervention for Stanford faculty to peer and national cohorts. Acad Med. 2014;89(6):904–11.
24. Program on Neotiation HLS. Harvard University; 2013.
25. Valerio A, Sawyer K. The men who mentor women. Harvard Business Review. 2016.
26. Turban S, Wu D, Letian LT. Research: When gender diversity makes firms more productive. Harvard Business Review. 2019.
27. Prince LA, Pipas L, Brown LH. Patient perceptions of emergency physicians: the gender gap still exists. J Emerg Med. 2006;31(4):361–4.
28. Tsugawa Y, Jena AB, Figueroa JF, Orav EJ, Blumenthal DM, Jha AK. Comparison of hospital mortality and readmission rates for medicare patients treated by male vs female physicians. JAMA Intern Med. 2017;177(2):206–13.
29. Delgado A, Lopez-Fernandez LA, Luna JD. Influence of the doctor's gender in the satisfaction of the users. Med Care. 1993;31(9):795–800.
30. McMurray JE, Linzer M, Konrad TR, Douglas J, Shugerman R, Nelson K. The work lives of women physicians results from the physician work life study. The SGIM Career Satisfaction Study Group. J Gen Intern Med. 2000;15(6):372–80.
31. Files JA, Mayer AP, Ko MG, Friedrich P, Jenkins M, Bryan MJ, et al. Speaker introductions at internal medicine grand rounds: forms of address reveal gender bias. J Womens Health (Larchmt). 2017;26(5):413–9.

32. Ruzycki SM, Fletcher S, Earp M, Bharwani A, Lithgow KC. Trends in the proportion of female speakers at medical conferences in the United States and in Canada, 2007 to 2017. JAMA Netw Open. 2019;2(4):e192103.

33. Kuhlmann E, Ovseiko PV, Kurmeyer C, Gutierrez-Lobos K, Steinbock S, von Knorring M, et al. Closing the gender leadership gap: a multi-centre cross-country comparison of women in management and leadership in academic health centres in the European Union. Hum Resour Health. 2017;15(1):2.

34. Jagsi R, Guancial EA, Worobey CC, Henault LE, Chang Y, Starr R, et al. The "gender gap" in authorship of academic medical literature – a 35-year perspective. N Engl J Med. 2006;355(3):281–7.

35. Jena AB, Olenski AR, Blumenthal DM. Sex differences in physician salary in US public medical schools. JAMA Intern Med. 2016;176(9):1294–304.

36. Bates C, Gordon L, Travis E, Chatterjee A, Chaudron L, Fivush B, et al. Striving for gender equity in academic medicine careers: a call to action. Acad Med. 2016;91(8):1050–2.

37. Dyrbye LN, Shanafelt TD, Balch CM, Satele D, Freischlag J. Physicians married or partnered to physicians: a comparative study in the American College of Surgeons. J Am Coll Surg. 2010;211(5):663–71.

38. Jolly S, Griffith KA, DeCastro R, Stewart A, Ubel P, Jagsi R. Gender differences in time spent on parenting and domestic responsibilities by high-achieving young physician-researchers. Ann Intern Med. 2014;160(5):344–53.

39. Ly DP, Jena AB. Sex differences in time spent on household activities and care of children among US physicians, 2003-2016. Mayo Clin Proc. 2018;93(10):1484–7.

40. Adesoye T, Mangurian C, Choo EK, Girgis C, Sabry-Elnaggar H, Linos E. Perceived discrimination experienced by physician mothers and desired workplace changes: a cross-sectional survey. JAMA Intern Med. 2017;177(7):1033–6.

41. Riska E. Towards gender balance: but will women physicians have an impact on medicine? Soc Sci Med. 2001;52(2):179–87.

42. Coe IR, Wiley R, Bekker LG. Organisational best practices towards gender equality in science and medicine. Lancet. 2019;393(10171):587–93.

43. McNamee S, MIller R. The meritocracy myth. 2nd ed. Landham: Rowman & Littlefield; 2009.

44. Thomas K, Mack D, Mantagliani A. The arguments against diveristy: are they valid? In: Stockdale MS, Crosby FJ, editors. The psychology and management of workplace diversity. Malden: Blackwell Publishing; 2004.

45. Harris C. Whiteness as property. Harv Law Rev. 1993;106(8):1707–91.

46. Markovitz D. How life became an endless, terrible competition. The Atlantic. Sept 2019.

47. Kang SK, Kaplan S. Working toward gender diversity and inclusion in medicine: myths and solutions. Lancet. 2019;393(10171):579–86.
48. Delgado A, Saletti-Cuesta L, Lopez-Fernandez LA, Toro-Cardenas S, Luna del Castillo J d D. Professional success and gender in family medicine: design of scales and examination of gender differences in subjective and objective success among family physicians. Eval Health Prof. 2016;39(1):87–99.
49. Maji S, Dixit S. Self-silencing and women's health: a review. Int J Soc Psychiatry. 2019;65(1):3–13.
50. Kay K, Shipman C. The confidence gap. The Atlantic. 2014. pp. 56–66.
51. Menendez A. The likeability trap. Harper Business: New York; 2019. 256 p.
52. Rodriguez JE, Campbell KM, Pololi LH. Addressing disparities in academic medicine: what of the minority tax? BMC Med Educ. 2015;15:6.
53. Fallin-Bennett K. Implicit bias against sexual minorities in medicine: cycles of professional influence and the role of the hidden curriculum. Acad Med. 2015;90(5):549–52.
54. Frankel LP. Nice girls still don't get the corner office. New York: Business Plus Books; 2014.
55. Zimmer L. Tokenism and women in the workplace: the limits of gender-neutral theory. Soc Probl. 1988;35(1):64.
56. Hu YY, Ellis RJ, Hewitt DB, Yang AD, Cheung EO, Moskowitz JT, et al. Discrimination, abuse, harassment, and burnout in surgical residency training. N Engl J Med. 2019;381(18):1741–52.
57. Dampier C, Lieff S, LeBeau P, Rhee S, McMurray M, Rogers Z, et al. Health-related quality of life in children with sickle cell disease: a report from the Comprehensive Sickle Cell Centers Clinical Trial Consortium. Pediatr Blood Cancer. 2010;55(3):485–94.
58. Tarbox K. Is #MeToo backlash hurting women's opportunities in finance? Harvard Business Review. 2018.
59. Brody DS, Miller SM, Lerman CE, Smith DG, Lazaro CG, Blum MJ. The relationship between patients' satisfaction with their physicians and perceptions about interventions they desired and received. Med Care. 1989;27(11):1027–35.
60. Martin A. Women benefit when they down play gender. In: Torres N, editor. Defend your research. Harvard Business Review; 2018.
61. Kanter R. Men and women of the corporation. New York: Basic Books; 1977.
62. Kanter R. A tale of "O" - on being different in an organization. New York: Harper Row; 1980.
63. Ibarra H, Carter N, Silva C. Why men still get more promotions than women. Harvard Business Review. 2010.
64. Johnson WB, Smith DG. How men can become better allies to women. Harvard Business Review. 2018.

65. Smith DC, Johnson B. Lots of men are gender-equality allies in private. Why not in public? Harvard Business Review. 2017.
66. Physicians Mom's Group (PMG) [Available from: https://www.facebook.com/groups/PhysicianMomsGroup/.
67. Bellock S. Research-based advise for women working in male-dominated fields. Harvard Business Review. 2019.
68. Zheng W, Kark R, Meister A. How women manage the gender norms of leadership. Harvard Business Review. 2018.
69. Ibarra H, Ely R, Kolb D. Educate everyone about second-generation gender bias. Harvard Business Review. 2013.
70. Wikipedia. Second-generation gender bias: Wikipedia; 2019. Available from: https://en.wikipedia.org/wiki/Second-generation_gender_bias.
71. Johnson SK, Hekman DR, Chan ET. If there's only ONe woman in your candidate pool, there's statistically no chance she'll be hired. Harvard Business Review. 2016.
72. Hall WJ, Chapman MV, Lee KM, Merino YM, Thomas TW, Payne BK, et al. Implicit racial/ethnic bias among health care professionals and its influence on health care outcomes: a systematic review. Am J Public Health. 2015;105(12):e60–76.
73. Gonzalez CM, Garba RJ, Liguori A, Marantz PR, McKee MD, Lypson ML. How to make or break implicit bias instruction: implications for curriculum development. Acad Med. 2018;93(11S Association of American Medical Colleges Learn Serve Lead: Proceedings of the 57th Annual Research in Medical Education Sessions):S74–81.
74. Johnson SK, Davis K. CEO's explain how they gender-balanced their boards. Harvard Business Review. 2017.
75. Bohnet I. How to take the bias out of interviews. Harvard Business Review. 2016.
76. Rivera L, Tilcsik A. One way to reduce gender bias in performance review. 2019.
77. Rotenstein L, Dudley JC. How to close the gender pay gap in U.S. medicine. Harvard Business Review. 2019.
78. Dermody SM, Litvack JR, Randall JA, Malekzadeh S, Maxwell JH. Compensation of otolaryngologists in the veterans health administration: is there a gender gap? Laryngoscope. 2019;129(1):113–8.
79. Maxwell JH, Randall JA, Dermody SM, Hussaini A, Rao H, Nathan AS, et al., editors. Pay transparency among surgeons in the veterans health administration: closing the gender gap. American College of Surgeons Clinical Congress. 25 Oct 2019. San Francisco.
80. Villablanca AC, Beckett L, Nettiksimmons J, Howell LP. Career flexibility and family-friendly policies: an NIH-funded study to enhance women's careers in biomedical sciences. J Womens Health (Larchmt). 2011;20(10):1485–96.
81. Shanafelt T, Goh J, Sinsky C. The business case for investing in physician well-being. JAMA Intern Med. 2017;177(12):1826–32.

82. Royce TJ, Davenport KT, Dahle JM. A burnout reduction and wellness strategy: personal financial health for the medical trainee and early career radiation oncologist. Pract Radiat Oncol. 2019;9(4):231–8.
83. J D. The White Coat Investor 2020. Available from: https://www.white-coatinvestor.com/.
84. Physician on FIRE (Financial Independence and Retire Early), 2020. Available from: https://www.physicianonfire.com/.
85. Koo B. Wealthy Mom MD. 2020.
86. Rohlfing J, Navarro R, Maniya OZ, Hughes BD, Rogalsky DK. Medical student debt and major life choices other than specialty. Med Educ Online. 2014;19:25603.
87. Pisaniello MS, Asahina AT, Bacchi S, Wagner M, Perry SW, Wong ML, et al. Effect of medical student debt on mental health, academic performance and specialty choice: a systematic review. BMJ Open. 2019;9(7):e029980.

Depression, Suicide, and Stigma

12

Pamela Frazier

Introduction

Serious and dedicated women practice the art of medicine using their hearts as well as their minds to do this work [1]. As a group, they have what might be called "gravitas" as in their practice of medicine they manage illness, adversity, despair, and defeat – including death – while maintaining hope and inspiration for their patients. These physicians often find themselves simultaneously bravely battling their own problems with mental health while trying to remain productive and effective in their clinical roles. Their symptoms may range from major depression with insomnia to stress arising from the role conflict experienced by many women physicians struggling to juggle the competing demands of work and home responsibilities. These are women with many strengths, which include their practical, proactive, and purpose-driven qualities. They live in a complicated world fraught with challenges related to demands placed on them as partners, mothers, daughters of aging dependent parents, or women living alone trying to manage work-life balance. Unfortunately, their concern about stigma often makes them reluctant to seek psychiatric help when they need it. Their personality strengths may cause them to go it

P. Frazier (✉)
Private Practice in Psychiatry and Psychotherapy, Scottsdale, AZ, USA

alone rather than to seek support and connection. In addition, they are profoundly affected by job-related problems and the inability to control their work schedules. Unfortunately, the literature to date is inadequate regarding women physicians and their unique difficulties. There is a great need for ongoing longitudinal studies of the risks of women physicians for mental illness. What is known about depression, suicidal ideation, suicide, and stigma regarding mental illness and its treatments for women physicians will be explored and illustrated in case vignettes.

Burnout: The Beginning of Mental Illness

Burnout has been described as a psychological syndrome characterized by exhaustion, reduced personal accomplishment, and the state of "depersonalization," or being disconnected from the self as one goes through the motions of living without feeling [2]. Later on, the description of burnout was refined to include cynicism as one of the cardinal signs of the syndrome [3, 4]. Self-reported physician burnout has grown from 40% in 2013 to 51% in 2017 with female physicians reporting a higher rate of burnout than men [5]. Burnout leaves its victims depleted with a negative, pessimistic, and misanthropic outlook on work and life which naturally leads to marginal productivity and diminished empathy which impacts success with both patients and staff. As a result, medical errors, compromised patient safety, and less optimal outcomes occur [5]. The symptoms of burnout constitute a danger signal. Often it can be difficult to differentiate the point where burnout stops and full-blown depression begins. Burnout appears to occupy space along a continuum between mental health at one pole and depression, substance abuse, and suicide at the other. In the center there exists healthy, resilient coping. However, the differentiating core feature of burnout appears to be stress at work. The concept of "job-induced depression" has been suggested as a more effective way to understand and intervene in this toxic syndrome [6, 7]. If it is recognized and treated early enough, progression to depression, substance abuse, and suicide should be preventable (Fig. 12.1).

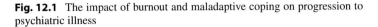

Mental Health   >   Stress   >   Burnout   >   Depression/SA/Suicide
Healthy coping   Adaptive coping Maladaptive coping   Psychiatric Illness and life risk

Fig. 12.1 The impact of burnout and maladaptive coping on progression to psychiatric illness

If left untreated, studies strongly suggest that burnout will lead to suicidal ideation and clinical depression in a subset of burnout sufferers. According to a 2006 to 2007 study of medical students, burnout is experienced by approximately 50% of medical students, 10% of whom experience suicidal ideation during medical school [8]. Since recovery from burnout is associated with a decline in suicidal ideation, there appears to be a strong correlation between burnout and suicidal ideation.

The practice of medicine involves making life and death decisions. This is a profession that is intense and demanding. Delay of gratification is necessary in order to achieve expertise over a lengthy education followed by internship and residency training. Because medicine is practiced at the battlefront of disease and death, doctors judge their own performance harshly and failure can have dire consequences. If the physician's personal limitations are added to the risks of practice, some stumbling blocks are inevitable for doctors as they navigate training, practice, and life.

Vignette 1: The prototype of a burned-out woman physician who later develops clinical depression

Dating back more than 20 years, I treated a 37-year-old depressed woman physician I'll call Dr. Rollins. She was my first physician patient with burnout. In addition to taking care of patients, she had an academic teaching role and administrative responsibilities. At our first appointment she complained that she needed to have her job "fixed," as if it were broken. Her job stress and the onus of responsibility she felt for her patients conflicted with her role at home as a wife and the mother of a 3-year-old daughter. When and how would she be ready to have another baby? During our initial consultation, she admitted she had been sneaking away from home on the weekends to catch up on progress notes for her practice. This was a secret she hid from her husband. Dr. Rollins was idealistic, caring, perfectionistic, and guilt-ridden. She believed patients and doctors had to have partnerships in order for healthcare to work. "Physicians must try to hear people in order to help people," she insisted. How her colleagues were seeing new patients for 30-minute evaluations while meeting with established patients for no more than 12-minute office visits confused her. She asked me, "How can they be doing all they should?" If something bad happened to a patient she blamed herself, soul searching while probing, "What could I have done better?" Honesty, integrity, and loyalty were all extremely important to her. When she began to experience intractable insomnia, she knew she had to get help. Her husband complained she was unavailable and preoccupied. There was more emotional distance between them than ever before in their 7 years together. It seemed like he was always angry at her. Because she felt unsupported at work, she was critical of office staff whom she did not trust to do enough for her patients. Only if she did everything herself could she be sure things would be done right. However, she was overwhelmed. Although she thought about suicide, she had never made a plan or attempted it. She would never abandon her daughter to be raised without a mother. Dr. Rollins felt there simply was not sufficient time to keep up with her own learning, teach residents, and see patients. Could she find a way to create time and space for herself, her work, and her family?

Dr. Rollins' treatment plan began with a leave of absence from work. No longer could she pretend to do it all alone. By the time she entered treatment, she was suffering from major depressive disorder with insomnia and was functioning poorly at both work and home. Treatments included SSRI antidepressant medication together with individual and marital therapy. Focusing on better resolution of the conflicts between work and family was essential [9, 10]. For the first time in their married life, she and her husband, working together constructively, decided to arrange for more help at home. The psychotherapy included work on improving her coping skills, reordering priorities, and decreasing her strong tendency toward self-criticism [11], perfectionism, and catastrophizing. Instilling a more realistic appraisal of herself and her capacities and limitations, as well as setting more attainable goals, was key to decreasing her stress. In the process, she made time for an abandoned hobby: playing tennis. When she returned to her practice after a 12-week medical leave, she was in remission from her depression, healthier, happier, and wiser.

Though not true for all, there exists a vulnerable subset of women physicians who are at risk for depression and other mental illnesses which, if untreated, may lead to serious symptoms and outcomes including suicide. Women physicians are growing in number and currently constitute over half of all medical school matriculants in the United States [12, 13] and one-third of the current physician workforce [14]. Many physicians who regard medicine as a satisfying career nonetheless report that it is stressful. As we look at women's burnout risks, we cannot ignore that women physicians react to and tolerate stress differently than do men. Also, women may have a higher subjective sense of medical practice as stressful compared to men [15]. Despite the fact that some women accept less than full-time pay and hours as they aim for a "lighter" professional workload, they actually spend more time connecting and communicating with patients, adding extra time to their days in the clinic, and sometimes putting them behind schedule [16]. Their responsibility and commitment to patients and to excellence propels them to extend themselves. Studies have revealed positive patient outcomes including lower mortality of patients treated by women physicians. This may reflect the greater time spent communicating and empathizing with their patients [17, 18]. Although all the reasons why women have a higher subjective sense of medical practice as stressful have not been elucidated, there is likely greater overall pressure on women, who usually have more stress outside the workplace, i.e., at home, than men do [15]. Women continue to bear more responsibility for the care of children than men. In fact, if the number of hours of unpaid labor at home is added to paid and unpaid hours at their jobs practicing medicine, the total number of hours per week worked by women physicians is far greater than those of their male physician counterparts [19].

On Self-Awareness and Acknowledgement of Mental Illness Among Physicians

Physicians are healers. They heal others while often ignoring their own needs and the reality that they are human beings with fallibilities and vulnerabilities. The practice of medicine demands courage and strength as doctors preside over serious and sometimes critical matters that involve life and death. The work evokes feelings and reactions which extract an emotional toll on the doctor. However, the profession of medicine, which until the past few decades has been predominantly male, has been critical of weakness in physicians, especially if they have psychiatric problems. Historically, substance abuse disorders have been more acceptable problems and better tolerated by the medical profession than mental illness. In addition, medical doctors have protected themselves and each other rather than confronted one another about signs and symptoms of mental illness and substance abuse. The stigma associated with mental illness has caused doctors to fear loss of respect in the medical community, trouble with state medical boards, and threats to their livelihood and income. There are multiple reasons why this culture has evolved [15, 20].

Fortunately, with the recent advent of more openness about psychiatric diagnoses, the medical profession has begun to witness a decline in stigma. Physicians' open acknowledgements of mental illness and its treatment appear to lead to greater public acceptance of the benefits of treatment. There is hope and optimism in the disclosures of doctors who have confronted mental illness. If established physicians get treatment, which allows for long, successful lives and careers in medicine, perhaps others will not fear diagnosis and treatment [20].

Vignette 2: About her own illness by Judith C. Engelman, MD

The following vignette was recently shared to a group of medical students by Dr. Engelman.

"I come from a family with bipolar disorder. My mother developed mood swings when I was ten or eleven. They got worse through my adolescence culminating in psychotic manic episodes and heartbreaking atypical depression by the time I was nineteen.

Because my mother refused psychiatric treatment, my physician father tried to treat her himself with antidepressants and tranquilizers to no avail. My mother committed suicide on August 8, 1971.

Mother's younger brother Marve was a grandiose, sociopathic, larger-than-life figure for as long as I can remember. He was married four times, constantly "borrowed" money from his parents which he never paid back. He was in debt to the mob and the IRS and around 1979, he too killed himself by taking an overdose.

My older brother Joel was very handsome and popular. Married with two wonderful daughters, at around age thirty-two, Joel became increasingly psychotic and found "special messages" he perceived were just for him from all kinds of sources. In 1980 he made four serious suicide attempts. Compassionately, my brother Mark moved Joel from Chicago to Arizona, where it fell to us to look after him for the next 28 years. Joel died at age 65 of a stroke as a complication of the type I diabetes he had developed from first generation antipsychotic medications.

Though as a child I was more outgoing, funny and engaging than many of my friends, my first real depression occurred when I was 19. I had been forced to transfer to Ohio State from Northwestern because of finances. I became depressed and paranoid, gained about 20 pounds and slept excessively. After a few months, the depression remitted without treatment. I married in 1970 at age 22 and once again became depressed. This time I got a referral to a psychiatrist, walked into her office and said, "my mother is going to die this year from suicide or homicide and I want you to help me get ready." Sadly, 5 months later, my prediction came true.

I was unhappy in my marriage and unfulfilled in my job. Once I decided to become a doctor, I returned to school to take pre-med courses and my mood steadily improved. I was accepted into medical school and my husband and I divorced in 1974 after 4 years of marriage.

One year later, I fell off a ten-speed bicycle and was, transiently, a quadriplegic! It took me 3 years to regain most of my function but I was left with some neurologic deficits. The year after the accident, I had a major depression with suicidal ideation.

I dropped out of medical school and returned to my psychiatrist who started me on medication, including lithium, to prevent mood swings. She was right, of course, to be concerned that I might develop the disease my mother had, but I was devastated. After 5 months of treatment in 1976, I returned to medical school, found a psychiatrist who took me off the drugs stating that anyone would have become depressed after such a catastrophic accident.

I remained depression-free for a few years. However, inevitably, I became depressed again and again until I finally capitulated to staying on an antidepressant. Though I suspected I had a variant of bipolar disorder, I denied it for years and my prescribers colluded in that denial, not wanting to label me with that "stigma." After my brother Joel died in 2009 I found myself constantly irritable. I finally went to a colleague and asked that lamotrigine be added to my antidepressant. Despite years of ups and downs before lamotrigine, I have felt stable and depression-free ever since starting it. Around 15 years ago, a wonderful child psychiatrist friend of mine suggested that I probably had attention deficit hyperactivity disorder. After further evaluation, I was started on medicine which has really helped me organize my thoughts and finish projects without the stress from procrastination. In addition, it has helped me to be on time for commitments!

As a result of my parents' troubled relationship, I made poor choices in men until I met and married my husband Harry 23 years ago who is "the wind beneath my wings". I also struggled with heartbreaking infertility but now have a wonderful stepson and a loving "daughter by choice" who was 15 when she came into my life.

In 1991, I became a certified Yoga teacher which has helped me with balance, strength and staying centered. I began to meditate in 1976 and I have maintained a meditation practice ever since. In addition, I credit years of therapy, rigorous self-examination, spirituality, a terrific husband and brother, many wonderful family members and great friends for gifting me with such a rich life.

Medicine has been the one constant through all these traumas. My career has always provided me with extraordinary colleagues and friends, joy, intellectual stimulation and a gratifying sense of "tikkun olam" which is Hebrew "for healing the world." As a physician, my personal struggles have definitely rendered me more empathic and optimistic that we human beings can supervene traumas and challenges with enough determination and support. I have learned that "disorder" does not equate with "dysfunction." I have learned that hope is the single most important gift we can give our patients and that resilience is a muscle we can develop as opposed to something with which we must be born. I have learned that everyone has challenges and that feeling ashamed and stigmatized because of my personal challenges is a waste of time and energy.

Finally, I have learned that sharing my story and/or the wisdom I've gained as a result of the traumas with medical students, residents and colleagues provides a powerful example of hope and triumph over tragedy."

Multiple studies have reported that medical students have high rates of depression and anxiety [8, 21–23]. Estimates are that approximately 11% of medical students experience suicidal ideation [22]. Interestingly, after Dr. Engelman's presentation, about 10% of the students who attended expressed interest in psychiatric treatment (albeit without specified reasons).

On Women's Greater Risk of Depressive Illness

Women in the general population have a 20% risk of suffering a depression in their lifetime in comparison to approximately half that number of men [10]. According to a large survey of women doctors, 19.5% self-disclosed a history of depression [24], virtually the same percentage as the risk for women in the general population. However, when self-reporting psychiatric symptoms, women doctors have a tendency to underreport because of stigma [10, 24, 25]. There is additional data that suggests a much higher risk of depression in women physicians. Among the data, including multiple databases, as high as 39% [25] to 46% [24] of women physicians have a history of depression or meet criteria for a diagnosis of depression [25]. Are women doctors truly more vulnerable to depression than the general population? Why are women so much more vulnerable to depression than men? There are multiple factors that place women at higher risk for depression, including neurobiological sex differences and environmental stressors [26–28]. In fact, women physicians have more depressive illnesses than their male counterparts [24].

It is worrisome that depression is higher among physicians than the general population, because depression inevitably affects the quality of a physician's work with patients [9]. The suicide rate for physicians is one of the highest in any professional group, as much as twice that of members of the general public [29]. Even though doctors die at a lower rate from major medical illness, they die from suicide at one of the highest rates of any professionals [30]. The suicide rate for female physicians has been estimated to be as high as four times the national rate for women in the general population [31].

Not exclusive to medical doctors, research reveals that there are higher rates of depression in professional women compared to women in the general public [24, 25, 32]. Potentially reflecting how gender differences may impact stress and mortality rates, a Danish study showed a positive relationship between greater life expectancy, high achievement, and higher social class in men but, disturbingly, not in women, for whom the opposite was true. Danish women who attained higher educational level with increasing social class had lower life expectancy [32]. Reasons for this are most likely multifactorial. High-functioning women who have attained greater education and success at work likely have more stress and it is speculated that role conflict and harassment at work are important factors, too [24]. Additional gender-specific stressors that may influence the risk of depression in women physicians include lack of social support, greater household responsibilities, and gender discrimination and isolation, particularly in fields that are predominantly male [19, 33, 34]. Women in medicine face unique challenges that impact their risk of depression. Patient care exposes them to disturbing cases, death and dying, and threats of physical injury or violence, for example, which are potentially traumatic experiences [35]. Studies have revealed that the divergence from the general population risk of depression begins in medical school where depression is estimated at 27% of both men and women, which is three times that of age-matched norms [36].

The risks for depression in women physicians can be considered by exploring the contributions of biological, psychological, and social factors:

- Cyclic hormone biology
- Trauma
- Neuroticism
- Family history of mental illness
- Risks for lesbian doctors
- Social roles
- The imposter syndrome

Cyclic hormone biology together with periods of radical changes in hormone status including puberty, the premenstrual period, the postpartum period, and perimenopause confer biological risks of mood disorders [37]. Estrogen is known to be psychoactive and to exert a cognitive-enhancing effect in the brains of both women and men [37]. Estrogen also interacts synergistically with both thyroid hormone and serotonin in the brain by binding and enhancing neurotransmitter activity [37, 38]. In some women, the monthly decline in the level of estrogen to its nadir prior to menses is associated with symptoms of irritability, insomnia, and depression during the week before her period. If this cyclic condition is pronounced and interferes with functioning, it is diagnosed as premenstrual dysphoric disorder or PMDD. Although PMDD remits when menses begin, some women, for whom symptoms are sufficiently severe, require treatment with an SSRI. For some, once-monthly premenstrual dosing during the week prior to her cycle eases PMDD. Estrogen and serotonin influence one another in the brain. The female hormones appear to regulate and enhance the serotonin system and response to SSRI medications. Conversely, the serotonergic system and serotonergic medications affect estrogen synthesis and enhance cellular binding of estrogen in the brain [39, 40]. In a similar fashion, treating depressed women who have high-normal TSH levels using thyroid hormone augmentation can boost the efficacy of antidepressant medication

[38]. It can be difficult to achieve remission from MDD for women whose TSH level is elevated at the high-normal end of the range. All women in the perimenopause and menopause have low estrogen levels commensurate with normal aging. A subset of these women may benefit from estrogen augmentation together with an antidepressant regimen [41]. The risks and rewards need to be assessed on an individual-by-individual basis, in particular in those women with family histories of breast cancer.

Vulnerability to *trauma* is greater in females than males and is highest among female children and adolescents. It is estimated that one-third or more of women with histories of intimate relationships have suffered sexual abuse by their partners [42]. Some of these women become physicians. In fact, out of a healthy yearning to master their trauma, histories of childhood abuse may draw some women toward careers in medicine. Physicians with problematic childhoods tend to have poor marriages, drug and alcohol abuse, and psychiatric problems [43]. The allure of treating and healing others is empowering, especially to women who have been vulnerable and without much voice in their own pasts. However, conflicted and unsatisfactory relationships at home and at work are warning signs. Intimate partner violence (IPV) can represent the perpetuation of a pattern of abuse dating back to childhood [44]. Those women physicians who have histories of childhood sexual or emotional abuse and neglect are at significant risk of depression in adulthood [42, 45]. Moreover, if indicated by symptoms of depression, women with current or childhood exposure to violence and trauma are strongly advised to consider evaluation for diagnosis of PTSD and treatment with psychotherapy or psychotherapy plus antidepressant. Psychotherapy is significantly more likely to lead to remission of depression in patients with childhood trauma by addressing and confronting the issues [45]. Additionally, if these women are also physicians, they will benefit from understanding their own histories of abuse and grow to become healthier doctors, partners, and mothers. Their children will benefit, too. Affluent mothers, who are stressed by work demands and are less connected to their children, have children with higher rates of psychopathology and drug abuse [46]. In one study, physician mothers under stress responded to increased support, including facilitated colleague support groups, which fostered not only their own well-being but positive parenting of their children [47].

Intelligence is usually considered a positive, protective factor, likely related to success and high performance at work and in life. Even in severe mental illness such as schizophrenia, high IQ is associated with improved functioning, specifically, better global functioning and insight, compared to typical schizophrenia [48], perhaps due to improved ability to problem-solve and cope with life's problems, including mental illness. On the other hand, evidence reveals that high verbal IQ predicts the tendency for *neuroticism*, i.e., to mull over and focus on doubts and concerns. Therein lies the potential for higher intelligence to increase the risk for developing anxiety disorders [49]. For example, more advanced levels of ego development in mothers failed to protect them from distress in their roles as mothers. Instead, these women had more rather than fewer psychological difficulties around conflicts in their roles as mother. These mothers demonstrated stronger negative reactions to their own critical feelings about their mothering [50].

For all women who have a *family history of mental illness* including depression, anxiety disorders, bipolar disorder, substance use disorders, or suicide, burnout may be a particularly dangerous step on the path toward onset of a mental illness, which in physicians usually presents as depression or substance use disorders or both [51]. Family histories provide crucial information about a person's risk of depressive illness. The offspring of depressed parents are at higher risk for depression themselves, with additional risks for persistent morbidity including recurrent depression, poor outcomes, and mortality, well into their middle years [52]. A history of childhood sexual abuse and/or emotional abuse and neglect are associated with increased risk of depression, especially chronic depression, in adulthood [45].

Risks for lesbian doctors. Limited data exists regarding lesbian physicians. Lesbian women physicians deserve special consideration because of their elevated risk for depression or sexual abuse compared to their heterosexual women physician colleagues [53]. Lesbian physicians reported being equally or even more satisfied with their medical careers than heterosexual women [53–55]. According to two sources, between 2 and 3% of female physicians are lesbian. Some studies, but not all, suggest a higher level of alcohol abuse or dependence histories among lesbian physicians. However, with regard to current alcohol consumption practices, there was no difference between lesbian and heterosexual female physicians according to one large comparison study [53]. Acknowledgment of a positive family history of alcohol abuse or dependence was a more frequent finding among lesbian physicians. Significantly, alcohol abuse has been correlated with social discrimination or family marginalization among younger lesbians and gays [53].

According to a study of 4501 women physicians, lesbian physicians were more likely to report histories of depression or sexual abuse than heterosexual women doctors. Lesbian physicians were three times more likely than heterosexual physicians to report histories of sexual abuse, too. For example, in one study, sexual abuse histories had occurred in the lives of 15% of lesbian women physicians compared to only 4% of heterosexual women physicians [53]. In contrast, as high as 20% of females in the general adult population had histories of sexual abuse. It is postulated that these data reflect the tendency for all women physicians to be psychologically healthier than women in the general population. Although some researchers posit that a history of sexual abuse may predispose some women to become lesbian, it is plausible that men may be more likely to abuse girls or women who are not stereotypically heterosexual. Additionally, sexual abuse history has been associated with increased risk of depression in adulthood, a risk which is higher in lesbian physicians in comparison with heterosexual women [45, 53].

Lesbians are more likely to report workplace harassment due to their sexual orientation. Since harassment is often associated with professional dissatisfaction in addition to personal distress, it is crucial to identify workplace harassment, prevent it, and intervene appropriately to sanction the perpetrators. Prior victimization, low self-esteem, and poor social support have been associated with depression in lesbians as well as gay men in the general population [53].

More research is needed in order to better understand the risks for lesbian women physicians, lesbian women in the general population, and women of different races, whether born within or outside the United States, since most data to date is specific to US-born and Caucasian women only [53].

Social roles of girls and women include the care of children and family members as well as friends and colleagues. For women physicians who are also mothers, their combined caretaking roles add more responsibility and can create conflict. Because women often hate saying "no," they are at increased risk for taking on too many patients, projects, and obligations and increasing their risks of burnout and/or resentment of family demands [25]. Women work a greater total number of hours every day performing unpaid labor for their families. If their work at home plus work at the clinic are totaled, women physicians work much longer hours than their male physician counterparts [42].

Depression is more common among women doctors who were not partnered and were childless [24]. According to the findings of the Women Physicians' Health Study [24], women physicians who developed depressive illness were more likely than nondepressed women physicians to also have the following:

- More stress at home
- Worse physical or mental health
- Concurrent history of obesity or chronic fatigue
- Alcohol substance use
- A household gun
- A comorbid diagnosis of an eating disorder or another psychiatric disorder [24].

In addition, other key risk factors for women doctors include working too many hours and having career dissatisfaction, high job stress, and less control of their work schedules [24].

Among women physicians, those who reported depression or suicide attempts had a higher likelihood of personal histories of the following:

- Cigarette smoking, or alcohol or substance abuse
- Sexual abuse or current domestic violence

– More severe harassment at work
– Psychiatric disorders in their families of origin [24].

The imposter syndrome (IS) is more common in women than in men and is characterized by feelings of being a fraud who is unworthy of successes gained because the sufferer believes she is not truly intelligent [56]. In contrast to men, who attribute their successes to their own abilities, women are more prone to believe their successes are due to luck or the transient efforts they have managed to put forth [57]. Historically, it has been found that IS begins to develop in girls due to the family's expectations of her, whether they are high or low. The family expectations have tended to mirror societal expectations of girls in comparison to boys [57]. As women are increasingly accepted into advanced professional education programs and professions such as medicine, it might be anticipated that IS will be less of a problem to girls and women in the future, but that is currently unknown. When the syndrome is present, IS provides insight into the inner struggle of the woman in the performance of her professional role. The symptoms of IS include cynicism, depersonalization, and emotional exhaustion, thus overlapping with, as well as leading to, increased risk for burnout. In the early career years of the developing professional, the imposter syndrome may be part of the normal transition to a new professional identity. As an example, upon graduating from medical school, she is no longer a medical student; now she is a doctor. However, that feeling of inauthenticity, phoniness, or pretense ought to disappear as the women gains experience and incorporates her professional identity into her whole identity.

If the woman doctor chronically believes herself to be less intelligent and less competent than other physicians, IS is likely to become a pathological state. Interestingly, as they progressed through their clinical years, male medical students were observed to grow in self-esteem but that was not true of the female medical students [51]. Male doctors have been observed to be more vulnerable than women doctors to insults or injuries to their sense of self-worth or narcissism [51]. Yet it has been observed that both patients and hospital staff react to male doctors with more respect and fewer challenges to their authority than is true for female doctors [51]. This respect that men receive from others buffers them from their insecure feelings of self-worth. Alarmingly, the same results have been borne out in a recent pilot project for evaluating emergency medicine (EM) residents. These results are discussed in a lively podcast interview with Dr. Jeannette Wolfe [58]. The results revealed that both male and female EM residents got similarly high grades at the end of PG year I, but by the end of PG year III, the male doctors had much higher evaluations in addition to stronger encouragement from evaluators [59, 60]. One would anticipate that IS would be worse if gender bias, communicated by less confidence in women's abilities and less respect for women as doctors, was routinely signaled to the female doctors. We might expect that a sense of inferiority would increase, despite greater experience, due to negative reactions toward women as doctors. In some specialties, like EM, quick decision-making and authoritative taking-charge are more important than thoughtful, deliberate interactions with patients over longer periods of time, such as the specialty of psychiatry requires.

To date, there is little or no research that compares women to men in medicine with respect to acceptance of criticism, their coachability, and reactivity or defensiveness. For both women and men physicians in training, feedback is more difficult to accept if it is derisive. Moreover, if feedback is excessively negative, it cannot be constructive and subsequently would not be expected to lead to desired growth and change in the physician in training. In addition, women have been socialized to be "communal" and cooperative at the expense of the more "masculine" attribute of "agentic." Consequently, women are trained to be less "aggressive" or decisive and can be penalized when they are, whereas the opposite is true for men [61]. Such experiences undermine women's feeling of mastery and self-esteem. Just as in burnout, individual strategies to cope and adapt are helpful, but understanding the organizational and cultural factors contributing to the higher incidence of IS among women physicians is critical to addressing the problem [62]. Group therapy has been found helpful to women with IS, and the experience of admitting their secret fear of being a fraud to other women who share the same fear has been found to be therapeutic in overcoming the syndrome [57].

Vignette 3: A depressed woman physician presenting with somatic features, an eating disorder, and anxiety with additional risk factors of a history of childhood psychological abuse, adolescent trauma with resulting PTSD, and being unpartnered

Presentation: Dr. Renata Renzi is a 46-year-old divorced woman cardiologist who presented with gastrointestinal complaints, insomnia, and anxiety. Her work in academic and clinical practice was stressful and she was deeply unhappy that she was still single, years after an early marriage and divorce in her 20s. However, she was consumed with her work, so she thought there was neither time nor energy for dating. Her problems with insomnia and early morning awakening began over the previous summer when she was diagnosed with irritable bowel disorder (IBS). In addition, she had lost ten pounds over that year, which led her to become obsessive about her food choices. Despite developing physical symptoms, she made it clear that she enjoyed her work and had close friendships that were important and rewarding to her.

Dr. Renzi was raised in Detroit, the second of three children, and only daughter in a Catholic family. Her father worked for a mortgage company and her mother had been a nurse until the couple started their family. Dr. Renzi's earliest memory was at 3 years old, the year her younger brother was born and her father had his first heart attack. The memory was a frightening one. She vividly recalled the emotional drama of the paramedics taking her father away. During her upbringing, her father was the dominant figure at home, a strict disciplinarian who expected nothing but academic excellence from all his children. Renata was the best student but rebellious during her adolescence. She was fearful of her father who yelled and was verbally abusive to all the children, often threatening to abandon the family. Her mother stayed out of the way while the father raged. Although her mother was referred to as "the calm and gentle one" of the family, as Renata told her story, it became clear that her mother had a tendency to distance herself emotionally from her children and her husband, thus emotionally abandoning her children. From her mother's example, Renata learned to distance herself emotionally, also. Many years later, she discovered that her mother had struggled with depression. When Renata got pregnant in her junior year of high school, her mother failed to notice that her oldest daughter was in crisis. Renata did not dare to confide in her parents and get their help. Instead, she found a way to get an abortion. From the symptoms she described following the abortion, it is likely she had an undiagnosed and untreated PTSD. She suffered insomnia, weight loss, and anxiety symptoms for 6 months after the abortion.

In young adulthood, Renata became the highest-achieving person in her family when she was accepted into medical school and fulfilled her dream to become a physician. Several years later, when she was in her residency, tragedy struck. Her youngest brother drowned in a boating accident, and with this sudden traumatic loss, Dr. Renzi's insomnia and anxiety returned. This time she entered psychotherapy and was treated with an SSRI. After she recovered fully, she abruptly decided to marry her college sweetheart. Initially it was happy, but her husband became verbally abusive toward her and she soon discovered he was unfaithful, too. Following completion of her residency, she divorced him. Claiming to have few regrets, she focused on embracing the future. By her late 30s, she had established a successful practice and was thriving. However, as she approached age 40, she was ambivalent about having a baby, having no desire to raise a child alone. She didn't acknowledge the loss of that opportunity. She just looked forward.

At our first meeting, Dr. Renzi was polite and cooperative but intensely private to the point of guardedness. She was careful in her use of words. Her mood was moderately depressed. Her face was expressionless with affect that was constricted and almost flat. What was most remarkable was her exclusive focus on her gastrointestinal symptoms. She stayed away from emotional material. Underneath her veneer of control, there was significant hurt. The history of her secret abortion in adolescence was central to understanding her core emotional issues. Out of "necessity," the accidental pregnancy was handled without the support of her parents. She voiced strong fears that her father, in his fury, would *have abandoned her. Dr. Renzi was diagnosed with major depression with somatic features and generalized anxiety disorder. The possible diagnosis of obsessive-compulsive personality disorder was considered due to her personality style and preoccupation with her health and diet. She had never abused substances.*

Dr. Renzi's preoccupation with medical and physical symptoms was an initial stumbling block to her psychotherapy. Owning her feelings and discussing emotions were hard for her. Because of her family history, she needed emotional distance in order to feel safe. Medication was the key first step in helping her get better. Her insomnia responded to low-dose trazodone at 25 mg at bedtime plus prn lorazepam, which she needed for only a few weeks. As soon as an SSRI began to exert its antianxiety and antidepressant effects, her depression lifted and the anxiety lessened. Only then, did her fixation on physical symptoms cease. She started to make significant progress with processing her emotional pain and grief. As her appetite returned and she ate less restrictively, she gained back some weight. Over time, she was able to express emotions including sadness about being alone and having no children. She also had lingering anger toward her father. There continued to be significant benefit for her gastrointestinal, mood, and anxiety symptoms from the antidepressant medication. She clearly felt supported in the trust and safety of psychotherapy. In addition, in psychotherapy she had a place to share her secrets, so she did not have to bear them alone. During the period of remission, she began to feel ready to start dating again.

Personality Characteristics of Women Physicians

Physicians have certain personality characteristics which are desirable and highly selected for by medical schools and the profession of medicine [32]. Moreover, these same characteristics may put physicians at higher risk for developing depression. The characteristics include the following:

- Perfectionism and compulsiveness
- A need for control and mastery
- An exaggerated desire for achievement

- A need to please
- A reluctance to say "no"
- Difficulty asking for help
- Self-sufficiency and reliability
- An excessive, distorted sense of responsibility for others and for circumstances beyond their control.

Obsessiveness and compulsiveness as personality traits can be adaptive, for example, as in the case of the doctor who worries about her patients and consequently commits fewer errors in their treatment. However, when exaggerated, these traits are maladaptive and can constitute an illness. The diagnosis of obsessive-compulsive personality disorder (OCPD) is made when there is a marked degree of either or both tendencies accompanied by clinically significant distress or impairment of functioning [63]. In turn, those feelings may lead to depression or anxiety symptoms. With high levels of perfectionism, there is often a tendency to feel guilty for failing to attain one's ideals. In addition, there is inevitable self-doubt in individuals who are always striving for perfection, which exacerbates both obsessiveness and compulsivity.

The need for mastery carries over to their personal lives, too. When the physician mother attempts to balance family and career, the person who comes last is usually herself. Women physicians tend to suppress and ignore their own feelings and may have difficulty making time for themselves [64]. Failure to prioritize self-care is frequent in women doctors. An example is the woman physician patient who confided to her psychotherapist: "I haven't had a drink of water or gone to the bathroom all day!"

Setting their own needs aside and denying themselves self-care must become a priority to avoid the inevitable consequences of burnout and depression. There is often a belief that they should not be vulnerable themselves. They should be able to do it all. Practical solutions, such as hiring a nanny to take care of the kids or asking their partners to start dinner, are essential for these physician mothers. If they can lighten their loads, these women feel less stressed and helpless so they can be better doctors, wives, and attentive mothers to their children.

In addition to their altruism and evolved moral compass, women physicians are often intellectually smart, inventive, and action-oriented, which in combination may cause them vulnerability to developing existential depression. If the life's work of these idealistic women gets derailed from a core sense of purpose – whether that is caring for patients or doing research – these doctors may soul-search and question themselves, "Why did I go to medical school?"

The following two measures of personality have been found to be common among physicians:

(a) Need for approval (also referred to as dependency)
(b) Self-critical perfectionism.

Both of these traits are associated with dysfunctional beliefs and, in turn, developing depression. In research conducted in Norway, physicians' "need for approval" and "perfectionism" were assessed via a survey and use of a scale called the Dysfunctional Attitudes Scale (DAS). Interestingly, men doctors more frequently fell into the perfectionistic/self-critical type, whereas female doctors were most often in the dependency/need for approval type [51]. Significantly, the presence of high levels of self-criticism as students was associated with depressive illness at 2 and 10 years later, especially in male doctors. Self-criticism is pernicious if not harnessed because it affects the regulation of self-esteem, also referred to as narcissism. In male medical students and interns, vulnerability to their concept of self predicted the development of problem drinking. In other words, they drank more alcohol because they felt bad about themselves [51]. In turn, the doctors with less harsh self-assessment ultimately developed fewer depressive illnesses. Doctors do bear a heavy burden in caring for others. Yet, since they are human, doctors can and do make errors. If self-esteem and sense of self-worth are only as strong as everyday success and validation, self-confidence is likely to be more fragile. This fragility and development of feelings of worthlessness may lead to vulnerability for both depression and suicide.

In the other group, predominantly women doctors with high needs for approval, disturbances in interpersonal relationships were associated with depressive symptoms. For example, a break-up with a boyfriend might be the trigger for depression. It has been postulated that medicine, because it is a helping profession, likely attracts students with higher dependency needs [51]. The high level of interpersonal connection with patients in medical practice may satisfy the doctors' needs for approval. In addition, there are inherent rewards in having satisfying relationships with patients. For some individuals with self-esteem issues, pursuit of an advanced degree, such as an MD, may be partially motivated by the wish to prove to one's self and the world that, ultimately, they are worthy of respect and admiration. Additionally, identity as a physician appears to be central to the self-worth of many physicians. For women physicians, the gender bias problem is problematic since women doctors do not enjoy as much respect from patients and colleagues as men do, especially within certain disciplines [19].

The Effects of a Toxic Workplace

The work environment has become a focus of concern for practitioners of medicine, in particular regarding women physicians. Work stress associated with the profession of medicine has consequences for the quality of healthcare in addition to the impact on the well-being of physicians and their ability to do their work [27]. Very significantly, a physician who commits suicide is more likely to have had a job-related problem than any other problem including the death of a loved one or a non-work-related crisis [21].

In the past, many doctors practiced medicine in the setting of a solo private practice. Increasingly, today's doctors work in salaried practice within medical practice groups or institutions, in particular women doctors [27]. Consequently, there is more regimentation of procedures and there is greater emphasis on administrative duties. In particular, the requirements of documenting medical treatment have grown and become dependent on the electronic medical record (EMR) [3]. Insurance companies together with hierarchical medical care institutions are setting the standards of both care and documentation which leads to conflict about how best to utilize limited time.

Four job-related stressors have been found to predict high levels of job dissatisfaction:

- Demands of the job and patients' expectations
- Interference with family life
- Constant interruptions at work and at home
- Lack of mental well-being about work [65].

The stress of working long hours is associated with higher rates of sleep disorders to which female physicians are more vulnerable than male physicians [66]. In addition, suicidal thinking is increased in physicians who are working long hours or are enduring degrading experiences or harassment [67]. Among female physicians, recent suicidal thoughts, and thinking about the methods by which to commit suicide, were found to be predictive of suicide risk [68]. This study's finding is in keeping with other research on suicidal ideation which has found a sensitive connection between suicidal ideation and the risk of committing suicide. Since physicians are more likely to underreport than overreport suicidal ideation because of fears of stigma, these findings may underrepresent actual suicidal thinking among doctors. In contrast, for both women and men physicians, high job satisfaction was associated with fewer work stressors and, consequently, more positive attitudes toward medical practice and the delivery of healthcare [27]. For women physicians, adequate time for their families and their personal lives was an important predictor of overall satisfaction with their work. Both men and women reported that time pressures in their practice were a source of considerable stress. That includes not only the total number of hours they worked, but, in addition, the time needed to take call, to keep up with professional knowledge [27], and to make time for their families. For women, having enough time with both patients and colleagues was an additional predictor of job satisfaction [27].

There are key protective factors which predict job satisfaction in women doctors:

- a manageable-sized workload, the ability to flexibly control the work schedule, and
- access to social support, specifically, participation in meetings to discuss stressful situations at work [68]

It is crucial that the sources of social support be confidential and nonjudgmental. The subjective perception of workplace stress is important. As an illustration, in a study of Italian doctors, *control of their work schedule* was more important to job satisfaction than the actual number of hours worked. Significantly, Italian physicians who were able to set their own work hours, influence the amount of work assigned to them, and confidentially discuss work-related problems had a lower risk of suicidal thinking. Even with higher work demands, long work hours, and less vacation, doctors fared better if they had more control over scheduling their work hours and the amount of work they were responsible for completing [67]. Consequently, it appears that it is the inability to control the work schedule that jeopardizes the mental health of practitioners. Women physicians who work their preferred number of hours are able to achieve the best balance of work and personal goals. For married women physicians in dual-career marriages, working their desired number of hours, whether they were full time or part time, was the most important factor in achieving positive outcomes. These women who worked their ideal number of hours had better job role quality, better marital role quality, lower burnout, and higher life satisfaction [69].

There is a useful model and formula available, the demand-control-support (DCS) model, which measures stress on individual physicians [67]. It provides a useful way to assess stress levels using the following factors that affect a physician's workload:

- Demand for work
- Control of the workload and schedule
- Social support in the workplace

Analysis of the DCS model results highlights that conflicting responsibilities and demands in the workplace are associated with feelings of less control, higher psychological demands, and job strain. It is job strain that confers a significant risk for the development of mental illness [67].

There may, however, be sex differences in the impact of any given type of social support. In a study of opposite sex twin pairs, men and women showed different responses to social support [70]. Among women, higher levels of support were strongly related to decreased risk for major depressive disorder (MDD), whereas that relationship was modest and nonsignificant for the men. It was a consistent finding that interpersonal relationships are more central to women and valued more highly by women than is true for men. It has been postulated that the explanation for these differences could be related to how female children are reared. Alternatively, it could be a sex-specific evolutionary adaptation. Females appear to both need and provide more social support than do males. This fact holds true with other mammals, too. In experiments with rats, the neurobiological and behavioral effects of shocking the feet of female rats were attenuated by social housing. If the female rats had companions in the cage with them during the shock trauma, the rats fared better. This benefit did not extend to the male rats who dealt no better with the trauma of shock when alone in their cage or in the company of fellow rats [20].

Just as social support can decrease the risk of depression in women, harassment can increase its risk. Studies of female physicians at work reveal a striking finding associated with harassment. Consistently, recent degrading experiences in the workplace were associated with suicidal thoughts [68]. This finding was not exclusive to doctors. Notably, bullying and harassment, also called mobbing, are associated with increased risk of suicide in the general population at work, too [67].

The existence of gender bias in some medical specialties and some departments represents yet another layer of stress for women doctors in certain fields, especially male-dominated fields like surgery and emergency department medicine [33, 58]. A woman physician's risk of developing depression becomes greatly elevated if there is a perfect storm of genetic risk, an abusive family history, current abuse, certain personality characteristics, and current workplace stress and harassment.

There is clearly a need for more research in this area and there are many interventions which can change the course of events to steer women to better outcomes. In the treatment section of this chapter, interventions that can interrupt unhealthy outcomes and lead women doctors to better support and treatment will be explored.

Suicide and Understanding Suicide Risk for Women Doctors

Women in the general population attempt suicide two to three times more frequently than men. In contrast, women physicians make fewer attempts on their lives but succeed at killing themselves more often than other women [24]. This is true despite the fact that women physicians suffer depression at a 20% lifetime prevalence which is the same as other women. Why do women physicians have more success at committing suicide than other women? Simply, they have medical knowledge as well as access to lethal medications. Moreover, although chilling to contemplate, women doctors may have less ambivalence about killing themselves when they put their suicidal plans in motion. Ambivalence is that grain of doubt about ending it all that can, and does, save lives. It is psychiatric distress that can shatter hope. With or without a diagnosis of depression, psychological distress is shared by suicide victims [21].

Women physicians are much less likely to be in treatment for mental illness for reasons including failure of insight into their own illness or because they fear stigma. These are women who also possess a strong wish to overcome mental illness on their own [25]. Depending on licensure renewal requirements, which vary by state or country, the diagnosis of a mental illness could be potentially damaging to medical licensing [15, 64, 71]. In addition, physicians believe they should be able to avoid getting depressed. They should be strong enough and self-sufficient enough to manage independently [64]. Current depressed mood, defined as 2 weeks prior to death, is a risk factor for suicide even in the absence of a known depressive disorder. Toxicology data reveals that physicians who die from suicide show very low rates of treatment with antidepressants [21]. These results are strong evidence that physicians with depression go untreated [25]. Instead of getting appropriate treatment, as high as 20% of depressed women physicians admitted they had self-prescribed antidepressant medication which may be an underestimate. In addition, they may have a colleague prescribe to them [21] or have ready access to drugs at hospitals or clinics [25].

Depression increases professional stress at the same time as it decreases job satisfaction among physicians [72]. The converse is also true. Problems at work contribute to anxiety, depression, and suicidal ideation in physicians. Therefore, it follows that the combination of problems at work and depressed mood plays a central role in physician suicides [21]. Because the physician identity is so important to a doctor's core sense of self and self-esteem, disruption at work is very threatening and leads to distress. Suicide by poisoning is the most frequent means of suicide for women doctors, but self-inflicted gunshot wound is the most frequent cause of suicide among all physicians, as it is the preferred means of male physicians who outnumber women in completed number of suicides. Although the data from the National Violent Death Reporting System is the most comprehensive reporting on physician suicides to date, the number of women doctor victims was small, with only 15% of the total of 203 physician suicides recorded [21].

Depression alone does not adequately explain suicidal ideation and intent. Even among suicidal subjects from the general population of individuals who have neither history nor diagnosis of depression, psychological pain was most highly associated with both current and lifetime suicidal ideation and attempts [73]. Studies suggest that widening the risk factors to include a triad of factors provides better predictability of suicide risk: (1) psychological pain, (2) depression, and (3) hopelessness. Using three factors more accurately predicts suicide risk than using only two measures, for example, depression and hopelessness [73].

Interpreting Suicide Data

The suicide data available is shocking, but it is also confounding. Some research studies reveal that suicides of men and women physicians are two times that of the general population with a similar risk to both men and women physicians [74]. Other studies report alarmingly higher rates of suicide among women physicians. Among the findings is that women physicians commit suicide up to twice as often as men doctors [52] but as much as four times the rate of women in the general population [75]. Since deaths by suicide occur at younger ages than are usual for female life expectancy, the calculation of life expectancy of women doctors is affected [76]. Yet studies of both women and men doctors reveal they are healthier, take better care of their health, and die of medical diseases at a lower rate than is true of the general population [32, 77]. Since women are known to outlive men, it would be a glaring anomaly if the overall life expectancy of women physicians was 10 years shorter than that of men doctors. Yet some research makes claims that this is so [76]. In actuality, the death rate of women doctors is low except due to premature death from suicide. Suicide death data is usually captured in studies with small sample sizes of women compared to large pools of men doctors. Comparing small numbers of women to large numbers of men likely overestimates the suicide rate of women doctors [78]. Nor are the raw numbers necessarily age-corrected. The question is how to interpret these findings. Mistakes with data collection and interpretation are well known in epidemiology. *"Simple comparison of age at death is therefore not appropriate since the denominators for calculating the death rates of men and women are not the same."* Non-age-corrected rates of suicide are deceptive and may lead to faulty conclusions [19]. Larger studies are needed to help clarify whether women physicians' suicide rate is truly elevated compared to men physicians [78].

There is a big cost to our society and our health-care system as well as to families if women doctors are incurring increased risk of early death to suicide. Since more women doctors have entered medicine in the past several decades, the composition and the culture of medicine has been affected. How those women doctors are faring and how the general public of patients is adapting to more women physicians are important issues. It is likely that the practice of medicine has been positively affected by the women who have entered the field. In comparison to men doctors, women doctors appear to communicate and connect differently and/or better to their patients, not necessarily related to the amount of time spent with individual patients. This may reflect that patients feel more caring and empathy from female physicians but it is related to higher satisfaction with women doctors by patients [16, 18, 79]. Moreover, there is some evidence that patients treated by women physicians have better mortality and morbidity outcomes than patients of male physicians [17]. Women doctors are undoubtedly affected by their participation in the practice of medicine, often in positive ways since practice is highly rewarding to most women doctors. However, a particularly ominous result of practice may be that women doctors are highly stressed, which increases their risk of suffering from mental illness and suicide. There is variability of suicide risk according to practice specialties, too. Psychiatrists have the highest suicide rate and pediatricians have the lowest according to one study [71] and anesthesiologists have a relatively higher risk in some studies [77]. Being single increased the risk to five times that of a married or cohabiting colleague according to European and US suicide data [21, 74].

Since only Northern European and North American data were used in most studies, it is unknown whether the results can be generalized to more diverse ethnic, racial, and socioeconomic groups. Unfortunately, it is difficult to understand mortality data, because there are too few studies of rates and causes of death in women physicians. More epidemiological studies are needed to understand the severity of mental health problems and mortality by suicide of women physicians.

The Special Case of Preventing and Treating Suicide

In any patient experiencing suicidal thoughts, a consideration of psychiatric hospitalization is crucial in order to save the life of the patient. Combined treatment with psychotherapy and medication will likely be necessary. Antidepressant medication, mood stabilizers, antipsychotic medications, and ECT have all proved to be instrumental in saving lives and achieving remission while stabilizing suicidal symptoms. Accurately screening and identifying the individuals with high levels of psychological pain could be key to suicide prevention [80].

In the experience of many psychiatrists, suicidal ideation and its discussion in psychotherapy often offer an escape valve from the pain of living life. Talking about these feelings is freeing and can offer the person a way out of their psychological pain so they can tolerate living. "I don't have to live this life if I don't choose to," patients voice. It can be highly therapeutic to hear their doctor acknowledge that ultimate control of living or dying is under the patient's own control. As is true in any course of psychotherapy, the patient may need to reconceptualize how she thinks about living a life she wants while meeting life's obligations. Among the vulnerable population of doctors who aspire to be self-sufficient and who assess themselves with self-critical eyes and high standards, suicide offers a way out of psychological pain. Suicidal patients may harbor anger toward a spouse, a parent, or a therapist who will be punished by the patient's suicidal act. Does the patient feel unworthy or isolated, or have fantasies of martyrdom? A way to comprehend the act of suicide is to envision a final defeat when there is no escape or rescue possible. At that point there is only hopelessness [81, 82].

Suicide prevention using psychotherapy aims to attenuate harsh self-criticism, self-hatred, and disparagement and diminish suffering, restoring a sense of well-being. As mentioned above, these self-critical personality qualities are better addressed early in a medical career or during medical school in order to prevent depression later in life. Cognitive behavioral therapy (CBT) techniques are often helpful for these patients. Newer techniques which incorporate CBT, positive psychology, and mindfulness show promise [41].

Training programs are beginning to address talking about and responding to trainee suicide risk. An example is the online program described in Med Ed Portal [83]. Also, there are programs such as "QPR gatekeeper training" and "Mental Health First Aid" training that teach faculty, learners, and colleagues to recognize the signs and symptoms of depression or suicidal ideation in order to respond in ways that help affected individuals take steps to obtain appropriate treatment [84, 85].

Stigma

"I would never want to have a mental health diagnosis on my record," to quote from a survey of female physicians [86].

The definition of stigma is, "a mark of shame or discredit," according to Webster's Dictionary. Synonyms for stigma include smudge, stain, and taint, none of which most people want, especially doctors. Shame is a painful emotion which is suffered alone. Since shame leaves us feeling we are bad, trapped, and powerless, it is little mystery that people attempt to avoid it. It makes it difficult to own having an illness or a diagnosis, such as depression if it is accompanied by stigma. But what if she does have a mental health diagnosis? Does getting treatment for depression, seeing a psychiatrist, and taking psychoactive medications brand the doctor with stigma? We want doctors to take care of themselves and to get treatment so they can practice, take care of patients, and enjoy their personal lives, too. Therefore, it is imperative for the culture of medicine to address stigma in medical school and during training. Only if stigma is less will doctors fearlessly take the steps toward proper diagnosis and treatment of mental health disorders. In the following paragraphs, stigma and the noxious effects of shame are examined.

The Burden of Shame

"Like an unskilled doctor, fallen ill, you lose heart and cannot discover by which remedies to cure your own disease," the chorus in "Prometheus Bound" chants to the suffering god [87]. The earliest reference to "Physician, Heal Thyself" dates back to the sixth century BC in Classical Greek literature [87]. According to the myth, the god Prometheus saved humanity with his gift of fire

which he gave to mortal humans in defiance of the orders of Zeus, king of the gods. As punishment, Zeus chained Prometheus to a remote crag, where, like the physician who heals others but cannot heal herself, Prometheus, who had saved humanity, could not save himself.

Sadly, it is hypocritical for the doctor to ignore or neglect her own ailments. Multiple factors likely influence denial of illness or outright avoidance of one's own treatment, especially regarding mental health. These factors include the psychological defense of denial in addition to avoidance of shame and fear of censure.

Psychological Factors and Shame

Doctors have the training and consequently the power to treat and cure illness. In addition, it is deeply satisfying work to heal others. In general, most doctors prefer the role of healer to that of being the patient. Disease and illness are like enemies to be conquered or controlled, but disease and illness also represent the fallibility and weakness of the human body and mind which are more acceptable in our patients who are sick. Moreover, the doctor has superior status and power. Could aversion to illness in one's self be a component of the doctor's very attraction to the field of medicine? Phobic avoidance and intolerance for their own sickness may be operating in the psychology of some physicians [74]. The doctor must see herself as strong and powerful, not vulnerable and ill. Nor does she have time to be sick. Yet the first step toward recovery for the depressed physician must be an acknowledgement that she needs help. Also, she must accept that she cannot treat herself. It is crucial that she avoids getting antidepressant medication samples from a colleague. No hands-on treatment means there is no ownership of responsibility and no oversight of the treatment. Resistance to psychiatric treatment and denial of illness lead to inadequate and bad psychiatric treatment of physicians, a very real danger to the profession.

Avoidance of Shame

As little children learn right from wrong, they experience scolding for mistakes and praise for things well done. Either guilt or shame may follow the reprimands of one's parents. To distinguish between the two, shame is the feeling of humiliating disgrace which occurs after making a mistake. Shame leads to subsequent feelings of being flawed and unworthy of love and belonging [88]. Dr. Brené Brown argues that shame is destructive. On the other hand, guilt is adaptive. It develops when the child feels she deserves blame for mistakes or offenses because she has failed to uphold her own internalized values [88]. When guilt is assumed, there is no disgrace because responsibility for the error has been owned. The parents who scold their children to excess promote the shame response which leads to hiding mistakes rather than owning them. Consider what happens when a doctor makes a mistake of small or considerable consequence in the care of a patient. Let us say a resident wrote an order for the wrong dose of insulin in a hospitalized diabetic patient. The lab reports back a blood glucose either too low or elevated but, in this example, let us say the patient is not unduly harmed. This resident will need to own up to making this error while presenting on rounds where she will likely be questioned by her attending. Undoubtedly, she will be exposed. If she responds with a shame response, her reaction centers on feeling, "I am deficient." The healthier reaction of experiencing guilt allows her to own up to her mistake and move past it, while acknowledging to herself, "I can learn from this. I can do better next time." Dr. William Bynum's research regarding the shame experience among medical residents and medical students has drawn attention to the significant adverse physical and/or psychological effects that shame reactions cause in this population as they are learning to become a doctor [89, 90]. Shaming experiences, especially during transitional periods of medical training, contribute to harsh self-judgments and may play a role in the development of the imposter syndrome and an impaired sense of belonging [89]. Alarmingly, according to psychological research, suicidality has been associated with shaming experiences [89].

Most of us would much rather avoid shame than suffer it. Ultimately, being unworthy is what separates us from human connection. Without that, we are alone, isolated, and, as a consequence, alienated [88]. Dr. Brown's work extends to "shame resilience," which occurs when medical errors or mistakes in judgment are shared with colleagues. Shame resilience actually tames the shame response, making it less toxic and less likely to occur in the future. However, in order to open up and share, the individuals must make themselves vulnerable. Shame resilience theory can be used to help medical students reflect on their most challenging experiences. It requires recognition of shame and its triggers. Becoming aware, telling our stories, and speaking about errors lead to resilience [88–90].

Fear of Censure

What happens if the medical board learns that a physician has been receiving treatment for depression? Is the doctor required to admit treatment on her medical license renewal form? Will her license to practice be denied if she admits treatment? Different states have different standards. In recent years, these standards are evolving toward greater acceptance of treatment for mental illness in physicians and elimination of any questions about mental illness diagnosis and treatment on the medical license renewal form. Fear of losing one's license for having a mental illness often causes doctors to avoid getting diagnosed or treated [20]. It is imperative that a well-functioning, "fit for service" doctor who is undergoing treatment for depression be recognized as healthy, i.e., not pathological. As doctors increasingly share stories about their psychiatric treatment, stigma is decreasing. When treatment contributes to restoration of the physician's psychological health, it also prevents disability. The doctors who warrant the most concern are those who deny and hide their problems while avoiding treatment. Sticking one's head in the sand is not a solution.

On the other hand, if there is a medical board complaint for whatever reason, it can be very stressful. The following vignette is a vivid example of the stress that a medical board complaint or a malpractice suit brings into the life of the physician. The potential shame and stigma associated with being accused and questioned, in addition to threats to livelihood and income, are deeply problematic for physicians. After all, most doctors are individuals who are drawn to the profession of medicine by strong altruistic wishes to help others and make them well. Adverse events are troubling for both patient and doctor.

It is usual for doctors to strive to be good citizens who are worthy of the profession of medicine. In the case of malpractice suits or medical board complaints, when there is often the assumption of wrong-doing in the care of patient, doctors feel blamed even before any hearing takes place. Legal advice is usually necessary for guidance through the process of making a defense. Inevitably, standing up for oneself and avoiding shame become part of the doctor's objective. While these burdens are being dealt with, the physician continues to take care of obligations to her practice and patients. By the time the case has resolved, the doctor may be feeling jaded, cautious, and even paranoid toward her patients. "If a bad case can ruin my career," the doctor might posit, "am I at risk for another bad outcome?" She might wonder if she should continue working in her profession. Unless she can expect that her patients have as good intentions toward her as she has toward them, there can be no trust. Also, she wants to believe that her medical board is supportive of her as a physician. However, medical errors, poor outcomes, and complaints do occur. In turn, there may be emotional injury to the physician and the so-called "second victim" syndrome [3]. The medical culture is one in which errors are frowned upon and poorly tolerated because the stakes are so high in a field where lives are at risk. The culture is one of "no mistakes allowed" [3].

It is clear that when doctors are stressed, the best policy is for them is to reach out to colleagues and gain support and guidance. Yet shame causes people to hide, to keep secrets, and to go it alone which is the wrong tactic for the continued good health of the doctor, especially one who has to face a lawsuit or board complaint. It is likewise bad for the treatment of patients.

Vignette 4. Confronting shame and stigma: a case of a medical board complaint leading to distress, personal crisis, and burnout

Dr. Lindsey was a psychiatrist in private practice. She was in her late 30s and happily married with a teenage daughter. In addition, she looked out for her retired parents who lived nearby. She enjoyed the richness of her rewarding work at a busy psychiatry group practice with several close colleagues. She made time to attend evening professional programs and regularly met with her colleagues to discuss cases and share patient care. Many of her patients were physicians. Among them was a 36-year-old woman Internist, Dr. Scott, who had a mood disorder and ADHD and had been under the care of Dr. Lindsey for 2 years. She was compliant with the treatment plan and progressing well, meeting every 2 weeks for psychotherapy sessions which included medication management. On occasion, Dr. Scott requested that her fiancé accompany her to appointments. They were planning a wedding in the coming year and wanted to have a child together. When her fiancé suddenly broke off the engagement, Dr. Scott was distraught. She became anxious and developed insomnia. After imploring her fiancé to enter couples' therapy with her, he agreed. Dr. Lindsey referred them to a couple's therapist. Soon thereafter, Dr. Scott began to cancel or "no-show" for her appointments. Despite reminders from Dr. Lindsey's office, over an eight-week period Dr. Scott failed to come in for an appointment. Out of concern for her patient, Dr. Lindsey instructed her office to inform Dr. Scott that her stimulant ADHD medication, a controlled substance, could not be renewed without another appointment.

At that point, a drama began to unfold. In the middle of a busy afternoon during her office hours, Dr. Lindsey was interrupted by two officers from the DEA. They informed her that the DEA suspected Dr. Scott was forging prescriptions for controlled substances, including a stimulant. It was inconceivable to Dr. Lindsey that this was true! She trusted this patient who was a good physician and, she believed, a good person. The officers informed Dr. Lindsey that under no circumstances was she allowed to tell her patient about the DEA investigation. Naturally, this conflicted with her therapeutic alliance with her patient. What should she do and where could she turn for advice? She felt it was contrary to the principles of good patient care to hide this information from her patient. However, she was scared for herself. She called her malpractice insurer for advice about finding a lawyer to help navigate the issues. Also, she turned to several of her trusted colleagues. They did not know what advice to give her, but they did provide her with support. Within the next few days, the situation unraveled further. The patient's fiancé contacted Dr. Lindsey, revealing that Dr. Scott had made a suicide attempt with an overdose of alcohol and prescription medications. Would Dr. Lindsey meet her at the emergency department, her fiancé asked? Out of moral obligation she wanted to see her patient, despite her conflicted interests. In compliance with, but also out of fear of, the DEA officers Dr. Lindsey did not reveal the DEA officers' visit to her office. The patient was grateful to see her doctor and admitted to her that she had been in a state of confusion and regretted her suicide gesture. She did not want to die. That was the last time Dr. Lindsey saw her patient. Immediately, Dr. Scott was required to relinquish her license while she completed an inpatient program for impaired physicians. Within days of these events, Dr. Lindsey was notified by mail of a complaint registered with the medical board concerning her care in this case. When she inquired who had lodged the complaint, she was told that information could not be disclosed. The source of the complaint was held in confidence. This was shocking, but what she subsequently learned was devastating. Serendipitously, Dr. Lindsey was told, in confidence, that it was the patient herself who had made the complaint to the medical board. The patient whom she had helped through difficult times over a two-year treatment history had betrayed her. She struggled with an explanation for why her patient would want to wound her.

Dr. Lindsey worked with her lawyer to prepare a defense for herself at the medical board hearing. Her lawyer was knowledgeable and kind. First and foremost, he advised, they needed to gather expert opinions about state-of-the-art treatment of patients with ADHD and mood disorders. To the best of their ability, Dr. Lindsey and her lawyer demonstrated that the best treatment had been offered to this patient and that her patient had done well *until the point at which she stopped treatment. Through this frightening and difficult time over the next several months, she awaited her hearing. Although Dr. Lindsey was an optimistic, resilient woman, nothing she had been taught or experienced in medical school or her residency prepared her for this experience. Her strong conscience had always dictated that she perform to her best ability. In addition, she cared deeply for her patients. She knew herself as a person who needed approval, a personality characteristic which is typical of women physicians. However, this crisis caused her to feel deep disapproval of herself. In turn, these feelings led to existential questions about her career. She developed difficulties falling asleep at night. "What could and should she have done differently?," she asked herself. She recognized unwelcome emotions similar to those she had experienced in her early 20s with the sudden, traumatic death of her brother in a car accident. Similar to the emotions following her brother's death, she feared the threat of new losses: her reputation, her practice, her career, and her income. For the first time in her career, she felt negative about the practice of medicine and saw risks where she had never seen them before. Now she was forced to consider that her patients, the people she cared for and about, could become adversaries. Her husband, trusted colleagues, and a course of psychotherapy provided support and help as she worked through this crisis in her career. In addition, under advice from her lawyer, she learned more about defensive medicine and improving her documentation practices. If she had become more cynical about practice, she had also become less naive.*

The day of the hearing finally arrived. There, the medical board's accusers had a face. The panel was composed of all male physicians. She felt like she was being tried for the crime of being a bad doctor. To her great relief, the panel did conclude what she knew to be true: Dr. Lindsey had performed treatment of her patient up to the standards of care. She gradually moved forward with her life and returned to normalcy, once again enjoying her practice. Her sense of shame diminished over time. Although deeply affected by what had happened, she had a new awareness of risk. Eventually, Dr. Lindsey faced her sole regret about the case: she had failed to be open and genuine with her patient at the time of her patient's suicide attempt. That was a mistake Dr. Lindsey had to own and never repeat. She strongly suspected that the DEA officers who scared her into secrecy about the investigation had likewise scared Dr. Scott into a state of desperation. She would never know whether her patient had truly forged prescriptions, nor would she ever find out why Dr. Scott reported her to the medical board. Once the DEA was involved, Dr. Lindsey had to worry about herself first and put her patient last, a bad situation for both doctor and patient.

A medical board is composed of a panel of physicians. The hearings are outside the legal system, functioning like a private court which polices the medical profession in order to protect the public within each state. Historically, medical boards have taken harsh or even punitive stands against doctors while performing their duties. However, it is critically important for the medical profession to protect its physician members and ensure that medical boards are not only prudent, but judicious in their complex task of safeguarding the public while supporting doctors.

Prevention of Burnout and Depression and How to Build Resilience: Fostering the Practical, Proactive, and Purpose-Driven Qualities of Women Physicians

It is critical for medical schools and residency training programs to play a key role in the preparation of physicians for stable, lifelong practice [36, 91]. By decreasing unnecessary sources of competition and stress in medical school, such as moving to a pass/fail grading system [36, 92–94] and improving the learning environment with role models who provide mentorship in addition to supervision, resilience will be inspired and burnout averted [95]. Students and trainees are more likely to engage in self-care when the learning environment is supportive [96]. In turn, the care of patients will not become so burdensome if the doctor takes care of herself better and tends to her own needs. This is an ideal that should continue beyond medical school, promoting growth in addition to resilience in the physician's professional and personal life. Prevention is especially important as a cultural philosophy for the population of medical professionals who are the guardians of patients' health. Striving for good mental and physical health can become a natural part of the physician's role and provides a good example for patients.

Mentors can foster improved self-awareness in medical students and physicians in training by encouraging proactive self-care. As a group, physicians possess an exaggerated sense of responsibility and push themselves hard. When they have more to do, they may push still harder, sometimes at a high personal cost. Yet it is imperative that physicians do not defy their own needs. The poorly groomed physician is an example of failure to attend to herself. Patients notice. Likewise, physicians have an obligation to reach out to fellow physicians when changes in personality are witnessed, including abuse of alcohol or other substances and carelessness or disenchantment at work. These are among the warning signals that a colleague's mental health is in trouble. Reaching out to reassure a troubled colleague to seek help is important. We must all do it!

Physician well-being can be assessed and tracked anonymously in order to interrupt burnout and prevent depression and suicide [97]. From existing research, it is clear that relationships, religion/spirituality, self-care practices, work attitudes, and life philosophies are the five general strategies which have been used successfully by physicians to promote their own personal well-being [98]. A positive relationship has been found between employment of these strategies and achievement of well-being [99]. Meeting basic human needs and participating in their own self-care are essential to ensure that women physicians are secure, healthy, and high-functioning individuals. To summarize, those basic needs and wellness strategies include the following:

- Good nutrition.
- Restorative sleep of adequate duration, 7–9 hours each night with times of bedtime and rising fairly constant.
- Regular exercise of at least 150 minutes a week to improve physical fitness and cognitive functioning as well as to decrease stress and depression [100].

- Social and emotional support and sharing of feelings and responsibilities in positive relationships with family, friends, and colleagues. Intimate involvement with a spouse and family members effectively combats depersonalization [98].
- A sense of purpose in one's personal and professional life, which includes some measure of control over one's work schedule, setting limits as well as active participation in leadership at one's institution.
- Achievement of flow in one's work/life integration. For example, participating in hobbies or interests which involves the arts, sports, or research is associated with increased joy and satisfaction in life [101].
- Ensuring and planning for financial security.
- Finding spirituality and/or religion [101]. Self-awareness practices such as meditation, yoga, time spent outdoors in nature, and mindfulness exercises all promote conscious awareness, and wellness [99, 101, 102].
- Seeking out mentorship, support groups, or mental health services when difficulties occur including consulting with a psychiatrist when burnout, depression, or substance abuse become problems [21].

Organization-Focused Interventions to Prevent Burnout and Depression Are an Essential Part of the Solution

Although individual physicians can and must take steps to promote their own wellness and prevent burnout, it is not likely to be sufficient to prevent burnout and achieve a sustainable and productive career [5]. Organizations must also do their part to engage in a responsible process to create healthier work environments. Effective organizational strategies for change include having a supportive community, providing meaningful work, and creating an environment of fairness, choice, and control [5]. For overworked physicians, the temptation may be to opt out of serving on committees that can create change, but a study from the Mayo Clinic demonstrates that organizational changes are more sustainable if physicians are part of the leadership team involved in determining causes of burnout, implementing change, and monitoring outcomes [5]. Research on burnout and wellness is now moving toward exploring how individual-focused and organization-focused interventions may work synergistically to create a sustainable workforce of resilient and fulfilled physicians, who can provide their communities with the valuable healthcare they deserve [98].

Mentors and wellness officers within medical institutions are important sources of support for women doctors. Both kinds of relationships have the potential to enhance the resilience and career development of women doctors.

Mentorship relationships are increasingly seen as an essential part of the woman physician's support system and a source of role models. Lack of professional support has been pointed to as a major problem for women physicians [103]. There are fewer women in medicine to serve as mentors to younger and more junior women. Also, women experience more role conflict due to their multiple roles as mothers and wives as well as doctors [104]. Mentors provide the support of a more senior professional who can help with navigating career and balance of life questions, having already made their way through earlier-career times of confusion and distress about choices. Often women delay their career paths while having babies and raising children. The leadership examples provided by mature women mentors are especially important in academic medicine where there may be a "publish or perish" mentality and the reality of obstacles to attainment of senior leadership positions. Ultimately, building job satisfaction is key. As long as there is a fraction of a woman's time at work that fuels an interest or passion – whether in research, teaching residents, or the clinic – her overall job satisfaction improves substantially. In any profession there will be the routine "bread and butter" of a job which may be less interesting, but if the woman has control over her schedule and time in various job roles, she may be more content in her job, be able to direct a percentage of her time to meaningful work activities, and offer more to her institution. Although many women work equally well with either a male or female mentor in a traditional dyadic mentorship relationship, it is apparent that a supportive mentor-lead group model is advantageous for younger women mentees [103].

Chief wellness officers in large medical organizations have a clear-cut role to canvass, troubleshoot, and prevent distress in the doctors within their organizations [105]. It is important for women doctors to feel that their employer cares about them and their career progression and promotion in addition to the clinical work they do. Chief wellness officers must ensure that female talent is not lost to the organization. For example, what happens if the woman doctor's child is too sick for her day care center? Does the institution support her and help find her alternative care? Does the institution offer fair and creative solutions to competition for scarce opportunities or resources among medical staff? In addition, a recent study found that women document in the electronic medical record (EMR) during home hours more than men and have longer notes, likely another factor contributing to higher burnout in women [106]. Ways to save time for the doctors such as employing scribes for transcribing progress notes in the EMR or providing nursing or medical assistant staff to help triage and respond to inbox messages simultaneously improves the institution's medical care. By decreasing the administrative burden of physicians, there will be more time available for patient care. The role of the wellness officer must include solutions to systemic problems in the host institution such as morale and departmental infighting. A dissatisfied and distressed medical staff likely contributes to a toxic work environment. Having a dedicated wellness officer who proactively considers these problems, especially the problems facing women doctors, not only improves medical care, but it provides more opportunities for collegial collaboration and career satisfaction [101].

Treatments for Mental Illness

On the path between burnout and depression (Fig. 12.2), the physician must become a patient in order to get better.

Healthy MD	>	MD Under Duress	>	MD Should be a Patient	>	MD Must be a Patient
*good sleep & nutrition		*distracted		*cynicism; depersonalization		*worthless & hopeless
*exercise/meditation		*insomnia/fatigue		*mood disturbance		*impaired functioning
Active Self-Care	>	Stress Symptoms	>	Burnout	>	Major Depression

Fig. 12.2 A guide for evaluating symptoms of stress and mental illness: when to refer the doctor for treatment

In the process of caring for patients and getting involved in the problems of their lives, physicians are also simultaneously navigating their own problems. In order to do a good job, doctors need to be mentally and physically healthy. If personal problems become too big and unwieldy, doctors do not function optimally. Burnout emerges as the physician "comes undone," leading to cynicism, carelessness, and ineffectiveness at work. Since treating patients requires understanding their problems, caring for and about them requires compassion and mercy toward them. The philosopher Martha Nussbaum says it well in her description of how people become more human and merciful while they are reading fiction [86]. The concerned reader of a novel is drawn into the lives of the characters and, in the process, develops deep understanding. The reader puts on the skin of the characters and enters their minds in an attempt to understand them and their dilemmas. The reader gets involved personally. Likewise, for physicians, as we listen closely to the problems of our patients, we identify with them and come to appreciate the "complex narrative of human effort in a world full of obstacles" [86]. Dr. Abraham Verghese captured this idea when he wrote, *"I've never bought this idea of taking a therapeutic distance. If I see a student or house staff cry, I take great faith in that. That's a great person, they're going to be a great doctor."*

Women physicians are practical, proactive, and purpose-driven human beings. These three essential qualities empower women physicians to find solutions and solve problems. These qualities are necessary for taking care of others. For many physicians, medicine is a calling. But the path to becoming a doctor often takes every ounce of what the woman has. The resolve and commitment of women doctors are enormous. After graduating from medical school, she may be dismayed with the complexities of today's corporate medicine which she views as inhumane and, perhaps, misogynous. However, when the doctor cannot do the job she was trained for, the job she may have felt born to do, existential despair may emerge. Her idealistic expectations may be unrealistic but reality may be daunting. During the third decade of life, while a woman is going through medical school, she will likely be searching for a partner, committing to a relationship and considering starting a family. Medical school teaches her to prioritize. It is not hard to imagine why ignoring one's own needs becomes expedient. The physician pays attention to the care of her patients ahead of her own needs. She may put the needs of her partner or child ahead of her own, too, and consequently have inadequate support. Alternatively, it may be a challenge for some woman physicians to relinquish management of all the details of her home life to a husband, partner, or extended family. Will she allow someone else to prepare the meals, help bathe the kids, and fold the laundry? Yet, if she can have the home life she wants and needs for stability and predictability, it will not only help to prevent her from burning out, it will make her a better doctor [21]. How she solves these problems depends on the support system available to her, how much money she can pay for outside help, whether she can work fewer clinic or administrative hours, and whether she needs to publish. If her family or a babysitter provides the extra support at home that she needs, she will function better.

Since the emergence of unhealthy coping patterns is more likely during periods of duress, recognizing personal challenges and psychological conflicts early can limit problems before they get too big. In this case, self-awareness constitutes prevention. Whether the problems are caused by family of origin and so-called "dysfunctional family" issues or genetic vulnerability for an illness like depression or alcoholism, admitting the risk gives the physician more control and better solutions. Individual psychotherapy can be used like a tool to help the physician patient avoid pitfalls. Although not every doctor requires psychotherapy, if there has been a history of trauma, abuse, or mental illness in the doctor or her family of origin, psychotherapy can expand her self-awareness allowing her to deal with maladaptive coping patterns, such as tolerating abusive interpersonal relationships at work or at home. In addition, psychotherapy aids the doctor's overall personal growth and development. At the beginning of any psychological treatment, the complex issue of who is in charge – the psychotherapist or the patient – must be confronted and navigated by the psychotherapist. In order to be treated, the woman doctor must surrender some measure of control to the therapist. In turn, the therapist becomes "the doctor" and the doctor becomes "the patient." This can feel alien and uncomfortable in the beginning. However, as the woman doctor, as patient, experiences a supportive therapeutic alliance with her psychotherapist, she will deepen her mastery over her own struggles and, in the process, develop trust. Physician mothers face different psychological challenges than women physicians who have no children. If she is single and alone, the woman doctor may need to find and build a supportive group of friends and colleagues in order to avoid loneliness and isolation. For those women who desire children but find themselves without, there may be a need to address disappointment and the loss of that chance to be a mother. Infertility and miscarriages of pregnancies may force the woman to enter therapy and work on resolving their disappointments. Charting a path forward in life, some women physicians with no children find that the mothering role is fulfilled by working with patients or actively participating in the lives of stepchildren or nieces and nephews. In addition, mentoring younger women doctors is deeply satisfying of these needs. Because psychotherapy fosters growth and change, it is highly beneficial to those women who are struggling with their roles or challenges in life [21].

The Role of Psychiatry

If a woman doctor becomes mentally ill, a psychiatric consult is essential to determine what caused the illness and how to treat it using psychopharmacology and/or psychotherapy.

Psychotherapy and Psychopharmacologic Treatments

Psychotherapy can improve coping strengths and prevent burnout even before there are signs of mental illness. What type of psychotherapy is best for an individual depends on multiple factors including the diagnosis, severity of symptoms, and the personality and cognitive style of the patient. If the patient is in crisis, emergency intervention and hospitalization may be necessary to stabilize the crisis before treatment can begin in a setting away from home and family. For those with mild depression, evidence-based psychotherapies like cognitive behavioral therapy or CBT [75] (see below) are the treatment of choice, without medication, although medication plus CBT is another alternative way to begin treatment even for mild depression. However, exercise added to CBT has been shown to ease the symptoms of mild-to-moderate depression [107]. Moreover, according to a recent large study, physical activity may help ward off depression [100]. If symptoms are more marked, moderate to severe, using antidepressant medication may be necessary before the patient is able to do psychotherapy work [107]. Together, antidepressant medication with psychotherapy has a high likelihood of improving patients' psychosocial functioning while decreasing their symptoms of depressed mood and additional symptoms such as irritability, anxiety, and insomnia. Although the level of experience of the psychotherapist may be a factor in the outcome of psychotherapy, it has been difficult to determine this is true in studies of outcomes to date. However, attainment of insight, an important component of psychodynamic psychotherapy work, but also cognitive behavioral therapy, does lead to improved patient outcomes and the achievement of beneficial change [108]. Personality disorders such as obsessive-compulsive (OCPD) complicate the treatment and outcome of patients with depression. Combining psychotherapy and antidepressant medication has been found to be more effective for this population with diagnoses of both personality disorder and mood disorder. In addition, the combined therapy helps sustain improvement over the long term [109].

The reduction of symptoms and attainment of remission from depression and anxiety are the goals of psychotherapy. In addition, it contributes to benefits in overall functioning of the patient and prevention of relapse, fostering growth in the capacity to cope more adaptively. All of the individual psychotherapies help individuals to become more integrated and authentic, capable of personal responsibility and improved relationships with others. In addition, the exploration of what in life has meaning to them, including within their work, is a key ambition of psychotherapy. Attaining more conscious awareness of oneself is key to growth. As people get healthier, they are able to maintain a view of the world that is more benevolent, i.e., less threatening, allowing a more honest and flexible self in relation to others [110]. The different psychotherapies listed below are ones which are likely to be most accessible and useful to women physicians. They are the techniques of psychotherapy which have been well-researched and found effective. Most well-trained therapists who are psychiatrists, psychologists (PhDs or PsyDs), and masters' level clinicians use a combination of theoretical principles and perspectives in their work with patients.

Cognitive behavioral therapy (CBT) targets maladaptive thoughts and behavioral patterns. It has potential benefit for individuals with mild to moderate depression and is recommended by the American Psychiatric Association (APA) as an initial treatment for these patients [109]. The aim of CBT is to alter depressive cognitive patterns such as pessimistic thinking. Cognitive therapy begins by identifying the distorted thinking so that a therapeutic reframing of the negative, distorted outlook may be possible. Cognitive behavioral therapy does not include close examination of emotional issues and confronts limited utility when deeper work is indicated for recovery.

Psychodynamic psychotherapy, also called insight-oriented or supportive-expressive psychotherapy [111], is especially beneficial to those individuals who need to explore past traumas or a history of abuse. It is also valuable to anyone who is maladaptively repeating patterns from earlier family dynamics in their current life. The aim of the work is to understand one's unique developmental and family history and one's emotions, relationships, and patterns of behavior that may be self-defeating. Successful treatment allows for the exploration of unconscious factors and leads to expanded self-knowledge, in turn diminishing unhappiness and conflicts. Mentalization, an important dimension of psychodynamic therapy, centers around developing and improving the capacity to "think about thinking" as a means to understanding oneself and others. It was first described in 1960 by the psychoanalyst, Peter Fonagy [112]. Evolving an ability to understand misunderstandings when they occur helps individuals to be empathic while navigating relationships and interpersonal conflict. However, individuals who have suffered physical, psychological, and sexual abuse may have a complicated and disorganized attachment to parents or caregivers and consequently [113] have difficulty maintaining a stable sense of self, which is a goal of mentalization therapy [110].

In addition, *relational psychotherapy* techniques may be particularly helpful to the women doctors who suffer from disconnection and isolation. As this form of therapy focuses on achieving satisfying, healthy relationships with others, it also helps with managing life stress. Because women are socialized to be nurturers, relationships are key to their psychological health. Benefits, such as understanding the behaviors which cause disconnection from others, lead to increased self-awareness and increased self-esteem. In addition, gaining greater awareness of power dynamics within relationships, including gender and racial issues, benefits women [114].

Group Psychotherapy and Support Groups

Group psychotherapy and support groups deserve special consideration for women physicians based on women's needs for supportive relationships with other women and the health benefits they derive from those connections. Since women are genetically and socially oriented to relationships, it makes sense that developing supportive networks within work or outside work could benefit the women, in addition to their families, their patients, their colleagues, and their institutions. The Authentic Connections

Groups (ACG) for medical professional mothers at the Mayo Clinic in Arizona demonstrated encouraging results that persisted and further improved 3 months after completion of the psychiatrist-led group therapy sessions. During the course of guided group therapy for 12 weeks, the women explored and discovered solutions to problems caused by the duality of motherhood and practicing medicine with consequent declines in their levels of the stress hormone, cortisol. During the group sessions, the mothers developed secure relationships of trust with fellow group members as they solved shared problems. Several women in each group also requested mental health referrals for themselves and/or their children. Many acknowledged that they would likely not have asked for additional help were it not for the group [47].

The high rates of burnout, anxiety, depression, and suicide in women physicians is often related to feelings of isolation and being overburdened [5]. It is perhaps unsurprising that stressed mothers might have stressed family systems and children as well.

A report, published in the American Psychological Association's Journal of Abnormal Psychology, looked at survey data from more than 600,000 adolescents and young adults [115]. Over the past decade, the rates of depression, anxiety, and suicidal ideation and attempts have increased alarmingly among people age 26 and younger with the highest increase being among children from higher-income families. Parental stress contributes to increased pressure on children to achieve as well as the isolation from their parents that these children experience. Furthermore, it was during their children's middle school years that mothers reported their lowest life satisfaction and lowest sense of fulfillment with their highest level of stress, loneliness, and emptiness [116].

For many ACG physician mother participants, it was their love for their children that inspired these mothers to invest in change. The ACG mothers' mandate was to develop a "go to committee" for support, mentoring, and validation. They were reminded of the evidence that it was the quality of their time with their children, not quantity, that contributed to the mental health of the children. Participants were encouraged to set up weekly "check-in" times with their committee to address their own needs and parenting concerns or just to share a glass of wine [117]. These four factors surfaced as critical in mitigating mothers' stress and they were independent of the mother's marital status:

- Unconditional acceptance
- Feeling comforted when needed
- Authenticity in relationships
- Friendship satisfaction

The fact that Mayo Clinic supported this intervention during regular working hours enabled these busy professional moms to participate in groups, which measurably decreased professional burnout. The results of this low-cost study benefited the mothers, their children and family, and the hospital. Tait Shanafelt, MD, the current chief wellness officer at Stanford, has documented the value to organizations of investing in physician well-being including positive business consequences [118]. Upwards of 54% of physicians experience burnout [119] with consequent increased physician turnover, poorly delivered healthcare, and decreased revenues. What is more difficult to quantify are the lives that are saved as a result of decreased isolation from proactive interventions. Additionally, satisfaction with marriage – not simply being married – was associated with maternal well-being. However, the most compelling factor overall in maternal well-being was satisfaction with friendships [97, 101]. These research-based insights can be utilized within supportive group-based interventions [99] aimed at fostering the resilience of mothers in their everyday lives. The Authentic Connections Group is a great example of the synergy created in the group therapy setting especially when it includes mentoring and support.

Support groups may provide benefits to women physicians whether they are struggling or highly functional. Unlike group therapy, there is no professional leader of the support group process. Instead, support groups bring together people with a common problem in an informal, protected space. Today, there are several programmatic and problem-focused support groups, the most well-known of which is Alcoholics Anonymous (AA), the first 12-step support group program. Al-Anon came later to provide a forum for families of alcoholics. These support groups can be helpful to individuals with psychiatric diagnoses like depression which are complicated by comorbid conditions such as alcoholism which confer risk not only to themselves, but to their family relationships and their jobs, too. Additional support groups exist for overeaters, sex addicts, gamblers, debtors, and the codependent. Parents Without Partners and groups for divorced or grieving individuals have sprung up because of the universal human need for support. Participating in a support group allows individuals to identify with others who have similar problems, giving voice to their struggles in a safe setting. As a consequence, the loneliness, isolation, and shame of a problem like overeating is diminished.

In a similar way, informal groups of women, particularly long-term groups where there are close connections, serve to protect women and provide them with trusted, authentic relationships within which they can be understood and supported. A group of ten women developed out of the need of one distressed professional woman who felt isolated in her job at a large male-dominated international firm. Twenty years ago, she invited women with different professional backgrounds – psychologists, psychiatrists, academics, lawyers, and women from the business world – to participate in a non-work-based group which met to discuss topics of mutual interest, in particular, women's personal and leadership challenges. Over the years, these busy women from different parts of the United States read books and watched movies in preparation for their meetings twice a year. In the process of these shared experiences, their children grew through adolescence and into young adulthood, their parents aged and died, and some of the women members got divorced and remarried. Relationships with significant others, colleagues, friends, and children were discussed along with the inevitable problems of living life. As a participant of this alliance, I can attest the bonds which developed among the women were strong ones because the group was authentic, voicing vulnerable feelings and getting validation. Meeting together became almost sacred because of the safety and truth of living life together.

Small groups of women physicians who meet for social purposes, to discuss books or to play tennis, will also share their worries about spouses, children, and work. If there is safety in their intimacy, the women will develop understanding and support for one another. This is what women physicians need: formal or informal support groups where there is no judgment and where life, support, and resources can be shared. What makes these groups work is the underlying hunger for connection. When women swap day care ideas while laughing together about the small frustrations of a sometimes clueless partner, they face the world with less stress, more joy, and more resourcefulness. When women laugh and cry together, they bare their souls and are no longer alone. That is what works [47].

There is also a place for physician support groups which focus on work and the care of patients. Instead of being alone, if the doctors can discuss stresses in the safety of a compassionate group, they can support one another while sharing difficult clinical cases and finding solutions. For example, Physician Engagement Groups have been demonstrated to decrease burnout in Mayo Clinic physicians [101]. Balint groups [71], the Schwartz Rounds® program [120], story-telling groups, and Doctoring to Heal programs are examples of groups that promote well-being by inviting participating physicians to expand their understanding and awareness of professional issues [101]. Balint groups originated in England with the psychoanalyst, Michael Balint. Their original purpose was to provide supervision for general practitioners who benefitted from discussing psychodynamic factors in the treatment of their patients. The general practitioners discussed with each other and Dr. Balint what caused anxiety and psychosomatic symptoms in patients. The aim was to decrease the number of futile and costly searches for medical explanations of symptoms while identifying causes of illness due to stress or psychiatric problems. This structure provides an example of collaborative care among physicians which improves care for the patient while the doctor receives more support and companionship in her work. Solving such problems as, "When do you fire a patient?" or "What do you do about a conflict of interest in treating someone?" If a doctor becomes afraid of a patient, is threatened by a patient, or feels the patient violates the doctor's boundaries, that doctor must turn to clinical peers for advice. At times, legal advice must be sought as well. This model provides an appealing example of how group therapy can support practitioners while stimulating the clinical work and fostering interest and pleasure in practice.

Conclusion

The practice of medicine is a calling for many of the women doctors whose altruism and idealism drew them to the field. However, for multiple reasons, women physicians may be at increased risk for burnout, depression, suicide, and stigma. Women physicians have similar risks to women in the general population for depressive illness, about a 20% lifetime risk, which is almost double the risk for men. It is true that all females, including women physicians, have an increased biological risk for depressive illness. That risk includes hormone changes due to the menstrual cycle, pregnancy, lactation, and menopause. Also, women are more vulnerable to the deleterious effects of childhood trauma and abuse which predispose them to depression and anxiety disorders later in life. In addition, all women have increased social risk factors for depression as a result of their burden of responsibility for the care-taking of children and parents. Lesbian women physicians have somewhat increased risk factors for depression compared to heterosexual women, including more family histories of depression, substance abuse, sexual abuse, and harassment.

Alarmingly, the risk of suicide for women physicians has been reported to be two to four times that of women in the general population and, according to different research findings, equal to [30] or twice that of male physicians [24, 25]. There are confounding epidemiological factors which complicate our deriving the true rate of suicide in women doctors. Because there are more men than women physicians in the United States, pools of data on women are small and comparison with the larger data on men physicians leads to distorted and sometimes invalid conclusions. Additionally, data available are exclusively about women from North America and Europe and do not include women born outside of the United States who are racially diverse. Moreover, women physicians appear to have a higher risk of suicide than other high-achieving professional women. Having expertise about medications and how to poison themselves, women physicians are more successful at completing suicides than other women. Once they put their suicidal plans into action, it appears that women doctors possess less ambivalence about ending their lives and more determination to do so. Consequently, identifying additional risk factors for women doctors is crucial so that intervention and treatment can prevent illness, disability, and untimely death. Psychological pain together with hopelessness and depression constitute the triad of factors which are key to understanding motivation for suicide. In addition, there are personality characteristics which increase the risks of depression and suicide in addition to job-related stresses and the dangers of a toxic work environment. The personality characteristics selected for in medicine include perfectionism and obsessiveness. Those characteristics are important because attention to detail saves patients' lives. High needs for approval are associated with feeling inauthentic, like an imposter. In fact, the imposter syndrome is more common in women. Other personality risk factors include a strong wish for control, mastery, and autonomy which may predispose women doctors to isolation, difficulty asking for help, and denial of their own needs, all of which culminate in higher levels of psychological pain and hopelessness. Stress at work, including onerous responsibilities to complete electronic medical records, long clinic hours, and little control of schedule, biases against women for promotion, and research opportunities, as well as harassment in the workplace, are of major significance because of their toxic effects on women. In the workplace, women appear to get less respect from patients and colleagues than men do, even during the training years of internship and residency. Moreover, the conflict between family and professional roles and responsibilities means women physicians work longer hours with more stress, especially if they have an inadequate support system at home.

Stigma is an important problem which prevents women doctors from acknowledging depression and getting psychiatric diagnosis and treatment. Clearly, more efforts must be made to diminish the stigma of mental illness and treatment. Recent increases in the number of physicians who openly reveal their own stories of depression are having a powerful effect on acceptance of treatment. Significant steps are underway in medical school curricula to educate medical students about the importance of early recognition and intervention when psychiatric illness presents. Identifying and discussing the role of shame when mistakes are made or poor outcomes occur in medical practice have a place in limiting the pain of shame and stigma, especially for women physicians who may be at heightened risk if censured by medical boards or if targeted in malpractice suits.

What appears to benefit women physicians most is increased social support, coaching, and mentoring including individual and group psychotherapy and authentic connections with other women colleagues and friends. Their intelligence, tendency to worry, and strong sense of idealism may make women doctors more vulnerable, but these characteristics also make them excellent candidates for successful psychotherapy treatment, coaching, and mentoring. The proactive, practical, and purpose-driven strengths of women physicians can be harnessed and redirected toward helping themselves – not only others. The positive results of group psychotherapy work with physician mothers and the anecdotal stories of individual psychotherapy treatment successes are examples of how resilient this population is when they have opportunities to improve their professional and personal coping skills and attain more balanced lives. Continuing research will better elucidate the risks for women doctors and lead to better prevention and earlier treatment of psychiatric illnesses. What is clear from current research is that women make great physicians. The patients of women doctors may fare better in morbidity and mortality than do the patients of male doctors. However, better support of women physicians in the workplace via organizational, cultural, and systemic change is called for in order to alleviate their stress and improve the professional satisfaction of this admirable population of women professionals.

Acknowledgments For their contributions to this chapter, I want to thank Dr. Judith Engelman for her clinical knowledge and passion; the editors, Dr. Cynthia Stonnington and Dr. Julia Files, for their inspiration and friendship; and Mayo Clinic Alix School of Medicine student, Sabrina Syed, for her literature searches. I am particularly thankful to Dr. Laura Falduto for sharing her keen observations, her incisive insights and her wisdom.

References

1. Osler W. The practice of medicine is an art, not a trade; a calling, not a business; a calling in which your heart will be exercised equally with your head. 2014. Available at: https://stanfordmedicine25.stanford.edu/blog/archive/2014/10-Osler-isms-to-Remember-in-Your-Daily-Practice.html.
2. Freudenberger HJ. Staff burn-out. J Social Issues. 1974;30(1):159–65. Available   at: https://spssi.onlinelibrary.wiley.com/doi/abs/10.1111/j.1540-4560.1974.tb00706.x.
3. Stehman CR, Testo Z, Gershaw RS, Kellogg AR. Burnout, drop out, suicide: physician loss in emergency medicine, part I. West J Emerg Med. 2019;20(3):485–94.
4. Maslach C. Maslach burnout inventory-human services survey (MBI-HSS) for medical personnel. 1981. Available at: https://nam.edu/valid-reliable-survey-instruments-measure-burnout-well-work-related-dimensions/.
5. Callahan K, Christman G, Maltby L. Battling burnout: strategies for promoting physician wellness. Adv Pediatr. 2018;65(1):1–17.
6. Bianchi R, Schonfeld IS, Vandel P, Laurent E. On the depressive nature of the "burnout syndrome": a clarification. Eur Psychiatry. 2017;41:109–10.
7. Bianchi R, Schonfeld IS. Defining physician burnout, and differentiating between burnout and depression-I. Mayo Clin Proc. 2017;92(9):1455.
8. Dyrbye LN, Thomas MR, Massie FS, Power DV, Eacker A, Harper W, et al. Burnout and suicidal ideation among U.S. medical students. Ann Intern Med. 2008;149(5):334–41.
9. Firth-Cozens J. Interventions to improve physicians' well-being and patient care. Soc Sci Med. 2001;52(2):215–22.
10. Andrew LB, Brenner BE. Physician suicide. 2018. Available at: https://emedicine.medscape.com/article/806779-overview. Medscape.
11. Spataro BM, Tilstra SA, Rubio DM, McNeil MA. The toxicity of self-blame: sex differences in burnout and coping in internal medicine trainees. J Womens Health (Larchmt). 2016;25(11):1147–52.
12. KFF. State health facts: demographics and the economy. Available at: https://www.kff.org/other/state-indicator/allopathic-medical-school-graduates-by-gender/?currentTimeframe=0&sortModel=%7B%22colId%22:%22Location%22,%22sort%22:%22asc%22%7D.

13. AAMC. 2018 Fall Applicant and matriculant data tables. 2018. Available at: https://www.aamc.org/system/files/d/1/92-applicant_and_matriculant_data_tables.pdf.

14. AAMC. 2016 Physician specialty data report executive summary. 2016. Available at: https://www.aamc.org/system/files/reports/1/2016physician specialtydatareportexecutivesummary.pdf.

15. Dyrbye LN, West CP, Sinsky CA, Goeders LE, Satele DV, Shanafelt TD. Medical licensure questions and physician reluctance to seek care for mental health conditions. Mayo Clin Proc. 2017;92(10):1486–93.

16. Roter DL, Hall JA, Aoki Y. Physician gender effects in medical communication: a meta-analytic review. JAMA. 2002;288(6):756–64.

17. Tsugawa Y, Jena AB, Figueroa JF, Orav EJ, Blumenthal DM, Jha AK. Comparison of hospital mortality and readmission rates for medicare patients treated by male vs female physicians. JAMA Intern Med. 2017;177(2):206–13.

18. Bertakis KD, Helms LJ, Callahan EJ, Azari R, Robbins JA. The influence of gender on physician practice style. Med Care. 1995;33(4):407–16.

19. Jolly S, Griffith KA, DeCastro R, Stewart A, Ubel P, Jagsi R. Gender differences in time spent on parenting and domestic responsibilities by high-achieving young physician-researchers. Ann Intern Med. 2014;160(5):344–53.

20. Gold KJ, Andrew LB, Goldman EB, Schwenk TL. "I would never want to have a mental health diagnosis on my record": a survey of female physicians on mental health diagnosis, treatment, and reporting. Gen Hosp Psychiatry. 2016;43:51–7.

21. Gold KJ, Sen A, Schwenk TL. Details on suicide among US physicians: data from the National Violent Death Reporting System. Gen Hosp Psychiatry. 2013;35(1):45–9.

22. Rotenstein LS, Ramos MA, Torre M, Segal JB, Peluso MJ, Guille C, et al. Prevalence of depression, depressive symptoms, and suicidal ideation among medical students: a systematic review and meta-analysis. JAMA. 2016;316(21):2214–36.

23. Maser B, Danilewitz M, Guerin E, Findlay L, Frank E. Medical student psychological distress and mental illness relative to the general population: a Canadian cross-sectional survey. Acad Med. 2019;94(11):1781–91.

24. Frank E, Dingle AD. Self-reported depression and suicide attempts among U.S. women physicians. Am J Psychiatry. 1999;156(12):1887–94.

25. North CS, Ryall JE. Psychiatric illness in female physicians. Are high rates of depression an occupational hazard? Postgrad Med. 1997;101(5):233–6, 9–40, 42.

26. Cahill L. Sex- and hemisphere-related influences on the neurobiology of emotionally influenced memory. Prog Neuro-Psychopharmacol Biol Psychiatry. 2003;27(8):1235–41.

27. Richardsen AM, Burke RJ. Occupational stress and job satisfaction among physicians: sex differences. Soc Sci Med. 1991;33(10):1179–87.

28. Goldman B. Two minds: the cognitive differences between men and women. Stanford medicine: sex, gender and medicine. 2017.

29. Vogel L. Physician suicide still shrouded in secrecy. CMAJ. 2016;188(17–18):1213.

30. Lindeman S, Laara E, Hirvonen J, Lonnqvist J. Suicide mortality among medical doctors in Finland: are females more prone to suicide than their male colleagues? Psychol Med. 1997;27(5):1219–22.

31. Pompili M, Mancinelli I, Girardi P, Tatarelli R. Letter to the editor on female physicians committing suicide. MedGenMed. 2004;6(2):60.

32. Juel K, Mosbech J, Hansen ES. Mortality and causes of death among Danish medical doctors 1973-1992. Int J Epidemiol. 1999;28(3):456–60.

33. Salles A, Awad M, Goldin L, Krus K, Lee JV, Schwabe MT, et al. Estimating implicit and explicit gender bias among health care professionals and surgeons. JAMA Netw Open. 2019;2(7):e196545.

34. Ly DP, Jena AB. Sex differences in time spent on household activities and care of children among US physicians, 2003-2016. Mayo Clin Proc. 2018;93(10):1484–7.

35. Belkic K, Nedic O. Workplace stressors and lifestyle-related cancer risk factors among female physicians: assessment using the Occupational Stress Index. J Occup Health. 2007;49(1):61–71.

36. Dyrbye LN, Sciolla AF, Dekhtyar M, Rajasekaran S, Allgood JA, Rea M, et al. Medical school strategies to address student well-being: a national survey. Acad Med. 2019;94(6):861–8.

37. Albert PR. Why is depression more prevalent in women? J Psychiatry Neurosci. 2015;40(4):219–21.

38. Cohen BM, Sommer BR, Vuckovic A. Antidepressant-resistant depression in patients with comorbid subclinical hypothyroidism or high-normal TSH levels. Am J Psychiatry. 2018;175(7):598–604.

39. Barth C, Villringer A, Sacher J. Sex hormones affect neurotransmitters and shape the adult female brain during hormonal transition periods. Front Neurosci. 2015;9:37.

40. Hudon Thibeault AA, Sanderson JT, Vaillancourt C. Serotonin-estrogen interactions: what can we learn from pregnancy? Biochimie. 2019;161:88–108.

41. Maki PM, Kornstein SG, Joffe H, Bromberger JT, Freeman EW, Athappilly G, et al. Guidelines for the evaluation and treatment of perimenopausal depression: summary and recommendations. Menopause. 2018;25(10):1069–85.

42. Prosman GJ, Jansen SJ, Lo Fo Wong SH, Lagro-Janssen AL. Prevalence of intimate partner violence among migrant and native women attending general practice and the association between intimate partner violence and depression. Fam Pract. 2011;28(3):267–71.

43. Vaillant GE, Sobowale NC, McArthur C. Some psychologic vulnerabilities of physicians. N Engl J Med. 1972;287(8):372–5.

44. Barrios YV, Gelaye B, Zhong Q, Nicolaidis C, Rondon MB, Garcia PJ, et al. Association of childhood physical and sexual abuse with intimate partner violence, poor general health and depressive symptoms among

pregnant women [published correction appears in PLoS One. 2015;10(3):e0122573]. PLoS One. 2015;10(1):e0116609.

45. Negele A, Kaufhold J, Kallenbach L, Leuzinger-Bohleber M. Childhood trauma and its relation to chronic depression in adulthood. Depress Res Treat. 2015;2015:650804.

46. Luthar SS, Becker BE. Privileged but pressured? A study of affluent youth. Child Dev. 2002;73(5):1593–610.

47. Luthar SS, Curlee A, Tye SJ, Engelman JC, Stonnington CM. Fostering resilience among mothers under stress: "authentic connections groups" for medical professionals. Womens Health Issues. 2017;27(3):382–90.

48. Cernis E, Vassos E, Brebion G, McKenna PJ, Murray RM, David AS, et al. Schizophrenia patients with high intelligence: a clinically distinct sub-type of schizophrenia? Eur Psychiatry. 2015;30(5):628–32.

49. Nolen-Hoeksema S. Women who think too much: how to break free of overthinking and reclaim your life. New York: Henry Holt and Company, LLC; 2003.

50. Luthar SS, Doyle K, Suchman NE, Mayes L. Developmental themes in women's emotional experiences of motherhood. Dev Psychopathol. 2001;13(1):165–82.

51. Vaglum P, Falkum E. Self-criticism, dependency and depressive symptoms in a nationwide sample of Norwegian physicians. J Affect Disord. 1999;52(1–3):153–9.

52. Weissman MM, Wickramaratne P, Gameroff MJ, Warner V, Pilowsky D, Kohad RG, et al. Offspring of depressed parents: 30 years later. Am J Psychiatry. 2016;173(10):1024–32.

53. Brogan DJ, O'Hanlan KA, Elon L, Frank E. Health and professional characteristics of lesbian and heterosexual women physicians. J Am Med Womens Assoc (1972). 2003;58(1):10–9.

54. Brogan D, Frank E, Elon L, O'Hanlan KA. Methodologic concerns in defining lesbian for health research. Epidemiology. 2001;12(1):109–13.

55. Harcourt J. Current issues in lesbian, gay, bisexual, and transgender health. New York: Routledge; 2011.

56. O'Brien McElwee R, Yurak T. The phenomenology of the impostor phenomenon. Individ Differ Res. 2010;9(3):184–97.

57. Clance PR, Imes SA. The impostor phenomenon in high achieving women: dynamics and therapeutic intervention. Psychother Theory Res Pract. 1978;15(3):241–7.

58. Wolfe J. Sex and why. 2018. Available at: https://www.sexandwhy.com/sex-why-episode-9-gender-differences-in-resident-evaluation/ [Internet]; Podcast.

59. Dayal A, O'Connor DM, Qadri U, Arora VM. Comparison of male vs female resident milestone evaluations by faculty during emergency medicine residency training. JAMA Intern Med. 2017;177(5):651–7.

60. Mueller AS, Jenkins TM, Osborne M, Dayal A, O'Connor DM, Arora VM. Gender differences in attending physicians' feedback to residents: a qualitative analysis. J Grad Med Educ. 2017;9(5):577–85.

61. Brescoll VL. Who takes the floor and why: gender, power, and volubility in organizations. Adm Sci Q. 2011;56(4):622–41.
62. Mullangi S, Jagsi R. Imposter syndrome: treat the cause, not the symptom. JAMA. 2019;322(5):403–4.
63. Perry JC. Cluster C Personality disorders. Desk reference to the diagnostic criteria from DSM-5: APA Press; 2013. p. 328. Available at: https://psychiatryonline.org/doi/10.1176/appi.books.9781585625048.gg73.
64. Myers MF, Gabbard GO. The physician as patient: a clinical handbook for mental health professionals: American Psychiatric Publishing, Inc. Arlington, USA; 2008. 252 p.
65. Cooper CL, Rout U, Faragher B. Mental health, job satisfaction, and job stress among general practitioners. BMJ. 1989;298(6670):366–70.
66. Gyorffy Z, Dweik D, Girasek E. Workload, mental health and burnout indicators among female physicians. Hum Resour Health. 2016;14:12.
67. Fridner A, Belkic K, Minucci D, Pavan L, Marini M, Pingel B, et al. Work environment and recent suicidal thoughts among male university hospital physicians in Sweden and Italy: the health and organization among university hospital physicians in Europe (HOUPE) study. Gend Med. 2011;8(4):269–79.
68. Fridner A, Belkic K, Marini M, Minucci D, Pavan L, Schenck-Gustafsson K. Survey on recent suicidal ideation among female university hospital physicians in Sweden and Italy (the HOUPE study): cross-sectional associations with work stressors. Gend Med. 2009;6(1):314–28.
69. Carr PL, Gareis KC, Barnett RC. Characteristics and outcomes for women physicians who work reduced hours. J Womens Health (Larchmt). 2003;12(4):399–405.
70. Kendler KS, Myers J, Prescott CA. Sex differences in the relationship between social support and risk for major depression: a longitudinal study of opposite-sex twin pairs. Am J Psychiatry. 2005;162(2):250–6.
71. Miller NM, McGowen RK. The painful truth: physicians are not invincible. South Med J. 2000;93(10):966–73.
72. Schwenk TL, Gorenflo DW, Leja LM. A survey on the impact of being depressed on the professional status and mental health care of physicians. J Clin Psychiatry. 2008;69(4):617–20.
73. Troister T, Holden RR. Comparing psychache, depression, and hopelessness in their associations with suicidality: a test of Shneidman's theory of suicide. Pers Individ Dif. 2010;49(7):689–93.
74. Aasland OG, Ekeberg O, Schweder T. Suicide rates from 1960 to 1989 in Norwegian physicians compared with other educational groups. Soc Sci Med. 2001;52(2):259–65.
75. DeRubeis RJ, Siegle GJ, Hollon SD. Cognitive therapy versus medication for depression: treatment outcomes and neural mechanisms. Nat Rev Neurosci. 2008;9(10):788–96.
76. Hem E, Haldorsen T, Aasland OG, Tyssen R, Vaglum P, Ekeberg O. Suicide among physicians. Am J Psychiatry. 2005;162(11):2199–200.

77. Hawton K, Clements A, Sakarovitch C, Simkin S, Deeks JJ. Suicide in doctors: a study of risk according to gender, seniority and specialty in medical practitioners in England and Wales, 1979-1995. J Epidemiol Community Health. 2001;55(5):296–300.

78. Schernhammer ES, Colditz GA. Suicide rates among physicians: a quantitative and gender assessment (meta-analysis). Am J Psychiatry. 2004;161(12):2295–302.

79. Wallis CJ, Ravi B, Coburn N, Nam RK, Detsky AS, Satkunasivam R. Comparison of postoperative outcomes among patients treated by male and female surgeons: a population based matched cohort study. BMJ. 2017;359:j4366.

80. Ducasse D, Holden RR, Boyer L, Artero S, Calati R, Guillaume S, et al. Psychological pain in suicidality: a meta-analysis. J Clin Psychiatry. 2018;79(3). https://doi.org/10.4088/JCP.16r10732.

81. Williams JMG. Cry of Pain: Understanding Suicide and Self-Harm. London: Penguin Books; 1997, pp. 1–272.

82. Baumeister RF. Suicide as escape from self. Psychol Rev. 1990;97(1):90–113.

83. Nagy C, Schwabe D, Jones W, Brown A, Shupe M, Mancone A, et al. Time to talk about it: physician depression and suicide video/discussion session for interns, residents, and fellows. MedEdPORTAL. 2016;12. Available at: https://www.mededportal.org/publication/10508/esr/.

84. Mental Health First Aid. Available at: https://www.mentalhealthfirstaid.org.

85. Quinnett P. QPR gatekeeper training for suicide prevention: the model, theory and research. 2012. Available at: https://qprinstitute.com/uploads/qpr-theory-2017.pdf.

86. Aviv R. The philosopher of feelings: Martha Nussbaum's far-reaching ideas illuminate the often ignored elements of human life – aging, inequality, and emotion. The New Yorker, Profiles. 2016.

87. Smyth HW. Prometheus bound – Aeschylus – Ancient Greece – classical texts library, lines 473–5. Available at: www.ancient-literature.com/greece_aeschylus.

88. Brown B. Daring greatly: how the courage to be vulnerable transforms the way we live, love, parent, and lead: Arlington, USA, Gotham Books; 2012.

89. Bynum WE, Artino AR Jr, Uijtdehaage S, Webb AMB, Varpio L. Sentinel emotional events: the nature, triggers, and effects of shame experiences in medical residents. Acad Med. 2019;94(1):85–93.

90. Bynum WE, Adams AV, Edelman CE, Uijtdehaage S, Artino AR Jr, Fox JW. Addressing the elephant in the room: a shame resilience seminar for medical students. Acad Med. 2019;94(8):1132–6.

91. Voltmer E, Kieschke U, Schwappach DL, Wirsching M, Spahn C. Psychosocial health risk factors and resources of medical students and physicians: a cross-sectional study. BMC Med Educ. 2008;8:46.

92. Spring L, Robillard D, Gehlbach L, Simas TA. Impact of pass/fail grading on medical students' well-being and academic outcomes. Med Educ. 2011;45(9):867–77.

93. Rohe DE, Barrier PA, Clark MM, Cook DA, Vickers KS, Decker PA. The benefits of pass-fail grading on stress, mood, and group cohesion in medical students. Mayo Clin Proc. 2006;81(11):1443–8.

94. Kim S, George P. The relationship between preclinical grading and USMLE scores in US allopathic medical schools. Fam Med. 2018;50(2):128–31.

95. van Vendeloo SN, Prins DJ, Verheyen C, Prins JT, van den Heijkant F, van der Heijden F, et al. The learning environment and resident burnout: a national study. Perspect Med Educ. 2018;7(2):120–5.

96. Anonymous. In my experience: how educators can support a medical student with mental illness. Acad Med. 2019;94(11):1638–9.

97. Dyrbye LN, Satele D, Sloan J, Shanafelt TD. Utility of a brief screening tool to identify physicians in distress. J Gen Intern Med. 2013;28(3):421–7.

98. Quill TE, Williamson PR. Healthy approaches to physician stress. Arch Intern Med. 1990;150(9):1857–61.

99. Weiner EL, Swain GR, Wolf B, Gottlieb M. A qualitative study of physicians' own wellness-promotion practices. West J Med. 2001;174(1):19–23.

100. Choi KW, Chen CY, Stein MB, Klimentidis YC, Wang MJ, Koenen KC, et al. Assessment of bidirectional relationships between physical activity and depression among adults: a 2-sample Mendelian randomization study. JAMA Psychiat. 2019;76(4):399–408.

101. Shanafelt TD, Sloan JA, Habermann TM. The well-being of physicians. Am J Med. 2003;114(6):513–9.

102. Kabat-Zinn J. 9 Powerful meditation tips. Available at: https://themindfulnesssummit.com/sessions/9-powerful-meditation-tips-jon-kabat-zinn/.

103. Mayer AP, Files JA, Ko MG, Blair JE. Academic advancement of women in medicine: do socialized gender differences have a role in mentoring? Mayo Clin Proc. 2008;83(2):204–7.

104. Ducker D. Research on women physicians with multiple roles: a feminist perspective. J Am Med Womens Assoc (1972). 1994;49(3):78–84.

105. In a first for U.S. academic medical center, Stanford Medicine hires chief physician wellness officer. 2017. Available at: https://www.google.com/search?client=safari&rls=en&q=In+a+first+for+U.S.+academic+medical+center,+Stanford+Medicine+hires+chief+physician+wellness+officer,+Jun+22+2017,+med.stanford.edu/news/all-news/2017/06/Stanford-medicine&ie=UTF-8&oe=UTF-8 [press release].

106. Gupta K, Murray SG, Sarkar U, Mourad M, Adler-Milstein J. Differences in ambulatory EHR use patterns for male vs. female physicians: case

study. 2019. Available at: https://catalyst.nejm.org/ambulatory-ehr-patterns-physician-gender/.

107. Gelenberg AJ, Reus VI. APA practice guidelines for the treatment of patients with major depressive disorder. 2010. Available at: http://www.psychiatryonline.com/pracGuide/pracGuidTopic_7.aspx.

108. Jennissen S, Huber J, Ehrenthal JC, Schauenburg H, Dinger U. Association between insight and outcome of psychotherapy: systematic review and meta-analysis. Am J Psychiatry. 2018;175(10):961–9.

109. Chand SP, Ravi C, Chakkamparambil B, Prasad A, Vora A. CBT for depression: what the evidence says. Curr Psychiatry. 2018;17(9):14–6, 20–3.

110. Choi-kain LW, Unruh BT. Mentalization-based treatment: a common-sense approach to borderline personality. 2016. Available at: www.psychiatrictimes.com/special-reports/.

111. Luborsky L. Principles of psychoanalytic psychotherapy: a manual for supportive-expressive treatment. New York: Basic Books, Inc.; 1984.

112. Wallin DJ. Attachment in psychotherapy. New York: Guilford Press; 2007. 366 p.

113. Bateman A, Fonagy P. Mentalization-based treatment. Psychoanal Inq. 2013;33(6):595–613.

114. Jordan JV. A relational approach to psychotherapy. Women Therapy. 1995;16(4):51–61.

115. Bahrampour T. Mental health problems rise significantly among young Americans. J Abnormal Psychol. 2019;

116. Luthar SS, Ciciolla L. What it feels like to be a mother: variations by children's developmental stages. Dev Psychol. 2016;52(1):143–54.

117. Luthar SS, Ciciolla L. Who mothers mommy? Factors that contribute to mothers' well-being. Dev Psychol. 2015;51(12):1812–23.

118. Shanafelt T, Goh J, Sinsky C. The business case for investing in physician well-being. JAMA Intern Med. 2017;177(12):1826–32.

119. Messias E, Flynn V. The tired, retired, and recovered physician: professional burnout versus major depressive disorder. Am J Psychiatry. 2018;175(8):716–9.

120. Lown BA, Manning CF. The Schwartz Center Rounds: evaluation of an interdisciplinary approach to enhancing patient-centered communication, teamwork, and provider support. Acad Med. 2010;85(6):1073–81.

Addictions

13

Amanda E. Sedgewick, Hilary S. Connery, and Shelly F. Greenfield

Clinical Vignette

Dr. Susan F. is a 49-year-old emergency medicine physician, divorced almost 1 year ago, and mother to David, age 19, a freshman at a school in another state, and Samantha, age 16, a 10th grade honor roll high school student who is also captain of her high school soccer team. Susan has felt stressed at work for the last 7 years since her department appointed a new chair who has been focused on clinical productivity, quality improvement, and measurement using a dashboard of metrics ascertained through the electronic health record. Susan notices that over the last 7 years, she has felt more emotionally overextended at work.

Around the same time her new chair came on board, Susan's former husband began traveling more for his position in a

A. E. Sedgewick (✉) · S. F. Greenfield
Division of Women's Mental Health and Division of Alcohol, Drugs and Addiction, McLean Hospital, Belmont, MA; Department of Psychiatry, Harvard Medical School, Boston, MA, USA
e-mail: asedgewick1@partners.org; sgreenfield@mclean.harvard.edu

H. S. Connery
Division of Alcohol, Drugs and Addiction, McLean Hospital, Belmont, MA; Department of Psychiatry, Harvard Medical School, Boston, MA, USA
e-mail: hconnery@mclean.harvard.edu

© Springer Nature Switzerland AG 2020
C. M. Stonnington, J. A. Files (eds.), *Burnout in Women Physicians*,
https://doi.org/10.1007/978-3-030-44459-4_13

technology sales company leaving her with more demands on her time at home just as their children's sports, high school academics, and college preparatory activities intensified. She found herself stretched thin in both domains of work and home life with little support from home as her former husband sometimes traveled for 3–5 days at a time often to other states at great distance from their home. When he returned on weekends, he was exhausted and she found him less supportive of her both emotionally and logistically. Susan also noted that her mother who was widowed when Susan was 40 and is now 75 years old was having increasing medical problems. She lives in another state near to Susan's brother and sister. They are both very supportive of their mother but work in non-medical fields and Susan finds herself providing medical back-up and advice at each of her mother's medical emergencies, as well as needing to schedule time to visit her mother for which she has taken vacation days.

At work, Susan finds that she is increasingly distracted. She finds herself doing more administrative work and medical record charting in the EHR with less time spent seeing patients, and when she does she is more rushed. Her days are longer as the administrative burden continues to increase, and she has also had less time to supervise and teach the emergency medicine residents and fellows from other specialties. Teaching and seeing patients are the two activities she has enjoyed the most, and these feel more squeezed between administrative meetings and work on the EHR documenting patient care and outcomes as requested by her chair. She feels as if she is going through the motions with patients in the emergency department and this has also diminished her satisfaction with work. She feels very tired, emotionally exhausted, and irritable when she leaves work each night.

Susan is trying to be as responsive to her 16-year-old daughter as possible and feels lucky that she is an independent high school student who needs little reminding to get her school work done. At night, Susan has been drinking some of her favorite wine to relax after work and also with dinner. She has always enjoyed wine and she and her former husband put together a nice wine cellar through the years most of which she kept in their divorce settlement. As a reward for her stressful day, each night she picked a bottle of wine she liked and would begin drinking as soon as she came home. Before her separation, she would have one glass of wine with dinner with the family as did her husband. After their separation, she increased that to one glass before dinner and one with dinner. In the last 6 months, Susan has been drinking one bottle of wine each night. She has been having more trouble sleeping and recently has opened a second bottle to have another glass right before bedtime. In the past month, she has had increased difficulty getting out of bed in the morning. One afternoon, she missed an important soccer game she had planned to attend and did not remember that her daughter had reminded her the night before. She left work early as her calendar indicated but did not recall the game. Instead she went home and began drinking. When her daughter arrived home, she confronted her mother about her drinking and expressed great anger and frustration about her absence at the game and her general absence emotionally. Susan felt greatly ashamed and promised she would get help.

As you read this chapter, there are several questions to consider regarding this clinical case. These will be addressed at the conclusion of the chapter:

(1) What are the stressors contributing to Susan's current mental and emotional state? (2) Is Susan having burnout at work? If so, how would you describe it? (3) What do you think are Susan's likely diagnoses? (4) What are the next steps for intervention for Susan?

Section 1: Substance Use in Women

Introduction

Sex and gender differences are increasingly recognized as an important factor in many aspects of substance use disorders (SUDs) including disease trajectory, risk factors, treatment access and outcomes, and rates and type of co-occurring disorders. While the prevalence of SUDs remains higher in men, there is a concerning pattern of gender convergence, especially notable in recent generations, which continues to highlight the need for further research specific to women and SUDs.

When compared to men with SUDs, women with SUDs have been shown to advance more rapidly from use, to regular use, and then to first treatment episode. They are more vulnerable to the physiologic effects of many substances and have more health-related issues earlier during the course of illness, compared with men. Women with substance problems are more likely to have co-occurring psychiatric disorders, such as depression and anxiety, than men with substance problems, further complicating their treatment response.

Epidemiology

While the prevalence of alcohol and drug use continues to be higher in men than women, the gender gap continues to narrow. The National Survey on Drug Use and Health conducted in 2017 [1] noted past-year alcohol use for individuals 12 years and older was 62% for females and 67% for males. Twenty-five percent of females reported cannabis use in the past year (versus 34% of males) and 20% of females reported cigarette use (versus 26% of males). Past-year opiate use is reported as 0.1% in females versus 0.2% in males. An even smaller gap is reported between the sexes in past-year cocaine use (1% females versus 1.3% males) and these gaps are narrowing more quickly in younger cohorts. Figure 13.2 depicts the use of these substances in the past year separated by gender.

Alcohol

Alcohol use disorders (AUDs) continue to be a significant and widespread public health problem in the United States. Although more severe AUDs generally affect more men than women, a growing body of research suggests that women are more vulnerable to the physiologic consequences of alcohol and are more likely to develop alcohol-related medical conditions [2] with lower levels of alcohol consumed over a briefer duration.

Several concerning trends have emerged from recent studies looking at sex and gender differences in patterns of alcohol use over time. Studies have identified targets such as past 12-month alcohol use, high-risk drinking, diagnosis of AUD, and binge drinking all increasing by alarmingly higher percentages in women than in men. Grant and colleagues published data from the National Epidemiological Survey on Alcohol and Related Conditions which reported a 16% increase in 12-month alcohol use in women (versus 7% in men), 58% increase in high-risk drinking (exceeding daily drinking guidelines at least weekly in past year) (versus 15% in men), and an 84% increase in diagnosis of AUD in women (versus 35% increase in men) between the survey period of 2001–02 and 2012–13 (See Fig. 13.1) [3]. The SAMHSA 2017 National Survey on Drug Use and Health reports the 12-month alcohol use in young women (ages 12–17) has now surpassed that of young men, with 23.9% of young women and 20% of young men reporting use of alcohol in the past 12 months. This data shows that alcohol use remains higher in men in all other age groups [4]. A 2018 study by Johnston and colleagues

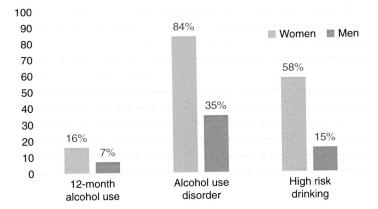

Fig. 13.1 Percent increase in alcohol related disorders from 2001–02 to 2012–13 from the National Epidemiological Survey on Alcohol and Related Conditions (NESARC). (Data from Grant et al. [3])

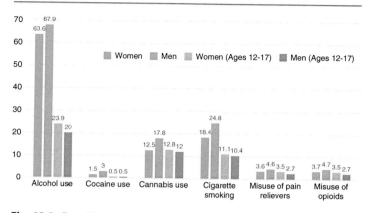

Fig. 13.2 Past 12-month substance use data (percentages) from the SAM-HSA 2017 National Survey on drug use and health. (Data from SAMHSA [4])

reports the gap has closed for binge drinking in adolescents, and now the rate of binge drinking in women is higher than in men for 8th, 10th, and 12th grade populations [5]. Figure 13.2 shows the epidemiology of past 12 month use of all substances separated by gender in the younger age cohort (12–17).

Earlier studies comparing multiple national surveys on alcohol use reported higher rates of AUD in younger age cohorts of women (born after World War II) compared with older birth cohorts (women born before WWII), as well as lower rates of abstinence from alcohol [6]. Data from the Centers for Disease Control released in 2013 revealed the highest prevalence of binge drinking (4 or more drinks on one occasion) in women was among younger age groups (19.8% in high school girls, 24.2% in women aged 18–24 years, and 19.9% in women aged 25–34 years) [7, 8]. Recent studies have shown a sharp increase in alcohol-related liver disease in younger females (adolescents and young adults) which could be a reflection of the increased use of alcohol in this age group and is consistent with previous evidence that suggests women experience health-related consequences earlier in the progression of the disease [9, 10]. A 2018 meta-analysis of 6 major national surveys revealed a significant and much sharper increase in past-year alcohol use in woman versus men, and a larger increase in binge drinking in middle aged and older adult women than in men [11].

Stimulants

The number of women using cocaine has been increasing significantly over the last several decades. The SAMHSA 2017 National Survey on Drug Use and Health reports past-year cocaine use to be 3% in men and 1.5% in women, but equal (0.5%) in men and women in the younger cohorts aged 12–17. Lifetime cocaine use is reported at 18.8% in men and 11.2% in women, and in 12–17 year old cohort women have surpassed men at 0.8% versus 0.6%, respectively [4]. A recent study by John and Wu published in 2017 indicated that past-year cocaine use in women had increased by 32% while increasing by 17% among men between 2011 and 2015. It also identified older adults' (50+ years old) weekly cocaine use as having increased by 228%. Weekly cocaine use in women increased by 60% (compared to 46% in men) although these trends were less significant. Weekly cocaine use was also strongly associated with heavy alcohol use [12].

Tobacco

Nearly half (48%) of the 42 million Americans who reported smoking cigarettes in the 2012 survey by the Department of Health and Human Services were women. Although fewer women than men report smoking cigarettes, this study suggests women are as likely to die from smoking-related diseases as are men. Females who smoke also have a greater risk of developing chronic obstructive pulmonary disease (COPD) and coronary artery disease (CAD) than men who smoke [13, 14]. Women smokers develop nicotine dependence more quickly than men from initial use, and also have a more difficult time quitting [15, 16]. Cigarette smoking in younger cohorts (adolescents) has declined overall, but the gender gap in this age group now reveals a minimal gender difference in report of past 30-day smoking [5]. The SAMHSA

2017 National Survey on Drug Use and Health (NSDUH) reports the prevalence of cigarette smoking in men and women between the ages of 12 and 17 to be 11.1% and 10.4%, respectively, the gap more narrow than the previous year, with 12.4% of males versus 10.8% of females [4]. Nicotine vaping has become an area of increasing concern in this population with past 30-day use of 16% in tenth graders and 19% in 12th graders [5].

Cannabis

The SAMHSA 2017 NSDUH reports past-year cannabis use of 17.8% in men and 12.5% in women; however, in the youngest age cohort of 12–17 year olds, the prevalence in females (12.8%) exceeds males (12.0%). Past-month cannabis use is reported as 11.9% in men and 7.3% in women, but this gender gap has closed in the 12–17 year old cohort with females having surpassed males at 6.6% versus 6.3%, respectively [4]. The 2018 study by Johnston et al. identified a significant increase in report of past 30-day cannabis use in 10th and 12th grade high school students (7% and 9% increase, respectively) since 1991. This reported use was higher in 10th grade males in 1991 (10.1% compared to 7.3% females), became roughly equal in 2013, and by 2017 reported use was higher in females (15.8% versus 15.3% in males). The difference in prevalence between genders in 12th grade students was 5% in 1991 and decreased to a 3% difference in 2017 (21% female versus 24% male). It should be noted that cannabis vaping is an area of increasing concern in this population with report of past 30-day use at 8% in 10th graders and 10% in 12th graders [5].

  Cannabis use is also significantly associated with tobacco use. A 2018 study found use of cannabis between 2002 and 2014 was 10 times higher in non-daily or daily smokers than in non-smokers, and by 2014 that its use was increasing most quickly in former smokers. Interestingly, in terms of gender differences, this study showed a three-fold increase in cannabis use among females who had never smoked compared with men in this category, but no gender differences in the smoking or former smoking groups [17].

Opioids

Recent studies have identified significant gender differences in regard to opioid use (both heroin and prescription opioid use). The SAMHSA 2017 National Survey on Drug Use and Health reports past-year misuse of pain relievers to be 4.6% in men and 3.6% in women, but 2.7% in men versus 3.5% in women in the younger cohorts aged 12–17. Similarly, misuse of opioids have been reported as 3.7% in women and 4.7% in men overall, but in the younger cohort aged 12–17 the proportion is 3.5% in females and 2.7% in males. The gap has notably narrowed in 18–25 year old group as well, with 7.4% of men reporting misuse of opioids in the past year and 7.2% of women [4]. Women's use of heroin has been steadily increasing since the 1960s and by 2010 was roughly equal to heroin use by men [18]. Overall trends for opioid use in the USA have shown decreasing use of prescription opioids and increasing use of heroin for both genders; however, the rate at which females are increasing their use of heroin is faster than men, and the rate at which they are decreasing their use of prescription opioids is slower than men [19]. Overdose deaths in women have increased five-fold in the past decade and are increasing at a faster rate than men [20, 21]. The 2019 CDC Morbidity and Mortality Weekly Report highlighted a 492% increase in opioid-involved overdose deaths in women aged 30–64 years. More specifically, rates of overdose deaths of women in this age group involving synthetic opioids increased by 1643%, heroin by 915%, and benzodiazepines by 830% [22]. One study showed that women were three times less likely than men to receive naloxone during EMS resuscitation attempts [23].

Physiology and Adverse Consequences

Physiologic factors may contribute to sex differences in substance use. Hormonal changes involving the menstrual cycle, pregnancy and lactation, and menopause can influence substance use in women. Neuroactive gonadal steroid hormones (estradiol, testosterone, and progesterone) have been shown to alter the release of dopamine, which in turn plays a significant role in the effects of many drugs of abuse on individuals' behavior and responses to different substances [24–26]. For example, several studies have noted that higher testosterone and estradiol levels in women are associated with a greater likelihood of current alcohol use [27, 28].

Physiologic factors related to sex differences and alcohol use have been well studied. Women may have higher blood alcohol levels than men after consumption of similar amounts of alcohol due to variations in levels of enzymes involved in alcohol breakdown (alcohol dehydrogenase and aldehyde dehydrogenase) [29]. In addition, women may have lower percentages of total body water which may result in greater blood alcohol concentrations when the same absolute amount of alcohol ingested, producing greater intoxication [30] at the same number of grams of alcohol ingested. These higher blood alcohol concentrations may be one reason women may have more severe medical consequences related to AUD than their male counterparts including alcohol-related liver disease, alcohol-induced cancers, brain damage, functional brain abnormalities, and cardiomyopathy [31–34]. Women also experience more sedation and sleepiness at similar blood alcohol levels when compared to men, and report increased sexual dysfunction [35].

Sex differences have also been studied in other SUDs. Activity of the liver enzyme that metabolizes nicotine (CYP2A6) is higher in woman than in men. In addition, women taking estrogen-containing oral contraceptives were found to metabolize nicotine even faster than woman not taking oral contraceptives or on progesterone-only oral contraceptives [36].

Sex differences in side effects and efficacy of medications used to treat SUDs have been studied. For example, women experience more side effects from nicotine replacement therapy than men in treatment of tobacco use disorder [37]. Converging evidence demonstrates that sex-related differences affect behaviors in smoking as well as response to nicotine replacement therapy (NRT) and other medications used for treatment.

Similarly, for treatment of opioid use disorder and AUD, women experience more side effects from naltrexone (including hormonally influenced increases in cortisol and prolactin) than men [38]. Women also were found to have higher blood concentrations of buprenorphine when given equivalent doses for treatment of opioid use disorder [39].

Results of earlier studies varied looking at different phases of the menstrual cycle and how this might affect cravings and experiences while using drugs/alcohol. Some studies have found that the follicular phase is more strongly associated with pleasant subjective effects of drug use when compared to the luteal phase [40, 41] while others have found no difference in subjective effects across the menstrual cycle [42–46]. A 2015 meta-analysis noted insufficient research to determine the impact of menstrual cycle phase/ovarian hormones on most outcomes related to smoking and cessation [47].

Several studies have shown that exogenous administration of progesterone in certain populations has been effective in lowering cravings and relapse. Fox et al. in 2013 and Milivoievic et al. in 2014 showed that progesterone administration in cocaine-dependent individuals is associated with decreases in cravings for cocaine [48, 49]. Progesterone administration has also been shown to reduce smoking behavior in women [50]. Further studies have been done in post-partum populations and have associated exogenous progesterone administration with decrease relapse on cocaine [51] and nicotine [52, 53].

There is a growing body of literature on sex differences in preclinical animal models of addiction that was recently reviewed in 2016 by Becker and Koob. In animal models, the female phenotype is associated with faster acquisition and self-administration of drugs and alcohol, more rapid escalation of drug taking with extended access, more motivational withdrawal (dysphoria, malaise, irritability, sleep disturbances, hypersensitivity to pain) versus drug-specific physical withdrawal, and greater reinstatement (craving/relapse) [54].

Course of Illness

There are sex and gender differences in the course of illness for SUDs. The course of illness for women is often described as "telescoping," which means women progress faster between landmarks of their disorder (from first use, to first substance-related problems, to first treatment episode), leaving shorter time windows for intervention opportunities. Women with SUDs have greater prevalence of co-occurring psychiatric disorders and substance-related medical issues and experience substance-related consequences at a greater rate than men [55, 56]. The telescoping course of illness has been demonstrated for many substances including alcohol, prescription opioids, cannabis, and cocaine. However, there is conflicting data for telescoping in opioid use disorder for those using heroin, as well as one population-based study on alcohol use. With respect to this discrepancy in this population-based study of AUD compared with treatment-seeking women, it has been hypothesized that studies demonstrating this effect are capturing a greater severity or higher risk subset of women (i.e., cohorts of women in treatment programs) and this effect may dissipate when including all women in the population [57].

Other studies have identified gender differences in dependence liability, or the transition from use to dependence, in which patterns vary by substance. For example, women have been shown to have a greater dependence liability for nicotine while men have a greater dependence liability for cannabis and to a lesser extent, alcohol. For other substances, such as cocaine, some studies have shown little difference between genders in human studies and dependence liability is similar in males and females [58–60].

Co-occurring Disorders

Co-occurring psychiatric disorders can complicate many aspects of substance use disorder course including diagnosis and treatment and can also affect treatment outcomes and there are significant gender differences. Women report more frequent use of substances to reduce negative affect [61] and women experience a higher rate of mood and anxiety disorders while men experience a higher rate of conduct disorder and antisocial personality disorder [62]. Co-occurring psychiatric disorders are more prevalent in women than men with SUDs and this has been suggested as an important focus for tailoring integrated treatments [63].

Mood and Anxiety Disorders

A 2012 study indicated that more women than men with AUD have co-occurring mood disorders, specifically major depressive disorder and bipolar 1 disorder [64]. Another study found that depression increases the risk of SUD in females while ADHD and conduct disorder increases this in males [65]. Data has variably identified gender differences in outcomes for men and women with co-occurring depression, with some studies showing disparities between genders. One study showed that having depression and an increasing number of stressors including abuse, homelessness, and decreased social support, among others, led to worse treatment outcomes in both residential and outpatient treatment settings for women [66]. Others showed that gender in itself is not a predictor of return to drinking following inpatient alcohol treatment; however, co-occurring major depressive disorder predicted decreased time to first drink following treatment and women had twice the risk of having major depression [67]. The authors concluded that untreated co-occurring major depression is a risk for relapse following alcohol treatment and that this risk is important for women given the increased prevalence rate compared with men. A 2012 study of cognitive behavioral therapy for SUDs noted poorer outcomes in women with a diagnosis of a current or lifetime anxiety disorder [68]. Interestingly, another study has shown that women with high levels of depression in an intensive case management model of treatment were more likely to engage in treatment and had fewer drinking days in a 24-month follow-up period than those in usual care [69].

Post-Traumatic Stress Disorder (PTSD) and Trauma

Chronic traumatic stress is a vulnerability factor for developing a substance use disorder. Reviews of the literature estimate the rates of co-occurring PTSD and SUD ranging from 14% to 60% [70–72]. There are several prospective studies examining the link between childhood sexual abuse and development of a substance use disorder later in life. One co-twin study concluded that childhood sexual abuse is associated with an increased risk of psychiatric co-morbidity including substance use disorder [73]. Another study showed that women with a history of having a violent partner have worse treatment outcomes [66]. Another study found that sexual abuse history was associated with shorter times to first drink and relapse. While women were more likely than men to have this history, there was no gender difference in the negative association between this history and women and men's treatment outcomes. In addition, after controlling for associated other baseline characteristics such as lower education, unemployment, depression diagnosis or other co-occurring disorder, and unmarried status, the association of sexual abuse history and treatment outcomes were no longer significant [74].

There is an overall convergence of data demonstrating that PTSD and SUD treatment should be integrated rather than sequential. Seeking Safety is a group therapy for women with PTSD and SUD [75]. The largest multi-site randomized trial of Seeking Safety versus Women's Health Education showed improvement in PTSD symptoms, but not in outcomes for SUDs. A secondary analysis of these data showed that reduction in severity of PTSD symptoms was associated with subsequent improved outcomes for substance use. This study concluded that trauma-informed treatment was superior in this sub-population [76, 77]. Results from the Women, Co-occurring Disorders and Violence Study (WCDVS) showed that comprehensive, trauma-informed, integrated services providing treatment to women with co-occurring substance use, psychiatric disorders, and victimization was successful in improving outcomes in both PTSD symptoms and alcohol and drug use at the 6-month follow-up [78]. At the 12-month follow-up, no effect was found for the improvement of substance use disorder symptoms, but a small effect on improvement of mental health symptoms [79]. A 2015 systematic review concluded that individual trauma-focused interventions alongside substance use treatment is beneficial in decreasing symptoms of both PTSD and substance use disorder [80]. Furthermore, randomized controlled trials with increased sample sizes that focus particular attention to specific characteristics of these integrated programs (i.e., incorporating understudied evidence-based treatments, innovative ways to engage patients, etc.) are necessary to determine the effectiveness of integrated versus non-integrative treatment as the current state of the literature is limited [81].

A 2005 review by Hien et al. detailed the literature on the connections between victimization, PTSD, and substance use disorder and specific approaches to further our understanding of the pathway from early trauma to development of a SUD. This review highlighted the "self-medication model" which suggests that some patients with PTSD use substances to avoid or manage distressing symptoms and to relieve painful emotions and intolerable physical sensations [72].

Eating Disorders

There is a high rate of co-morbidity between substance use and eating disorders, namely bulimia nervosa or anorexia nervosa binge/purge type but not restricting type. A 2003 review considered studies looking at these co-occurring diagnoses and identified interesting patterns. Studies of women in treatment for SUDs were found to have a higher than expected rate of eating disorders with binge/purging behaviors while men had a much lower rate. While eating disorders are more prevalent in women, the rate found in the population with co-occurring substance use was significantly higher than that in the general population. Other studies looked at additional co-occurring diagnosis such as borderline personality disorder and/or affective disorders and sought to identify causal relationships without clear success. One highlighted finding was that patients' frequency of laxative abuse was strongly associated with a co-occurring substance use disorder. The association between these disorders suggests that clinicians managing these related conditions should be well-versed in treatment of substance use disorder [82, 83]. A 2010 study by Cohen et al. examined binge eating symptoms in a group of women in a treatment study for co-occurring PTSD and SUDs. They found the group with these co-occurring binge eating symptoms had significantly less improvement. The authors proposed that screening for symptoms of binge eating may help tailor treatment interventions and ultimately enhance outcomes in this population [84].

ADHD

Co-occurring ADHD with substance use disorder is a significant issue for both genders. Prospective studies have shown that having ADHD increases risk up to five-fold for developing a substance use disorder, and that risk may be higher in women than men [85]. Women were found to have other co-morbidities which may have been confounders and were also found to have other factors that were contributors to worse outcomes such as higher risk for developing schizophrenia, admission to an inpatient unit, increased mortality, and being more likely to be perceived as less impaired [85, 86].

While the literature focused on co-occurring disorders has increased over the past three decades, there is still much work to be done to determine directionality and relationships among SUDs and other psychiatric co-morbidities. Identifying factors that predict specific treatment outcomes, including functional outcomes, for both women as well as men, could identify potential targets for treatment development to improve outcomes for women in treatment of SUDs.

Treatment Outcomes and Predictors for Women with Substance Use Disorders

The growing literature and awareness of gender differences in SUDs has led to a change in terminology in more recent years. In the 1990s the term "gender-responsive" emerged and is defined as treatment that addresses issues specific to women that may affect their treatment outcomes such as co-occurring disorders, exposure to trauma, relationships and responsibilities to children and intimate partners, and physical health issues, among others [87].

Two reviews published in 2017 on treatment outcomes for women with SUDs and sex and gender differences in SUDs by Sugarman et al. and McHugh et al., respectively, built upon a 2007 comprehensive review by Greenfield et al. and identified a growing literature noting gender as a key factor in study design, analysis, and reporting [57, 63, 88]. These reviews summarize the converging evidence that women are less likely to enter substance use treatment than their male counterparts, but once in treatment, that gender alone is not a predictor of outcome. They noted several gender-specific factors that did predict outcomes and found that treatments addressing these factors (e.g., co-occurring disorders, victimization in childhood and adulthood, responsibilities in caring for children, lack of financial and other resources, fear of discrimination and stigma, among others) showed greater success. These reviews specifically discussed findings focused on treatment, including gender-specific treatment (women-only treatment programs). Although certain outcomes were not necessarily improved, many studies identified improvements in women's experience of and attitudes toward treatment [63, 89]. This is important, because substance use treatment is underutilized by women and more recent population-based studies identified that women with AUD are more likely to perceive stigma as a barrier to treatment [90, 91]. Treatments that improve satisfaction and acceptability may also improve utilization.

Studies that have looked at the effect of having a partner with alcohol misuse or AUD on outcomes for women's substance abuse have identified vulnerabilities for women. Dawson et al. published the results of a large retrospective, cross-sectional study from NESARC data in 2007, indicating that having a partner with alcohol problems left women more likely to experience victimization, injury, mood and anxiety disorders, and worse health outcomes than women whose partners didn't have problems with alcohol [92]. In addition, the ways in which people are introduced to substances varies by gender, with women more likely to be introduced by a male partner and men more likely to be introduced by a friend [93].

Although there is variability among studies of gender differences in SUD treatment outcomes, most recent large-scale randomized controlled trials have noted no significant gender differences in main treatment outcomes. This includes two large randomized trials of pharmacotherapy for alcohol and prescription opioid dependence [61, 94]. However, investigators also point out that analyses for subgroups may show gender differences and that large RCTs rarely look at other outcomes such as functional status, which varies by gender [61].

Clinicians should know that important gender differences have been documented in treatment outcomes for nicotine dependence. Effectiveness of nicotine replacement is greater in men than in women, but effectiveness of treatment outcomes with bupropion and varenicline is greater in women than men [15, 37, 95]. A meta-analysis of randomized clinical trials of tobacco cessation noted better outcomes in smoking cessation in women versus men demonstrating that varenicline is 46% more efficacious for women at the end of treatment and 34% more effective 6 months post-treatment compared with men [96], whereas a 2008 study showed the transdermal patch to be 40% more effective in men than women [97]. Another study showed that decreasing nicotine in cigarettes was more effective for women than men in achieving abstinence [98]. A larger metanalysis revealed comparable efficacy of varenicline versus placebo in men and women, but women had greater benefits to varenicline compared to transdermal nicotine replacement and bupropion [95]. Significant gender differences have not been consistently demonstrated in other pharmacotherapies such as naltrexone, disulfiram, buprenorphine, or methadone for treatment of SUDs.

Several studies from the early 2000s identified gender differences in outcomes for treatment in AUD. One prospective study by Timko et al. published in 2006 examined factors in 16-year mortality for patients initiating help-seeking treatment for AUD (47% women). This study revealed several factors that predicted a higher likelihood of death, which included being older and unmarried, and having greater symptoms of alcohol dependence at baseline. They found that patients who had better 1-year drinking outcomes paired with either a shorter duration of inpatient/residential care or a longer duration of outpatient level care or Alcoholics Anonymous attendance were less likely to die in the following 16-year period. They concluded that future efforts should be made to help identify those who are not responding positively to short-term care and focus on motivation for longer-term outpatient or AA participation [99]. Another study by Satre et al. published in 2007 showed better 7-year addiction treatment outcomes for older women than men, with 76% of older women reporting 30-day abstinence compared to 54% of older men. They found that longer treatment lengths of stay predicted abstinence more significantly than gender [100].

Because of known gender differences in baseline clinical characteristics and treatment outcomes, gender-specific treatment programming for women has been a focus of investigation. Multiple reviews have focused on characteristics and components of women's SUD treatment programs and have noted that many provided specific services for domestic violence, pregnancy and post-partum issues, childcare, as well as opportunities for children to co-reside with women in residential treatment [101–103]. The 2008 review by Grella details multiple approaches such as empowerment and supportive models, trauma-informed models, and models attending to co-occurring disorders and social issues common to women [101]. This review and two others [102, 103] identified and summarized common factors that were related to successful treatment outcomes across 35 and 38 studies, respectively, of SUD treatment for women. Among the factors identified were: child care, prenatal care, women-only program composition, supplemental services and workshops that address women-focused topics, mental health services and case management, and comprehensive programming including provision of individual counseling [102, 103]. It also identified shortcomings of the studies reviewed including lack of standardized measures, randomized assignment to conditions, consistent outcomes and measures, and thorough statistical analysis, among others [101]. More recently, the Substance Abuse and Mental Health Services Administration (SAMHSA) provided guidance on gender-responsive components of care for mixed-gender SUD treatment programs [104].

Gender-specific treatments have also been identified that have resulted in decreased utilization of mental health services, criminal activity, and incarceration [105]. Other studies of specific sub-populations such as mothers and children [106] and women with co-occurring psychiatric disorders such as Borderline Personality Disorder [107], and PTSD [75, 77], and women in the criminal justice system [108, 109] have all demonstrated better outcomes for gender-specific treatments.

Another treatment developed specifically for women with SUDs is the Women's Recovery Group (WRG), which is an empirically supported manualized, gender-specific group therapy that when delivered in a closed-group format showed better outcomes at 6-months post-treatment compared with mixed-gender group therapy [110]. A larger randomized trial implemented in community treatment with rolling group format (i.e., open admissions) showed clinically meaningful reduction in substance use during and 6 months after treatment, which was as effective as mixed-gender treatment [111]. In addition, women who experienced the highest level of group affiliation in the WRG group had superior treatment outcomes compared with other women in the study [112]. Other important outcomes such as greater satisfaction with treatment, enhanced comfort and feelings of safety, and increased continuity of care following discharge have been identified in the WRG treatment [89, 113, 114] and in other women-only treatments [115]. Seeking Safety targeting co-occurring PTSD and SUDs [75] has been studied in multi-site trials which have shown reduction in PTSD symptoms in particular although reductions in substance were not necessarily superior to the control condition [77].

Section 2: Substance Use in Women Physicians

Overview

Women physicians are vulnerable to SUDs, as are women in the general population; however, many questions characterizing this vulnerability remain [116]. The prevalence of SUDs in female physicians is increasing, and patterns specific to substance use among women physicians are emerging. Compared with their male physician colleagues, a lower percentage of female physicians present for substance use treatment. When they do present, they do so at a younger average age and they have higher rates of co-occurring psychiatric disorders [117]. At treatment presentation, either for primary psychiatric or substance use issues, they are more willing to engage in voluntary treatment and some evidence shows increased rates of sustained abstinence following treatment [118].

What has not yet been well-studied is the specific experience of women physicians who develop a substance use disorder (SUD). What are the problems they present with medically, psychiatrically, and psychosocially? Does a medical school education and career as a physician protect females against certain experiences or experiences that co-occur with addiction such as intimate partner violence or, or does this make them more vulnerable given the high demands on multiple fronts (challenges in the workplace and at home)? Is it more difficult for them to seek treatment and what might be potential barriers? When women physicians do seek treatment, what is the type and quality of treatment that they receive? Are they more or less successful in treatment and what are the factors that predict this? There is a growing body of research investigating these questions for women in the general population, but less is available for the specific population of women physicians. In 2015, women were 34% of the physician work force but a 2018 survey demonstrated that 60% of physicians under age 35 are women [119]. Because there are and will continue to be an increasing number of women in the physician workforce [120], with this growth will come the statistical likelihood of a higher prevalence of SUDs in this population and a greater demand for answers to these questions in order to more effectively address the treatment needs of women physicians with SUDs.

Epidemiology

Data used to estimate the prevalence of SUDs in female physicians has been sparse and inconsistent since initial studies were published on physicians with SUDs in the 1980s. Prior to this time, publications commenting on this were made without reference to data and thus accurate prevalence of substance use in the physician population was uncertain. Since the 1980s multiple studies estimating prevalence have been published [117, 121–124]. Results are limited by inconsistent definitions of substance use, "abuse," and identification of substance-related consequences and health harms as self-reported by physicians or detected by their treating clinicians. Few studies used any standardized measures of substance use disorder or included control groups for comparison. The early consensus hypothesis was that prevalence of SUDs among physicians might not differ from the rest of the population [125].

Multiple studies have looked at groups of physicians who receive treatment for SUDs in various treatment settings and had either a primary diagnosis of a substance use disorder or a primary diagnosis of co-occurring psychiatric disorder. Characteristics of physicians in specialized treatment for SUDs during the 1980s and 1990s identified an increasing number of female physicians receiving care over time (13.7% in the 1990s versus 8.9% in the 1980s), which may reflect the growth of women in the physician workforce during this time interval rather than any absolute increase in SUD prevalence among female physicians.

Most recently, in 2012, a cross-sectional study of 7,197 individuals estimated the prevalence of AUD among US surgeons to be 15.4% [123]. Of significance, this study identified a concerning gap between male and female prevalence of AUD of 13.9% in male surgeons and 25.6% in female surgeons. The prevalence of AUD in female surgeons exceeded the prevalence of all SUDs in the general population at the time (9.4%) and certainly differed by gender in the general population where males were twice as likely as females to have met criteria for AUD in the year prior (10.5% versus 5.1%) [123], demonstrating a five-fold greater prevalence of AUD in female surgeons compared to women in the general population.

A follow-up cross-sectional study in 2015, inclusive of all US physicians ($n = 7288$ with a 27% response rate), identified a prevalence of AUD of 15.3%, with similar findings of differences between male and female physicians (12.9% male versus 21.4% female) (See Fig. 13.3) [124]. This study demonstrates a female-to-male ratio of AUD of 1.7:1 among physicians, nearly the inverse of the general population male-to-female ratio for AUD of 2.1:1. Put another way, women physicians may be 4 times as

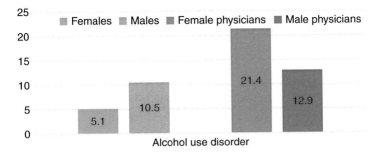

Fig. 13.3 Estimates of prevalence for AUD in physicians versus the general population, by gender. (Data from Oreskovich et al. [124])

likely to have AUD than women in the general population (21.4% versus 5.1%).

Data on prevalence of SUDs other than alcohol in physicians is sparse, and most come from studies of physicians in treatment, or at the entry into treatment. In a 1995 study of 92 physicians admitted to a psychiatric hospital (16 of whom were female), the pattern and type of substance use varied by gender. Of those patients admitted with substance use disorder, 54% of male physicians had AUD compared to 14% of female physicians, whereas sedative hypnotic use disorder was present for 43% of female physicians and 15% of male physicians. In addition, it was also found that female physicians were more likely to have opioid use disorders than male physicians (29% and 19%, respectively). Stimulant use disorders were found to be roughly equal in both genders (%) [117].

Most recent studies conclude that substance use disorders in physicians are not as common as previously thought. Of those reporting use of other substances with alcohol, cannabis was the highest reported at 2.7%. Additionally, only 1.3% of respondent physicians reported either illicit or improper use of prescribed opioids [124]. There has been no recent epidemiological data reporting on the misuse of other substances, including sedative/ hypnotics or stimulants, in the physician population.

Characteristics of Women Physicians with Substance Use Disorders

There are several common characteristics noted for women physicians with SUDs including co-occurring disorders/psychiatric symptoms, patterns of substance use, and characteristics of treatments. Characteristics such as burnout, quality of life rating, and relationship status have been found to be associated with SUDs in physicians but have not yet been looked at in women physicians specifically with further detailed analyses or in larger data sets. Perhaps this is due to limitations in the number of women physicians in treatment, or the general lack of data on physicians with SUDs in general. Given data that supports the increasing number of women, both affected by SUDs and participating in physician treatment programs, the characteristics specific to all physicians with SUDs will be summarized and the gap in analysis by gender noted in order to promote further investigation and gender-specific analyses of past and future data.

Co-occurring Disorders and Psychiatric Symptoms

Multiple small studies from the 1990s found physicians with SUDs to have a high prevalence of mood disorders (major depressive disorder, bipolar disorder, and dysthymic disorder) and personality disorders (narcissistic, dependent, mixed/atypical, antisocial) as is consistent with the general population of individuals with SUDs who also have a higher prevalence of these disorders than individuals without SUDs. Regardless of the primary diagnosis on admission to a private inpatient psychiatric facility (primary substance versus primary axis I psychiatric diagnosis), one study found around 90% of physicians admitted were given a diagnosis of an affective illness. In addition, 59% of physicians were diagnosed with personality disorders (most commonly obsessive-compulsive personality disorder and personality disorder, not otherwise specified, less commonly cluster B personality disorders such as narcissistic personality disorder, borderline personality disorder, and antisocial personality disorder). These data were not reported by gender [117].

An interview study from the 1980s entitled One Hundred Alcoholic Women in Medicine interviewed women physicians (and five medical students) who were self-described alcoholics, active in Alcoholics Anonymous, and reported at least 1 year of sobriety. Seventy-three percent of those interviewed reported serious suicidal ideation prior to achieving sobriety, and 26% reported this continued after sobriety. Thirty-four women reported serious suicide attempts (twice as many as their male counterparts). The group of women who reported a history of addiction to narcotics were more likely to report a suicide attempt. Thirty-three subjects reported a serious overdose with a sedative drug other than alcohol [126].

Since the 1980s, epidemiological data has remained consistent regarding the prevalence of mood or anxiety disorders in females in the general population. The prevalence among female physicians remains consistent with the general population and is almost twice that of males [127].

One of the first studies to extensively review the limited literature on female physicians and addiction was a 2007 study of 969 "impaired" physicians, 125 of whom were female. This study revealed that female physicians with substance use disorder who were entering treatment had more co-occurring psychiatric and medical problems, were more likely to report past or current suicidal ideation, and were five times more likely to have had a suicide attempt under the influence and ten times more likely to have had a suicide attempt not under the influence of substances [116].

Patterns of Substance Use

In the 2015 study of 7288 US physicians, those who had AUD were not very likely to abuse either prescription drugs or other illicit substances. Cannabis was the most common co-occurring substance present (2.7%) and 1.3% of physicians acknowledged misuse of opioids either illicitly or as misuse of a medication prescribed to them. The more specific data in this study were not reported by gender [124]. Earlier studies identified alcohol as the consistent primary substance in physicians with substance use disorder, although polysubstance use with opioids is reported to have increased since at least the 1980s [122].

The 2007 study of women physicians and addiction reported that although alcohol was the primary substance of abuse for all physicians, female physicians were twice as likely to abuse sedative hypnotics than their male physician colleagues [116].

One earlier study by Nace and colleagues of 92 physicians entering treatment showed female physicians to be younger by 5 years (on average) than male physicians when entering treatment [117]. They were much less likely to have had prior treatment, and their length of stay was longer. In contrast to the study of surgeons and the national study of all physicians, in this treatment study, women physicians were found to be less likely to have AUD (14% versus 49%), and much more likely to be diagnosed with sedative/hypnotic use disorder than males (43% to 15%). The same study also showed females to be more likely to have opioid use disorder (29% versus 19%). This study had a small sample, and may not be representative of all physicians presenting for treatment. Nevertheless, lifetime rates of prescriptions of sedative hypnotics and opioids are higher for women than men in the general population [128].

The interview study, One Hundred Alcoholic Women in Medicine, revealed that only 40% were addicted to alcohol alone and abuse of other drugs was common [126]. Reporting in this study was individual, and subjects who reported having an "addiction" to a substance were taken at their word, though efforts were made to discriminate between use of the drug and addiction where there was uncertainty. Thirty percent of women interviewed reported addiction to cannabis. Eighteen of the 100 women reported ever injecting narcotics, while 13 reported having been addicted. Twenty-eight of the 100 interviewees had tried cocaine and 10 reported addiction, while 14 reported history of addiction to oral narcotics. Of the 75% of women who had been regular cigarette smokers, 50% had stopped smoking at the time of the interview. This study also highlighted that marital instability was common and many reported multiple marriages, divorce, and involvement with alcoholic men as well as children who were alcoholics. More than half of the women identified at least one alcoholic parent and 52% of those with siblings identified at least one alcoholic sibling. Many women reported that drugs of abuse were obtained from work, while several reported being given medication by physician-husbands, and two reported becoming addicted after being given drugs in childhood by their physician fathers.

This 1987 study was among the only one found to have studied the prevalence of domestic violence in this population. Twenty-two women physicians reported they had been physically assaulted (though rarely shared with anyone or sought help via law enforcement or other supports). Twenty-one women reported they had beaten spouses, lovers, fathers, and one reported having beaten her grown son. Two women reported being strangled by their husbands, one woman reported having choked her lover, with these episodes happening infrequently and usually when drugs or alcohol were involved. Thirty-eight women reported histories of emotional abuse, while 20 reported histories of physical and/or sexual abuse [126].

Patterns in Treatment and Treatment Outcomes

The first Physician Health Programs were developed in the 1970s to target SUDs in physicians with a goal of preventing poor outcomes in patient care related to psychiatric and SUDs in physicians. Physicians are usually referred to programs by colleagues or regulatory agencies, and enrollment includes formal acknowledgement of impairment and acceptance of a treatment contract with highly structured monitoring. Outcomes of these programs are relatively well studied and thought to have about a 75% rate of favorable outcome defined by completion of treatment and resumption of practicing under supervision and follow-up testing [129]. These physician health programs are available in some states but not all, and they do not provide treatment services; rather, physician health programs contract with or provide referrals to treatment, including 60–90 day residential treatment followed by outpatient treatment with prolonged oversight and monitoring [130]. Less is known about the specific curricula in participating programs and whether there is inclusion of any gender-specific treatment offered to either female or male physicians participating, but most treatment centers offer a version of a comprehensive evaluation, individual and group treatment, family involvement, and a component of long-term monitoring, although they vary state-to-state.

Female physicians may receive treatment for SUDs in a psychiatric setting as demonstrated in one study that found it was more common for female physicians to be admitted primarily for psychiatric symptoms (63%) than primarily for substance use problems (37%). By contrast, in male physicians this percentage was reversed (61% substance use versus 39% psychiatric) [117]. A more recent study found that compared with male physicians, female physicians with SUDs were younger on admission to treatment programs, more likely to be admitted for a primary psychiatric disorder, more likely to be self-referred, and may be better able to sustain abstinence from substances following treatment [127].

Qualitative studies such as "One Hundred Alcoholic Women in Medicine" study highlight the different paths that these patients take that are potentially being missed in more recent studies done only in treatment settings. This study showed that many achieved abstinence through AA alone (21%) whereas others sought longer-term residential treatment (23%) and most did not get to treatment via therapist referral or intervention by impaired-physician committees. A total of 72% reported receiving some kind of treatment for their substance use whether medical or psychiatric, but many described difficulty accessing treatment and delayed referrals from providers. It should be also noted that these women were asked if, retrospectively, they believed they would have benefited from gender-specific treatment for their substance use disorder. Many commented that they would have preferred or benefited from a completely female treatment or at least gender-based component, but also noted that at the time they may have needed some convincing to participate [126]. It is important to note that at the time of this study, pharmacotherapy for AUDs consisted only of disulfiram while current practice includes other approved medications such as naltrexone and acamprosate. Medication treatment for AUD was therefore not included in these earlier studies.

A newer pilot study examined treatment experiences of 73 physicians (10 female and 63 male) and found that post-treatment, women were more likely to use marital/family/and individual psychotherapy treatment modalities and were less likely to have been previously psychiatrically hospitalized. The authors identified the issue of access to treatment and that it varies both in likelihood of presenting for treatment (women are less likely) and by precipitant (women present voluntarily and for more subjective distress whereas men present more often from work-related referrals). The authors also discussed that women may be more private in their substance use (e.g., using alone rather than in social settings) and therefore may be less likely to come to the attention of others [131]. The fact that fewer female physicians present for SUD treatment yet have a higher prevalence of the illness in the population is concerning. It highlights the need for a multipronged approach to promote female physician wellness (while at the same time decreasing judgment and stigma), as well as improving policies for full and partial medical leaves and coverage when female physicians are faced with challenges such as these. Despite the differences described in addiction treatment between male and female physicians, it has generally been shown that once in treatment, outcomes for both genders were positive and similar [131].

Physician Specialty

Rates of AUD have been shown to vary by specialty. Dermatology, orthopedic surgery, and emergency medicine physicians showed higher rates of AUD, while pediatricians and neurologists were among those specialties with the lowest rates [124].

A 2016 chart review of physicians being treated in physician health programs for SUDs found that alcohol use was highest in surgeons, while rates of any opioid use with or without alcohol as well as rates of non-opioid drug use was highest in family practice physicians. This study also found histories of intravenous drug use to be highest in anesthesiologists compared with other specialties [132].

An older, small study of physicians in treatment for substance use disorder found the specialties of physicians to vary by gender. The specialties of female physicians in treatment were representative of US physicians, but specialties of male physicians in treatment for SUDs were over-represented by family practice, emergency medicine, and psychiatry [118].

Section 3: Substance Use and Relationship with Burnout in Women Physicians

Physician Burnout and Substance Use Disorders

Professional burnout is gaining visibility as a major issue for US physicians and has received increased attention in recent years with more research focused on understanding etiology as well as prevention and treatment. In 2012, a large study revealed high rates of burnout in US physicians, and a follow-up study in 2015 showed worsening of burnout through 2014 and that nearly half of US physicians reported experiencing professional burnout [133, 134]. The Maslach Burnout Inventory-Human Services Survey (MBI-HSS), which measures emotional exhaustion, depersonalization, and perceptions of personal accomplishment, is the tool typically used to assess burnout. High levels of burnout are also thought to amplify physicians' individual vulnerabilities, which may present as mental health symptoms, substance use problems, and worsening medical issues, among others.

In the 2012 study of 7,197 US surgeons and the 2015 follow-up study of 7,288 US physicians, alcohol abuse/dependence was shown to be strongly associated with female gender, high levels of burnout, co-occurring depression, and poor rating on quality of life scales. In addition to female gender, alcohol abuse/dependence was more likely in those physicians who were younger and in a current relationship. For those with alcohol abuse or dependence who were in a relationship, it was more common for the physician to report dissatisfaction with the relationship and also report having no children. The fewer years in practice, the more likely the physician was to report AUD. Physicians with AUD were more likely to be working 40–60 hours per week [123].

These studies also report a significant relationship between depression, burnout, suicidal ideation, quality of life, and career satisfaction. Physicians who screened positive for AUD more commonly reported burnout, positive screening for depression, and lower quality of life. In terms of burnout, they more commonly reported emotional exhaustion and depersonalization, and also were more likely to report that they would not become a physician again if given the choice. More than 8% of physicians with AUD reported they had suicidal ideation in the previous year. This data was not reported by gender [123, 124].

Another recent study on burnout and alcohol abuse/dependence among US medical students concluded that in this population, burnout was also strongly related to alcohol problems, as was depression and low mental and emotional quality of life measures. They also found that increased amount of education debt (>$50,000) was a predictive factor for high risk of AUD. Interestingly, there was no association found between gender and alcohol abuse/dependence in this population of student doctors [135]. Another recent cross-sectional study of 1,841 Danish physicians (4,000 surveys sent, 46% response rate) found a significant association between risky alcohol use and all dimensions of burnout, including emotional exhaustion, depersonalization, and low levels of personal accomplishment [136]. In contrast to the previous studies, one 2011 study of anesthesiologists ($N = 206$) who participated in a webinar and survey did not identify a significant relationship between burnout and substance use [137].

Conclusions and Recommendations

There are important gender differences in SUDs in terms of epidemiology, physiology, co-occurring psychiatric disorders, trauma histories, and treatment preferences. Data suggests an increase in alcohol, cannabis, and opioid use disorders in women in the USA as well as a narrowing gender gap in younger age cohorts. Women physicians reflect a subgroup of the general population and though the prevalence of SUDs in this population is understudied, some studies suggest an alarming increase in SUDs, and especially AUDs, in women physicians.

Physician burnout is associated with depression, exhaustion, depersonalization, lower perceptions of personal accomplishment, and lower ratings of quality of life. AUDs seem among the most prevalent of all substance problems in physicians, perhaps mirroring the prevalence rates of AUD in the general population. Women with alcohol and other SUDs in the general population have twice the prevalence of depression. The co-occurrence of depression and alcohol problems among women presenting for treatment is common and often reflects the use of alcohol by women as a maladaptive coping strategy to manage depression or relieve stress. It would not be surprising if women physicians with burnout experiencing depression and exhaustion were at higher risk for drinking related problems. Additional research in this area would assist in understanding the vulnerabilities of women physicians experiencing burnout to depression, alcohol, and other SUDs.

Among the most important and easily implemented recommendations is a form of regular screening for women physicians for substance use problems. Detecting problems when they are mild allows for effective and less-intensive interventions with excellent potential outcomes. The National Institute on Alcohol Abuse and Alcoholism (NIAAA) *Helping Patients who Drink Too Much: A Clinicians Guide* [138] provides screening tools and approaches to assisting patients in cutting down on their drinking. This Guide uses the 10-question AUDs Identification Test (AUDIT) [139] which is a common screening tool that can be implemented in all health-care settings and detecting the likelihood of mild, moderate, and severe AUDs. Briefer versions of the AUDIT including a one question AUDIT [140] and the 3-question AUDIT-C [141] are also effective at screening for alcohol problems. The 17-question Brief Addiction Monitor (BAM) [142] can be used for screening for alcohol, drugs, and associated problems. The World Health Organization's screening tool for alcohol, drug, and tobacco problems, the ASSIST, is another tool that could be used [143].

For women physicians who screen positive, it will be necessary to provide follow-up assessments to determine whether there is a substance use disorder as well as to assess for other co-occurring psychiatric disorders, especially anxiety and depression, as well as other stressors and life circumstances that may be contributing to the clinical picture.

Conversely, screening for other mental health disorders in female physicians such as depression and anxiety can be useful in assessing physicians who may already be experiencing burnout or are vulnerable to burnout. In addition, those female physicians with depression, anxiety, or other psychiatric disorders are at increased risk for alcohol and other drug use disorders.

Women physicians assessed as having substance and co-occurring other psychiatric disorders will require appropriate access and referral to mental health treatment. Ideally, referrals to providers or groups with specialized training in treatment of physicians with these illnesses might be most helpful. Women physicians may also benefit from gender-specific treatment programs or perhaps mixed-gender programs that focus on physicians and/or other professionals.

Given that women physicians have reported more concern regarding shame and stigma as a barrier to seeking help, it is necessary that these screening and treatment referrals be handled in a confidential manner, with clear outlined goals and benchmarks for measuring substance impairment and ability to continue to care for patients and/or return to work. Many women physicians will likely be seeking help by choice for both a substance use disorder and/or co-occurring disorder (versus coerced/forced treatment by employer due to being in legal trouble, poor outcomes, etc.), so we must provide a comfortable and non-judgmental process for them to do so.

It will be important as the field progresses to work towards development of gender responsive and/or gender-specific treatment for women physicians that addresses both SUDs and also issues of burnout. This might include advocacy programs and/or development of treatment and return-to-work guidelines that can be adopted by administrators who are supporting physicians across the country. Providers treating physicians and physician health programs should pay close attention to physicians treated for burnout and mental health disorders and perform careful psychoeducation and screening for SUDs and vice versa.

Lastly, it is important that we continue to look at gender in physicians as we design studies investigating burnout and associated outcomes, as clear gender differences have been identified. More research is needed to more fully understand processes for prevention as well as the manifestations of burnout. While much of the current research is focused on physician wellness, it is quite clear that there are also gender differences in this area with many contributing factors. Improved study design and efforts to disseminate current information to physicians in programs across the country will likely generate further awareness and spark new program and treatment development as well as opportunities for funding to address and study these large-scale issues.

Follow-Up to Clinical Vignette

At the beginning of this chapter we described Dr. Susan F., a 49 year-old emergency medicine physician, and asked four questions to consider while reading this chapter. Considering each question in turn:

1. What are the stressors contributing to Susan's current mental and emotional state?
    Susan has had a confluence of factors in both the work and personal spheres. At work, changes in her department have increased her stress level. These have happened contemporaneously with important stressors and losses in her personal life including changes from the dissolution of her marriage, the change from living with a spouse to living only with her teenage children, having her first child leave for college, having little adult support at home since her separation, and stress of a parent living at distance with an unstable medical situation.
2. Is Susan having burnout at work? If so, how would you describe?
    Susan is clearly experiencing burnout at work with the triad of depersonalization, exhaustion, and diminished feelings of personal satisfaction and personal accomplishment. She is spending more time managing electronic health records as well as increased demands from her department chair to pro-

vide measures and metrics to demonstrate quality. This has decreased her time doing the two activities that provided her the greatest satisfaction: seeing patients and teaching residents. She leaves work exhausted and irritable each day.

3. What do you think are Susan's likely diagnoses?

It seems that burnout at work and stressors at home are related to the onset of major depressive disorder in which Susan has experienced tiredness, diminished pleasure, difficulty sleeping, low mood, and low energy every day for more than 2 weeks. As a maladaptive coping strategy for her depression, her work burnout, and her home stressors, Susan has tried to relieve these symptoms and internal experiences through the use of alcohol. She has seen her drinking increase from one glass of wine each night to 4–5 glasses each night. This culminated in a black out experience of not remembering her daughter's discussion with her the night before and not showing up for her athletic event. She also has had more difficulty getting out of bed. Susan's drinking has not yet caused problems at work but it has created stress with her daughter who is concerned about her drinking. It has also taken over time that she might have spent pursuing other leisure activities such as exercise, reading, and social engagement with friends. She most likely qualifies for a diagnosis of alcohol use disorder, moderate severity.

4. What are the next steps for intervention for Susan?

It will be important for Susan to see a psychiatrist or other physician or specialist who can perform a comprehensive assessment of her depression and alcohol use disorder as well as any other physical or mental health conditions and provide Susan with accurate diagnoses and a treatment plan. This could include an outpatient detoxification (depending on whether Susan has any signs of physical withdrawal), an intensive outpatient program for alcohol problems, or possibly outpatient psychiatry and therapy. It will be necessary for Susan to have treatment of her depression which could include pharmacotherapy or evidence-based psychotherapies such as cognitive behavioral therapy. Depending on her level of readiness to stop drinking alcohol, she will need an abstinence treatment plan (safest option for her health and recovery) or a drinking risk reduction treatment plan. In either case an alcohol use disorder medication such as naltrexone, a mu-opioid antagonist demonstrated to be effective for both targeted drinking reduction and alcohol abstinence, should be recommended along with counseling to support achieving and maintaining drinking reduction goals. Susan would likely benefit from supportive therapy to examine recent stressors, consider her feelings about the loss of her marriage, and how she can build new adaptive strategies to manage stress. In this setting, she may also examine approaches to work that might give her greater satisfaction. Susan has not had impairment at work as a consequence of either her depression or drinking and at this time does not need a referral to a Physicians Health Service program (if one exists in her state), but her therapist ought to describe this type of program and provide her information regarding how it is used to assist physicians. There may also be physician support groups for burnout, depression, and for substance use disorders including professional-led groups as well as physician or professional focused AA. In addition, women's groups for alcohol abstinence such as women-only AA or professional-led group treatment for women with depression or women with alcohol problems, such as the Women's Recovery Group, may provide Susan with greater support. Another consideration would be whether family therapy with her daughter would be beneficial and whether her daughter might also benefit from having a therapist as she has also had many stressors over the past several years.

References

1. Substance Abuse and Mental Health Services Administration. Key substance use and mental health indicators in the United States: results from the 2017 National Survey on Drug Use and Health (HHS Publication No. SMA 18–5068, NSDUH Series H-53). Rockville: Center for Behavioral Health Statistics and Quality, Substance Abuse and Mental Health Services Administration; 2018.

2. Greenfield SF. Women and alcohol use disorders. Harv Rev Psychiatry. 2002;10:76–85.
3. Grant BF, Chou SP, Saha TD, Pickering RP, Kerridge BT, Ruan WJ, et al. Prevalence of 12-month alcohol use, high-risk drinking, and DSM-IV alcohol use disorder in the United States, 2001–2002 to 2012–2013: results from the National Epidemiologic Survey on alcohol and related conditions. JAMA Psychiat. 2017;74(9):911–23.
4. SAMHSA. Overview of findings from the 2017 National Survey on drug use and health. SAMHSA, Center for Behavioral Health Statistics and Quality: Rockville; 2017.
5. Johnston LD, Miech RA, O'Malley PM, Bachman JG, Schulenberg JE, Patrick ME. Monitoring the future national survey results on drug use: 1975–2017: overview, key findings on adolescent drug use. Ann Arbor: Institute for Social Research, The University of Michigan; 2018.
6. Grucza RA, Bucholz KK, Rice JP, Bierut LJ. Secular trends in the lifetime prevalence of alcohol dependence in the United States: a re-evaluation. Alcohol Clin Exp Res. 2008;32(5):763–70.
7. Centers for Disease Control and Prevention. Vital signs: binge drinking among women and high school girls — United States, 2011. MMWR. 2013;62(1):9–13.
8. Centers for Disease Control and Prevention. Vital signs: binge drinking: a serious, under-recognized problem among women and girls: Centers for Disease Control and Prevention, National Center for Chronic Disease Prevention and Health Promotion, Division of Population Health; United States, 2013.
9. Doycheva I, Watt KD, Rifai G, Abou Mrad R, Lopez R, Zein NN, et al. Increasing burden of chronic liver disease among adolescents and young adults in the USA: a silent epidemic. Dig Dis Sci. 2017;62(5):1373–80.
10. Yoon YHC, C. M. Surveillance report #111: liver cirrhosis mortality in the United States: national, state and regional trends, 2000–2015. National Institue on Alcohol Abuse and Alcoholism, Services USDoHaH: Arlington; 2018.
11. Grucza RA, Sher KJ, Kerr WC, Krauss MJ, Lui CK, McDowell YE, et al. Trends in adult alcohol use and binge drinking in the early 21st-century United States: a meta-analysis of 6 National Survey Series. Alcohol Clin Exp Res. 2018;42(10):1939–50.
12. John WS, Wu LT. Trends and correlates of cocaine use and cocaine use disorder in the United States from 2011 to 2015. Drug Alcohol Depend. 2017;180:376–84.
13. Han MK, Postma D, Mannino DM, Giardino ND, Buist S, Curtis JL, et al. Gender and chronic obstructive pulmonary disease: why it matters. Am J Respir Crit Care Med. 2007;176(12):1179–84.
14. Maas AH, Appelman YE. Gender differences in coronary heart disease. Netherlands Heart J. 2010;18(12):598–602.

15. Greenfield SF, Back SE, Lawson K, Brady KT. Substance abuse in women. Psychiatr Clin North Am. 2010;33(2):339–55.
16. McKee SA, O'Malley SS, Salovey P, Krishnan-Sarin S, Mazure CM. Perceived risks and benefits of smoking cessation: gender-specific predictors of motivation and treatment outcome. Addict Behav. 2005;30(3):423–35.
17. Goodwin RD, Pacek LR, Copeland J, Moeller SJ, Dierker L, Weinberger A, et al. Trends in daily cannabis use among cigarette smokers: United States, 2002–2014. Am J Public Health. 2018;108(1):137–42.
18. Cicero TJ, Ellis MS, Surratt HL, Kurtz SP. The changing face of heroin use in the United States: a retrospective analysis of the past 50 years. JAMA Psychiat. 2014;71(7):821–6.
19. Marsh JC, Park K, Lin YA, Bersamira C. Gender differences in trends for heroin use and nonmedical prescription opioid use, 2007–2014. J Subst Abus Treat. 2018;87:79–85.
20. Jones CM. The paradox of decreasing nonmedical opioid analgesic use and increasing abuse or dependence – an assessment of demographic and substance use trends, United States, 2003–2014. Addict Behav. 2017;65:229–35.
21. Mack KA, Jones CM, Paulozzi LJ. Vital signs: overdoses of prescription opioid pain relievers and other drugs among women–United States, 1999–2010. MMWR Morb Mortal Wkly Rep. 2013;62(26):537–42.
22. VanHouten JP, Rudd RA, Ballesteros MF, Mack KA. Drug overdose deaths among women aged 30–64 years – United States, 1999–2017. MMWR Morb Mortal Wkly Rep. 2019;68(1):1–5.
23. Sumner SA, Mercado-Crespo MC, Spelke MB, Paulozzi L, Sugerman DE, Hillis SD, et al. Use of naloxone by emergency medical services during opioid drug overdose resuscitation efforts. Prehosp Emerg Care. 2016;20(2):220–5.
24. Becker JB, Perry AN, Westenbroek C. Sex differences in the neural mechanisms mediating addiction: a new synthesis and hypothesis. Biol Sex Differ. 2012;3(1):14.
25. Bobzean SA, DeNobrega AK, Perrotti LI. Sex differences in the neurobiology of drug addiction. Exp Neurol. 2014;259:64–74.
26. Becker JB, Hu M. Sex differences in drug abuse. Front Neuroendocrinol. 2008;29(1):36–47.
27. Lenz B, Muller CP, Stoessel C, Sperling W, Biermann T, Hillemacher T, et al. Sex hormone activity in alcohol addiction: integrating organizational and activational effects. Prog Neurobiol. 2012;96(1):136–63.
28. Martin CA, Mainous AG 3rd, Curry T, Martin D. Alcohol use in adolescent females: correlates with estradiol and testosterone. Am J Addict. 1999;8(1):9–14.
29. Chrostek L, Jelski W, Szmitkowski M, Puchalski Z. Gender-related differences in hepatic activity of alcohol dehydrogenase isoenzymes and aldehyde dehydrogenase in humans. J Clin Lab Anal. 2003;17(3):93–6.

30. Marshall AW, Kingstone D, Boss M, Morgan MY. Ethanol elimination in males and females: relationship to menstrual cycle and body composition. Hepatology (Baltimore, Md). 1983;3(5):701–6.
31. Nolen-Hoeksema S, Hilt L. Possible contributors to the gender differences in alcohol use and problems. J Gen Psychol. 2006;133(4): 357–74.
32. Mann K, Ackermann K, Croissant B, Mundle G, Nakovics H, Diehl A. Neuroimaging of gender differences in alcohol dependence: are women more vulnerable? Alcohol Clin Exp Res. 2005;29(5):896–901.
33. Caldwell LC, Schweinsburg AD, Nagel BJ, Barlett VC, Brown SA, Tapert SF. Gender and adolescent alcohol use disorders on BOLD (blood oxygen level dependent) response to spatial working memory. Alcohol Alcohol (Oxford, Oxfordshire). 2005;40(3):194–200.
34. Agabio R, Campesi I, Pisanu C, Gessa GL, Franconi F. Sex differences in substance use disorders: focus on side effects. Addict Biol. 2016;21(5):1030–42.
35. Arndt JT, Rohsenow DJ, Almeida AB, Hunt SK, Gokhale M, Gottlieb DJ, et al. Sleep following alcohol intoxication in healthy, young adults: effects of sex and family history of alcoholism. Alcohol Clin Exp Res. 2011;35(5):870–8.
36. Benowitz NL, Lessov-Schlaggar CN, Swan GE, Jacob P 3rd. Female sex and oral contraceptive use accelerate nicotine metabolism. Clin Pharmacol Ther. 2006;79(5):480–8.
37. Weinberger AH, Smith PH, Kaufman M, McKee SA. Consideration of sex in clinical trials of transdermal nicotine patch: a systematic review. Exp Clin Psychopharmacol. 2014;22(5):373–83.
38. Roche DJ, King AC. Sex differences in acute hormonal and subjective response to naltrexone: the impact of menstrual cycle phase. Psychoneuroendocrinology. 2015;52:59–71.
39. Moody DE, Fang WB, Morrison J, McCance-Katz E. Gender differences in pharmacokinetics of maintenance dosed buprenorphine. Drug Alcohol Depend. 2011;118(2–3):479–83.
40. Evans SM, Haney M, Foltin RW. The effects of smoked cocaine during the follicular and luteal phases of the menstrual cycle in women. Psychopharmacology. 2002;159(4):397–406.
41. Justice AJ, de Wit H. Acute effects of d-amphetamine during the follicular and luteal phases of the menstrual cycle in women. Psychopharmacology. 1999;145(1):67–75.
42. Holdstock L, de Wit H. Effects of ethanol at four phases of the menstrual cycle. Psychopharmacology. 2000;150(4):374–82.
43. Terner JM, de Wit H. Menstrual cycle phase and responses to drugs of abuse in humans. Drug Alcohol Depend. 2006;84(1):1–13.
44. Lammers SM, Mainzer DE, Breteler MH. Do alcohol pharmacokinetics in women vary due to the menstrual cycle? Addiction (Abingdon, England). 1995;90(1):23–30.

45. Kouri EM, Lundahl LH, Borden KN, McNeil JF, Lukas SE. Effects of oral contraceptives on acute cocaine response in female volunteers. Pharmacol Biochem Behav. 2002;74(1):173–80.

46. Gray KM, DeSantis SM, Carpenter MJ, Saladin ME, LaRowe SD, Upadhyaya HP. Menstrual cycle and cue reactivity in women smokers. Nicotine Tob Res. 2010;12(2):174–8.

47. Weinberger AH, Smith PH, Allen SS, Cosgrove KP, Saladin ME, Gray KM, et al. Systematic and meta-analytic review of research examining the impact of menstrual cycle phase and ovarian hormones on smoking and cessation. Nicotine Tob Res. 2015;17(4):407–21.

48. Fox HC, Sofuoglu M, Morgan PT, Tuit KL, Sinha R. The effects of exogenous progesterone on drug craving and stress arousal in cocaine dependence: impact of gender and cue type. Psychoneuroendocrinology. 2013;38(9):1532–44.

49. Milivojevic V, Fox HC, Sofuoglu M, Covault J, Sinha R. Effects of progesterone stimulated allopregnanolone on craving and stress response in cocaine dependent men and women. Psychoneuroendocrinology. 2016;65:44–53.

50. Sofuoglu M, Babb DA, Hatsukami DK. Progesterone treatment during the early follicular phase of the menstrual cycle: effects on smoking behavior in women. Pharmacol Biochem Behav. 2001;69(1–2):299–304.

51. Yonkers KA, Forray A, Nich C, Carroll KM, Hine C, Merry BC, et al. Progesterone reduces cocaine use in postpartum women with a cocaine use disorder: a randomized, double-blind study. Lancet Psychiatry. 2014;1(5):360–7.

52. Forray A, Gilstad-Hayden K, Suppies C, Bogen D, Sofuoglu M, Yonkers KA. Progesterone for smoking relapse prevention following delivery: a pilot, randomized, double-blind study. Psychoneuroendocrinology. 2017;86:96–103.

53. Allen SS, Allen AM, Lunos S, Tosun N. Progesterone and postpartum smoking relapse: a pilot double-blind placebo-controlled randomized trial. Nicotine Tob Res. 2016;18(11):2145–53.

54. Becker JB, Koob GF. Sex differences in animal models: focus on addiction. Pharmacol Rev. 2016;68(2):242–63.

55. Brady KT, Randall CL. Gender differences in substance use disorders. Psychiatr Clin N Am. 1999;22(2):241–52.

56. Hernandez-Avila CA, Rounsaville BJ, Kranzler HR. Opioid-, cannabis- and alcohol-dependent women show more rapid progression to substance abuse treatment. Drug Alcohol Depend. 2004;74(3):265–72.

57. McHugh RK, Votaw VR, Sugarman DE, Greenfield SF. Sex and gender differences in substance use disorders. Clin Psychol Rev. 2018;66:12–23.

58. Lopez-Quintero C, Perez de los Cobos J, Hasin DS, Okuda M, Wang S, Grant BF, et al. Probability and predictors of transition from first use to dependence on nicotine, alcohol, cannabis, and cocaine: results of the

National Epidemiologic Survey on alcohol and related conditions (NESARC). Drug Alcohol Depend. 2011;115(1–2):120–30.

59. Florez-Salamanca L, Secades-Villa R, Hasin DS, Cottler L, Wang S, Grant BF, et al. Probability and predictors of transition from abuse to dependence on alcohol, cannabis, and cocaine: results from the National Epidemiologic Survey on alcohol and related conditions. Am J Drug Alcohol Abuse. 2013;39(3):168–79.

60. Wagner FA, Anthony JC. Male-female differences in the risk of progression from first use to dependence upon cannabis, cocaine, and alcohol. Drug Alcohol Depend. 2007;86(2–3):191–8.

61. McHugh RK, Devito EE, Dodd D, Carroll KM, Potter JS, Greenfield SF, et al. Gender differences in a clinical trial for prescription opioid dependence. J Subst Abus Treat. 2013;45(1):38–43.

62. Conway KP, Compton W, Stinson FS, Grant BF. Lifetime comorbidity of DSM-IV mood and anxiety disorders and specific drug use disorders: results from the National Epidemiologic Survey on alcohol and related conditions. J Clin Psychiatry. 2006;67(2):247–57.

63. Greenfield SF, Brooks AJ, Gordon SM, Green CA, Kropp F, McHugh RK, et al. Substance abuse treatment entry, retention, and outcome in women: a review of the literature. Drug Alcohol Depend. 2007; 86(1):1–21.

64. Goldstein RB, Dawson DA, Chou SP, Grant BF. Sex differences in prevalence and comorbidity of alcohol and drug use disorders: results from wave 2 of the national epidemiologic survey on alcohol and related conditions. J Stud Alcohol Drugs. 2012;73(6):938–50.

65. Kuhn C. Emergence of sex differences in the development of substance use and abuse during adolescence. Pharmacol Ther. 2015;153: 55–78.

66. Comfort M, Sockloff A, Loverro J, Kaltenbach K. Multiple predictors of substance-abusing women's treatment and life outcomes: a prospective longitudinal study. Addict Behav. 2003;28(2):199–224.

67. Greenfield SF, Weiss RD, Muenz LR, Vagge LM, Kelly JF, Bello LR, et al. The effect of depression on return to drinking: a prospective study. Arch Gen Psychiatry. 1998;55(3):259–65.

68. Farris SG, Epstein EE, McCrady BS, Hunter-Reel D. Do co-morbid anxiety disorders predict drinking outcomes in women with alcohol use disorders? Alcohol Alcohol (Oxford, Oxfordshire). 2012;47(2): 143–8.

69. Kuerbis AN, Neighbors CJ, Morgenstern J. Depression's moderation of the effectiveness of intensive case management with substance-dependent women on temporary assistance for needy families: outpatient substance use disorder treatment utilization and outcomes. J Stud Alcohol Drugs. 2011;72(2):297–307.

70. Brady KT, Dansky BS, Back SE, Foa EB, Carroll KM. Exposure therapy in the treatment of PTSD among cocaine-dependent individuals: preliminary findings. J Subst Abus Treat. 2001;21(1):47–54.

71. Brady KT, Killeen TK, Brewerton T, Lucerini S. Comorbidity of psychiatric disorders and posttraumatic stress disorder. J Clin Psychiatry. 2000;61(Suppl 7):22–32.

72. Hien D, Cohen L, Campbell A. Is traumatic stress a vulnerability factor for women with substance use disorders? Clin Psychol Rev. 2005;25(6):813–23.

73. Kendler KS, Bulik CM, Silberg J, Hettema JM, Myers J, Prescott CA. Childhood sexual abuse and adult psychiatric and substance use disorders in women: an epidemiological and cotwin control analysis. Arch Gen Psychiatry. 2000;57(10):953–9.

74. Greenfield SF, Kolodziej ME, Weiss RD, Sugarman DE, Vagge LM. History of sexual abuse, sex differences, and drinking outcomes following discharge from inpatient alcohol treatment. Drug Alcohol Depend. 2000;60:S79.

75. Najavits LM, Weiss RD, Shaw SR, Muenz LR. "Seeking safety": outcome of a new cognitive-behavioral psychotherapy for women with posttraumatic stress disorder and substance dependence. J Trauma Stress. 1998;11(3):437–56.

76. Hien DA, Jiang H, Campbell AN, Hu MC, Miele GM, Cohen LR, et al. Do treatment improvements in PTSD severity affect substance use outcomes? A secondary analysis from a randomized clinical trial in NIDA's Clinical Trials Network. Am J Psychiatry. 2010;167(1):95–101.

77. Hien DA, Wells EA, Jiang H, Suarez-Morales L, Campbell AN, Cohen LR, et al. Multisite randomized trial of behavioral interventions for women with co-occurring PTSD and substance use disorders. J Consult Clin Psychol. 2009;77(4):607–19.

78. Cocozza JJ, Jackson EW, Hennigan K, Morrissey JP, Reed BG, Fallot R, et al. Outcomes for women with co-occurring disorders and trauma: program-level effects. J Subst Abus Treat. 2005;28(2):109–19.

79. Morrissey JP, Jackson EW, Ellis AR, Amaro H, Brown VB, Najavits LM. Twelve-month outcomes of trauma-informed interventions for women with co-occurring disorders. Psychiatric Serv (Washington, DC). 2005;56(10):1213–22.

80. Roberts NP, Roberts PA, Jones N, Bisson JI. Psychological interventions for post-traumatic stress disorder and comorbid substance use disorder: a systematic review and meta-analysis. Clin Psychol Rev. 2015;38:25–38.

81. Torchalla I, Nosen L, Rostam H, Allen P. Integrated treatment programs for individuals with concurrent substance use disorders and trauma experiences: a systematic review and meta-analysis. J Subst Abus Treat. 2012;42(1):65–77.

82. Spindler A, Milos G. Links between eating disorder symptom severity and psychiatric comorbidity. Eat Behav. 2007;8(3):364–73.

83. O'Brien KM, Vincent NK. Psychiatric comorbidity in anorexia and bulimia nervosa: nature, prevalence, and causal relationships. Clin Psychol Rev. 2003;23(1):57–74.

84. Cohen LR, Greenfield SF, Gordon S, Killeen T, Jiang H, Zhang Y, et al. Survey of eating disorder symptoms among women in treatment for substance abuse. Am J Addict. 2010;19(3):245–51.

85. Ottosen C, Petersen L, Larsen JT, Dalsgaard S. Gender differences in associations between attention-deficit/hyperactivity disorder and substance use disorder. J Am Acad Child Adoles Psychiatry. 2016;55(3):227–34.e4.

86. Dirks H, Scherbaum N, Kis B, Mette C. ADHD in adults and comorbid substance use disorder: prevalence, clinical diagnostics and integrated therapy. Fortschr Neurol Psychiatr. 2017;85(6):336–44.

87. Greenfield SF, Grella CE. What is "women-focused" treatment for substance use disorders? Psychiatric Serv (Washington, DC). 2009;60(7):880–2.

88. Sugarman DE, Reilly ME, Greenfield SF. Treatment outcomes for women with substance use disorders: a critical review of the literature (2010–2016). Curr Addict Rep. 2017;4(4):482–502.

89. Greenfield SF, Cummings AM, Kuper LE, Wigderson SB, Koro-Ljungberg M. A qualitative analysis of women's experiences in single-gender versus mixed-gender substance abuse group therapy. Subst Use Misuse. 2013;48(9):750–60.

90. Khan S, Okuda M, Hasin DS, Secades-Villa R, Keyes K, Lin KH, et al. Gender differences in lifetime alcohol dependence: results from the national epidemiologic survey on alcohol and related conditions. Alcohol Clin Exp Res. 2013;37(10):1696–705.

91. Verissimo AD, Grella CE. Influence of gender and race/ethnicity on perceived barriers to help-seeking for alcohol or drug problems. J Subst Abus Treat. 2017;75:54–61.

92. Dawson DA, Grant BF, Chou SP, Stinson FS. The impact of partner alcohol problems on women's physical and mental health. J Stud Alcohol Drugs. 2007;68(1):66–75.

93. Powis B, Griffiths P, Gossop M, Strang J. The differences between male and female drug users: community samples of heroin and cocaine users compared. Subst Use Misuse. 1996;31(5):529–43.

94. Greenfield SF, Pettinati HM, O'Malley S, Randall PK, Randall CL. Gender differences in alcohol treatment: an analysis of outcome from the COMBINE study. Alcohol Clin Exp Res. 2010;34(10):1803–12.

95. Smith PH, Weinberger AH, Zhang J, Emme E, Mazure CM, McKee SA. Sex differences in smoking cessation pharmacotherapy comparative efficacy: a network meta-analysis. Nicotine Tob Res. 2017;19(3):273–81.

96. McKee SA, Smith PH, Kaufman M, Mazure CM, Weinberger AH. Sex differences in varenicline efficacy for smoking cessation: a meta-analysis. Nicotine Tob Res. 2016;18(5):1002–11.

97. Perkins KA, Scott J. Sex differences in long-term smoking cessation rates due to nicotine patch. Nicotine Tob Res. 2008;10(7):1245–50.

98. Vogel RI, Hertsgaard LA, Dermody SS, Luo X, Moua L, Allen S, et al. Sex differences in response to reduced nicotine content cigarettes. Addict Behav. 2014;39(7):1197–204.

99. Timko C, Debenedetti A, Moos BS, Moos RH. Predictors of 16-year mortality among individuals initiating help-seeking for an alcoholic use disorder. Alcohol Clin Exp Res. 2006;30(10):1711–20.

100. Satre DD, Blow FC, Chi FW, Weisner C. Gender differences in seven-year alcohol and drug treatment outcomes among older adults. Am J Addict. 2007;16(3):216–21.

101. Grella CE. From generic to gender-responsive treatment: changes in social policies, treatment services, and outcomes of women in substance abuse treatment. J Psychoactive Drugs. 2008;Suppl 5:327–43.

102. Ashley OS, Marsden ME, Brady TM. Effectiveness of substance abuse treatment programming for women: a review. Am J Drug Alcohol Abuse. 2003;29(1):19–53.

103. Sun AP. Program factors related to women's substance abuse treatment retention and other outcomes: a review and critique. J Subst Abus Treat. 2006;30(1):1–20.

104. Substance Abuse and Mental Health Services Administration. Guidance document for supporting women in co-ed settings. Rockville: Substance Abuse and Mental Health Services Administration; 2016. Report No.: HHS Publication No. (SMA) 16–4979.

105. Hser YI, Evans E, Huang D, Messina N. Long-term outcomes among drug-dependent mothers treated in women-only versus mixed-gender programs. J Subst Abus Treat. 2011;41(2):115–23.

106. Slesnick N, Erdem G. Efficacy of ecologically-based treatment with substance-abusing homeless mothers: substance use and housing outcomes. J Subst Abus Treat. 2013;45(5):416–25.

107. Linehan MM, Schmidt H 3rd, Dimeff LA, Craft JC, Kanter J, Comtois KA. Dialectical behavior therapy for patients with borderline personality disorder and drug-dependence. Am J Addict. 1999;8(4):279–92.

108. Messina N, Calhoun S, Warda U. Gender-responsive drug court treatment: a randomized controlled trial. Crim Justice Behav. 2012;39(12):1539–58.

109. Messina N, Grella CE, Cartier J, Torres S. A randomized experimental study of gender-responsive substance abuse treatment for women in prison. J Subst Abus Treat. 2010;38(2):97–107.

110. Greenfield SF, Trucco EM, McHugh RK, Lincoln M, Gallop RJ. The Women's Recovery Group Study: a stage I trial of women-focused group therapy for substance use disorders versus mixed-gender group drug counseling. Drug Alcohol Depend. 2007;90(1):39–47.

111. Greenfield SF, Sugarman DE, Freid CM, Bailey GL, Crisafulli MA, Kaufman JS, et al. Group therapy for women with substance use disorders: results from the Women's Recovery Group Study. Drug Alcohol Depend. 2014;142:245–53.

112. Valeri L, Sugarman DE, Reilly ME, McHugh RK, Fitzmaurice GM, Greenfield SF. Group therapy for women with substance use disorders: in-session affiliation predicts women's substance use treatment outcomes. J Subst Abus Treat. 2018;94:60–8.
113. Sugarman DE, Wigderson SB, Iles BR, Kaufman JS, Fitzmaurice GM, Hilario EY, et al. Measuring affiliation in group therapy for substance use disorders in the Women's Recovery Group study: does it matter whether the group is all-women or mixed-gender? Am J Addict. 2016;25(7):573–80.
114. Greenfield SF, Kuper LE, Cummings AM, Robbins MS, Gallop RJ. Group process in the single-gender Women's Recovery Group compared with mixed-gender group drug counseling. J Groups Addict Recover. 2013;8(4):270–93.
115. Claus RE, Orwin RG, Kissin W, Krupski A, Campbell K, Stark K. Does gender-specific substance abuse treatment for women promote continuity of care? J Subst Abus Treat. 2007;32(1):27–39.
116. Wunsch MJ, Knisely JS, Cropsey KL, Campbell ED, Schnoll SH. Women physicians and addiction. J Addict Dis. 2007;26(2):35–43.
117. Nace E, Davis C, Hunter J. A comparison of male and female physicians treated for substance use and psychiatric disorders. Am J Addict. 1995;4(2):156–62.
118. McGovern MP, Angres DH, Uziel-Miller ND, Leon S. Female physicians and substance abuse. Comparisons with male physicians presenting for assessment. J Subst Abus Treat. 1998;15(6):525–33.
119. Johnson M. The healthcare future is female: Athenahealth, Inc.; 2018. Available from: https://www.athenahealth.com/insight/healthcare-future-female.
120. Association of American Medical Colleges (AAMC). Active physicians by sex and specialty, 2015: Table 1.3 number and percentage of active physicians by sex and specialty, 2015: AAMC; 2015. Available from: https://www.aamc.org/data/workforce/reports/458712/1-3-chart.html.
121. Hughes PH, Brandenburg N, Baldwin DC Jr, Storr CL, Williams KM, Anthony JC, et al. Prevalence of substance use among US physicians. JAMA. 1992;267(17):2333–9.
122. Angres DH, McGovern MP, Shaw MF, Rawal P. Psychiatric comorbidity and physicians with substance use disorders: a comparison between the 1980s and 1990s. J Addict Dis. 2003;22(3):79–87.
123. Oreskovich MR, Kaups KL, Balch CM, Hanks JB, Satele D, Sloan J, et al. Prevalence of alcohol use disorders among American surgeons. Arch Surg (Chicago, Ill: 1960). 2012;147(2):168–74.
124. Oreskovich MR, Shanafelt T, Dyrbye LN, Tan L, Sotile W, Satele D, et al. The prevalence of substance use disorders in American physicians. Am J Addict. 2015;24(1):30–8.
125. Brewster JM. Prevalence of alcohol and other drug problems among physicians. JAMA. 1986;255(14):1913–20.

126. Bissell L, Skorina JK. One hundred alcoholic women in medicine. An interview study. JAMA. 1987;257(21):2939–44.

127. Braquehais MD, Arrizabalaga P, Lusilla P, Valero S, Bel MJ, Bruguera E, et al. Gender differences in demographic and clinical features of physicians admitted to a program for medical professionals with mental disorders. Front Psych. 2016;7:181.

128. Maust DT, Lin LA, Blow FC. Benzodiazepine use and misuse among adults in the United States. Psychiatric Serv (Washington, DC). 2019;70(2):97–106.

129. McLellan AT, Skipper GS, Campbell M, DuPont RL. Five year outcomes in a cohort study of physicians treated for substance use disorders in the United States. BMJ (Clinical research ed). 2008;337:a2038.

130. DuPont RL, McLellan AT, Carr G, Gendel M, Skipper GE. How are addicted physicians treated? A national survey of physician health programs. J Subst Abus Treat. 2009;37(1):1–7.

131. McGovern MP, Angres DH, Shaw M, Rawal P. Gender of physicians with substance use disorders: clinical characteristics, treatment utilization, and post-treatment functioning. Subst Use Misuse. 2003;38(7): 993–1001.

132. Merlo LJ, Campbell MD, Skipper GE, Shea CL, DuPont RL. Outcomes for physicians with opioid dependence treated without agonist pharmacotherapy in physician health programs. J Subst Abus Treat. 2016;64:47–54.

133. Shanafelt TD, Boone S, Tan L, Dyrbye LN, Sotile W, Satele D, et al. Burnout and satisfaction with work-life balance among US physicians relative to the general US population. Arch Intern Med. 2012;172(18):1377–85.

134. Shanafelt TD, Hasan O, Dyrbye LN, Sinsky C, Satele D, Sloan J, et al. Changes in burnout and satisfaction with work-life balance in physicians and the general US working population between 2011 and 2014. Mayo Clin Proc. 2015;90(12):1600–13.

135. Jackson ER, Shanafelt TD, Hasan O, Satele DV, Dyrbye LN. Burnout and alcohol abuse/dependence among U.S. medical students. Acad Med. 2016;91(9):1251–6.

136. Pedersen AF, Sorensen JK, Bruun NH, Christensen B, Vedsted P. Risky alcohol use in Danish physicians: associated with alexithymia and burnout? Drug Alcohol Depend. 2016;160:119–26.

137. Hyman SA, Shotwell MS, Michaels DR, Han X, Card EB, Morse JL, et al. A survey evaluating burnout, health status, depression, reported alcohol and substance use, and social support of anesthesiologists. Anesth Analg. 2017;125(6):2009–18.

138. Helping patients who drink too much: a clinician's guide [Internet]. NIH Publication No 07–3769. 2007.

139. Saunders JB, Aasland OG, Babor TF, de la Fuente JR, et al. Development of the Alcohol Use Disorders Identification Test (AUDIT): WHO col-

laborative project on early detection of persons with harmful alcohol consumption: II. Addiction (Abingdon, England). 1993;88(6): 791–804.

140. Smith PC, Schmidt SM, Allensworth-Davies D, Saitz R. Primary care validation of a single-question alcohol screening test. J Gen Intern Med. 2009;24(7):783–8.

141. Bush K, Kivlahan DR, McDonell MB, Fihn SD, Bradley KA. The AUDIT alcohol consumption questions (AUDIT-C): an effective brief screening test for problem drinking. Ambulatory care quality improvement project (ACQUIP). Alcohol use disorders identification test. Arch Intern Med. 1998;158(16):1789–95.

142. Cacciola JS, Alterman AI, DePhilippis D, Drapkin ML, Valadez C, Fala NC, et al. Development and initial evaluation of the brief addiction monitor (BAM). J Subst Abus Treat. 2013;44(3):256–63.

143. Humeniuk R, Ali R, Babor TF, Farrell M, Formigoni ML, Jittiwutikarn J, et al. Validation of the alcohol, smoking and substance involvement screening test (ASSIST). Addiction (Abingdon, England). 2008;103(6):1039–47.

Influence of Hormonal Fluctuations, Pregnancy, and the Postpartum Period on the Career of the Female Physician

14

Jaya Mehta and Juliana M. Kling

Introduction

Female physicians experience significant physiologic events unique to women that if not addressed can adversely impact their careers. The reproductive years pose challenges that relate to changes in the hormonal milieu and physical demands of menstrual symptoms, pregnancy and the peripartum timeframe, breastfeeding, perimenopause, and ultimately menopause; experiences only faced by female bodied physicians. Hormonal fluctuations have both short- and long-term effects on the body due to the influence of sex chromosomes and sex steroids. Activational sex steroid hormonal effects include those that are non-permanent and reversible, which come at puberty and disappear at menopause, while organizational hormonal effects are perma-

J. Mehta
Internal Medicine, Mayo Clinic, Phoenix, AZ, USA

J. M. Kling (✉)
Women's Health Internal Medicine, Mayo Clinic, Scottsdale, AZ, USA
e-mail: Kling.juliana@mayo.edu

© Springer Nature Switzerland AG 2020
C. M. Stonnington, J. A. Files (eds.), *Burnout in Women Physicians*,
https://doi.org/10.1007/978-3-030-44459-4_14

451

nent and remain despite loss of hormone, such as the effects on breast tissue. Sex hormones act via steroid receptors throughout the body including in the central nervous system (CNS) resulting in changes of the brain that regulate mood, behavior, and cognition. In this chapter, the physiologic changes and biopsychosocial ramifications resulting from hormonal changes across a women's reproductive lifespan that may play a role in the careers of female physicians will be discussed. Solutions that may mitigate the symptoms and potentially prevent various ramifications will also be reviewed.

Hormonal Fluctuations Throughout a Woman's Life Span

Women go through remarkable changes during their life span that are characterized by significant fluctuations in circulating pituitary-ovarian hormones. Menarche, menstruation, pregnancy, and menopause represent times with wide variation in levels of the estrogens (estradiol, estrone, estriol), progesterone, androgens (testosterone, DHEA), as well as the pituitary hormones (follicle-stimulating hormone (FSH), luteinizing hormone (LH)). The neuromodulatory effects of these hormones can result in changes of mood, behavior, and cognition [1]. Sex hormones bind steroid receptors, both extra and intracellularly, ultimately resulting in regulation of gene expression [2], with both activational and organizational effects. Activational effects occur in the CNS by acting on GABAergic, serotonergic, and dopaminergic synapses, as well as in peripheral tissues through hormone-specific receptors [3, 4]. Central organizational effects include neural changes such as myelination and dendritic spine remodeling. Through cellular pathways, estrogen acts to activate anti-apoptotic and cell survival pathways, which help cells meet their energy demand and protect against neurodegeneration [1]. Peripherally, sex hormones act to develop secondary sex characteristics, as well as interact on peripheral tissues such as the vasculature and organs [5]. Differences in estrogen and testosterone levels across the life span mean that sex steroids influence the regulatory and structural aspects of the body differently in women and men [5].

Mood Disorders

Compared to men, postpubertal women worldwide are on average twice as likely to develop symptoms that meet criteria for major depression or anxiety during their lifetime [6, 7]. The underlying mechanisms explaining these differences are likely multifactorial and include biopsychosocial influences. Fluctuations in sex hormones throughout a women's life may be one contributor, as demonstrated by the fact that the risk of mood disorders can be higher around a woman's menstrual cycle, postpartum, and during the peri- and postmenopausal transition [1]. It has also been shown that sex hormone fluctuations affect various cognitive domains. For example, low levels of estrogen and progesterone during the menstrual cycle are associated with improved visual-spatial abilities and decreased verbal abilities; with opposite effect seen when estrogen and progesterone are high [8].

Vignette: A 27-year-old general surgery intern is on day 2 of her 7-day period. She knows this is the day she has the heaviest flow but feels uncomfortable alerting her senior resident and attending that she may need to scrub out of a case to change her tampon. Six hours into the case she realizes she has leaked through her tampon and must scrub out to change her scrubs and tampon. Her senior resident tells her not to scrub back in because they are almost done. When the attending returns at the end of the case, he sees she is no longer working on the case and wonders why, but does not bring it up. The following day she develops significant cramping and lightheadedness making it difficult for her to remain in another case. Due to the discomfort, she scrubs out again and her attending again wonders why she was absent. The senior resident relates these events to others in the program, and later the intern is advised by other senior residents that she has been viewed as unreliable and even unprofessional because she left the operating room.

Menstruation, Premenstrual Syndrome (PMS), and Premenstrual Dysphoric Disorder (PMDD)

Menarche heralds a major transition in a woman's reproductive life span. Menses become a monthly event for most women, and for some women it is associated with debilitating recurrent emotional and physical symptoms such as mood symptoms, dysmenorrhea, and menorrhagia [9].

PMS is defined as recurrent adverse symptoms present only in the luteal phase of the menstrual cycle [10]. Up to 90% of menstruating women suffer from at least one premenstrual symptom, and 5–8% suffers from severe symptoms with significant impairment [9, 11, 12]. Women may develop physical (breast tenderness, bloating), behavioral, or emotional symptoms (irritability, depressed mood, tearfulness) in response to hormonal fluctuations [9, 13]. While the etiology has not been fully elucidated, individual response to fluctuations in estrogens and progestogens and serotonin insufficiency offer possible explanations [14].

The diagnosis of PMDD, as defined by the Diagnostic and Statistical Manual of Mental Disorders, Fifth Edition (DSM 5), includes at least five symptoms with at least one symptom pertaining to affectively, lability, irritability, depressed mood, or anxiety, and at least five of the following symptoms must be present including appetite change, decrease interest in activities, concentration difficulty, feeling out of control, sleep disturbance, low energy, or physiologic symptoms including breast tenderness, increased weight, bloating, arthralgias, or myalgias [15]. The diagnosis of PMDD is more stringent than PMS. While it is difficult to accurately assess the epidemiology of PMDD, based on few community-based surveys, the prevalence of PMDD ranged from 1.2% to 6.4% and is ubiquitous worldwide [14].

Effects of PMS reach further than just physical symptoms and may lead to missed work or school, higher medical costs, and decreased quality of life [16]. As noted in the vignette above, menstrual symptoms including but not limited to menorrhagia, dysmenorrhea, and mood changes may interrupt work days and negatively impact work performance of the female physician or trainee.

Treatment for PMS and PMDD

Prior to initiating treatment, it is important to rule out other disorders that are common mimickers including depression or anxiety, hypothyroidism, or substance use disorders. Treatment for PMS and PMDD oftentimes includes a multifactorial approach including lifestyle measures, medications, supplements, and nonpharmacologic therapies [14, 16, 17]. Selective serotonin reuptake inhibitors (SSRIs), including sertraline, paroxetine, and fluoxetine, may be used as first-line pharmacologic therapy for both PMS and PMDD [14, 16, 17]. Although the evidence is not robust, studies have shown that combined hormonal contraceptives (CHC) may help with depressive symptoms associated with hormonal fluctuations [1, 13, 14, 16, 18, 19]. Additionally, calcium (1000–1200 mg per day) may improve depressive symptoms, fatigue, and appetite for those with PMS [14, 16]. Complementary alternative pharmacologic therapies that have been evaluated include vitamin B6, chasteberry, St. John's wort, *Ginkgo biloba*, and evening primrose oil [14]. Nonpharmacological therapies include acupuncture, exercise, a complex carbohydrate diet during the luteal phase, and cognitive behavior therapy with mixed results [14, 16]. For those with resistant symptoms, other therapies include GnRH agonists, surgery with bilateral oophorectomy, and hysterectomy [14]. Given the increased risk of long-term health consequences of premature surgical menopause, especially without hormone replacement therapy until the average age of menopause, use of this option is and should be rare [20].

Combined Hormonal Contraceptives (CHCs) and Long-Acting Reversible Contraceptives (LARCs)

CHCs regulate endogenous sex steroids by suppressing hypothalamic gonadotropin-releasing hormone (GnRH) and gonadotropin secretion from the pituitary, thus reducing ovarian hormone secretion [21]. Contraception is largely a result of inhibition of the midcycle surge of LH, but progestins also act at the endometrium and create cervical mucus that helps with contraception. Due to hormonal regulation, CHCs reduce menstrual variability and oftentimes lead to less severe premenstrual symptoms. Depending on the dosages of estrogen and progestins, potential side effects include emotional lability, bleeding irregularities, nausea, weight gain, breast tenderness, headaches, and sexual dysfunction [22]. Many of the side effects depend on the type and dose of the hormone used (Table 14.1). For example, lower ethinyl estradiol levels may be considered safe regarding VTE risk, but provide less endometrial stabilization [23, 24].

In addition to contraception, CHCs are often initiated for management of dysmenorrhea, menorrhagia, menstrual-related migraine, or polycystic ovarian syndrome. The benefit of CHC on reproductive regulation and quality of life for many menstrual-related conditions is large, and the risk appears low. For female physicians, the ability to partly control reproduction timing with CHCs helps to balance their career and reproductive life planning. Furthermore, CHCs have been shown to reduce the risk of both ovarian and endometrial cancer [25–29]. Although decreased with lower formulations of estrogen, risks of CHCs include cardiovascular vascular events, including venous thromboembolism, pulmonary embolism myocardial infarction, and cerebrovascular events. Breast cancer incidence is increased only slightly while taking CHCs and within 10 years of discontinuation [30].

LARCs are highly efficacious as a contraceptive and can help to mitigate some symptoms associated with the menstrual cycle including dysmenorrhea and menorrhagia. LARCs approved by the Federal Drug Administration (FDA) include five intrauterine devices (IUDs) and one subdermal progestin implant. The copper IUD contains no hormones and is safe for those who have contraindications to estrogen use. Some develop heavier menses with increased dysmenorrhea, an undesired side effect. Levonorgestrel-containing IUDs and subdermal progestin implants are also safe for those with contraindications to estrogen use. Both have the additional benefit of decreasing menstrual bleeding and sometimes causing amenorrhea, and both may result in irregular bleeding [31]. The Center for Disease

Table 14.1 Side effects related to the hormonal composition of combined hormonal contraception as well as various formulations available [15]

Hormone	Dosage	Side effect
Estrogen	Low (20 mcg EE)	Break through bleeding, amenorrhea
Estrogen	High (35 mcg EE)	Nausea/bloating, headache, breast tenderness
Progestins	Low[a]	Break through bleeding, dysmenorrhea, menorrhagia
Progestins	High[a]	Weight gain, depression
Androgenic progestins	Low	Low libido
Androgenic progestins	High	Acne, weight gain, hirsutism
Formulations		**Hormone combination**
High estrogen: high progestin: high androgenic		Ethinyl estradiol/norgestrel
High estrogen: high progestin: anti-androgenic		Estradiol valerate/dienogest
Medium estrogen: high progestin: anti-androgenic		Ethinyl estradiol/drospirenone
Medium estrogen: low progestin: low androgenic		Ethinyl estradiol/norgestimate
Medium estrogen: medium progestin: low androgenic		Ethinyl estradiol/norethindrone
Medium estrogen: medium progestin: medium androgenic		Ethinyl estradiol/levonorgestrel
Medium estrogen: high progestin: low androgenic		Ethinyl estradiol/desogestrel
Low estrogen: low progestin: low androgenic		Ethinyl estradiol/norethindrone
Low estrogen: medium/high progestin: medium/high androgenic		Ethinyl estradiol/norethindrone
Low estrogen: high progestin: low androgenic		Ethinyl estradiol/ethynodiol diacetate

EE ethinyl estradiol
[a]Dose levels dependent on type of progestin

Control and Prevention (CDC) publishes a summary of US Medical Eligibility Criteria for Contraceptive Use that can help tailor choice of contraceptive based on underlying medical conditions [32].

Noncontraceptive Benefits of CHC

Female physicians and physician trainees may benefit from both the contraceptive and noncontraceptive benefits of CHC and LARCs. While not FDA approved specifically for these indications, CHC helps treat dysmenorrhea, menorrhagia, hyperandrogenism, ovarian cysts, polycystic ovary syndrome (PCOS), endometriosis, and PMS [33]. In women over 40, data suggest CHC may help prevent cardiovascular disease and depression [34].

Given the additional burdens based on hours worked and disproportionate home burdens female physicians face, it is logical to conclude that addressing these disorders in female physicians can lead to improved quality of life. In addition, utilizing CHCs or LARCs to provide predictability in menstruation can be empowering to female physicians who at times have no control over other parts of their schedule. For example, in the above vignette the surgical resident could consider continuous CHCs to control menorrhagia and dysmenorrhea. Lastly, many aspects of medical training have to be planned, so having access to reliable contraception to facilitate reproductive life planning is crucial for many female physicians.

Vignette: A 35-year-old female family medicine resident became pregnant with her second child during her second year of residency. It had taken her a long time to conceive her first child, so the timing of the second pregnancy was a bit unexpected, but it was a wanted pregnancy. Her first trimester went well and she felt supported by her program director, who rearranged her second-year residency schedule to accommodate delivery and maternity leave. She was on an away rotation, which delayed her scheduled anatomy scan. At the anatomy scan, she learned her fetus had a severe congenital anomaly and the pregnancy could not be continued. She had to leave an inpatient rotation to receive the emergent required care. Her program continued to accommodate her during this time with days off for the procedure, but she was required to return to her inpatient rotation only a few days after the procedure. She later pursued genetic testing prior to attempting an additional pregnancy and sought counseling given the emotionally and physically taxing unexpected experience she had endured.

Pregnancy, the Postpartum Period, and Reproductive Life Planning

Motherhood can be a factor associated with significant stress and burden for female physicians for many reasons. Pregnancy takes a physical and emotional toll on the female body. During pregnancy, there are increases in chorionic gonadotropin, progesterone, and estradiol levels, which can result in multiple physical complaints that may impact activities of daily living. These include, but are not limited to, gastrointestinal symptoms such as nausea, vomiting and constipation, fatigue, breast tenderness, frequent urination, changes in appetite, back pain, pelvic pain, chronic nasal congestion, and sleep disturbances [35]. While causation has not been established, hormonal changes in progesterone, estrogen, prolactin, cortisol, oxytocin, thyroid hormone, and vasopressin after child birth may play a role in postpartum depression [36]. It is estimated that 7–15% of pregnant women suffer from depressive symptoms in developed countries and 19–25% of women in low-resource countries [37]. After pregnancy, up to 13–19% of women suffer from postpartum depression [38]. Fortunately, treatments for postpartum depression are effective and typically include use of standard antidepressants and psychotherapy. In addition, brexanolone, an intravenously administered synthetic allopregnanolone and a positive allosteric modulator of α-aminobutyric acid (GABA), was recently approved by the FDA specifically for postpartum depression [39].

The demands that accompany a physician's career may take a toll on pregnancy outcomes [35–39]. A study done by Takeuchi et al. found that female physicians in Japan who worked longer hours during the first trimester had a higher risk of threatened abortion and preterm birth [40]. In fact, women who worked ≥71 hours per week had a threefold higher risk of a threatened abortion compared to women who worked 40 hours or less per week. It may become a necessity for female physicians to disclose early on in pregnancy to their employer or training program given concerns such as radiation exposure (e.g., interventional radiology or cardiology) or scheduling conflicts (residency schedule). Women may already be concerned about risk for pregnancy complications or loss, and early reporting may further contribute to their emotional uneasiness or distress [41]. However, there would be presumably less emotional distress associated with reporting early in pregnancy if it were considered routine and accepted within the medical culture as demonstrated by an infrastructure that was able to accommodate the schooled disruption associated with pregnancy and delivery.

The stress of family planning and its effect on a female physician's career has been studied in multiple countries denoting the universality of this challenge [40, 42–44]. Female physicians oftentimes delay childbearing due to training requirements and commitments. A study conducted in Taiwan found that female physicians tend to give birth at an older age compared to nonphysician counterparts (approximately 34 vs. 31 years old) [42]. Maternity leave can contribute to a delay in training completion because there are minimum required days trainees must work during residency and fellowship [45]. In fact, being younger at the time of first childbirth has been associated with a delay in attaining specialty board qualifications [46]. Female physicians were more likely to attain their medical degree and/or specialty board with just a 1 year increase in age of first childbirth, and the likelihood was lower if they resigned work for childbirth instead of taking a maternity leave.

On average, female physicians take a shorter maternity leave than other working mothers. The Family and Medical Leave Act (FMLA) allows 12 weeks of unpaid leave for those with newborns or newly adopted children living in the United States, and the average maternity leave taken is 10 weeks [47]. For comparison, a group of female physician trainees at Mayo Clinic averaged only 5–8 weeks of maternity leave, and in the early 2000s the mean time taken for maternity leave among pediatric residents was a mere 3 weeks [48, 49]. Although a study found that 9 weeks or greater of maternity leave is associated with greater satisfaction with maternity leave and child birth timing, most female physicians did not take 9 weeks [50]. Female physicians may desire longer maternity leaves but feel pressure from their training, work, and colleagues to take a shorter leave [45, 48]. Factors that may allow more female physician trainees to have an adequate maternity leave include larger size training programs, more nonresident-run teams, and the increased hire of advanced practitioners [48]. The latter may also benefit maternity leave availability for practicing physicians.

Reproductive Life Planning

A reproductive life plan is a set of personal goals set by both men and women regarding the conscious decision whether or not to have children, and it includes the tools to achieve those goas; it is recommended by the CDC to promote preconception health [51, 52]. It allows one to accomplish reproductive life goals in the setting of personal values and access to resources (Box 14.1) [53]. For female physicians, their education trajectory may complicate this plan. For example, female residents have been found to delay pregnancy due to perceived threats to careers. Specifically, in surgical fields, women may have a longer delay in pregnancy compared to those in nonprocedural fields. Subsequently, there has been a higher rate of assisted reproduction and infertility. Nearly 25% of surveyed female physicians experienced infertility [54–56]. Another study looking at deferment of personal life decisions found that 64% of female physicians deferred personal life decisions such as marriage (28%) or buying a home (5%) and over 80% of them deferred childbearing. These deferrals may threaten career satisfaction. Of the women surveyed, fewer would elect to do medicine again of those who deferred personal life decisions compared to the group who did not defer life choices (71% vs 85%, $p < 0.0001$) [44]. Along with the potential emotional dissatisfaction that may come with delaying childbirth, there are numerous health consequences due to advancing maternal age including higher risk for stillbirths, miscarriage, ectopic pregnancies, and birth defects [57].

Box 14.1: Reproductive Life Planning [50]

A set of personal goals set by both men and women regarding the conscious decision whether or not to have children and includes the tools to achieve those goals. It allows one to accomplish reproductive life goals in the setting of personal values and access to resources.

Example of questions to create a RLP:

- "Do you want to have (more) children?"
- "How many (more) children would you like to have and when?"
- "How will you prevent childbirth until you are ready?"

The ideal biologic time for a woman to have a baby tends to coincide with periods of high demand in medical training and new career steps for women, such as starting fellowship or transitioning to a faculty position after training. This is even more salient for women who decide to subspecialize or continue training [48] and may influence the reason why a substantial proportion of female physicians reported regrets about family planning and career decisions [55]. Furthermore, despite taking primary responsibility for child care and domestic activities, female physicians are often left feeling inadequate in both their family and professional roles [58]. Responses from over 300 female residents surveyed at Mayo Clinic highlights some of the stressors associated with pregnancy and child birth during residency. The decision to have a child during residency influenced research output, alterations in rotations, program completion dates, and changes in previous career plans for women more when compared to male colleagues [48]. A study conducted in Hungary by Gyorffy et al. found that female physician burnout is a risk factor for high-risk pregnancies and miscarriages, and poor pregnancy outcomes are risk factors for female physician burnout [43]. Accommodating pregnancy and childbirth in a supportive way would clearly benefit the health and wellbeing of female physicians and trainees.

There is promising data that female residents perceive program directors and division chiefs as more supportive of pregnancy during residency than previously perceived. Over a 7 year span, these improvements were noted by residents spanning different subspecialities, and they noted that involvement of female program leadership was likely a positive factor contributing to a more supportive environment [59]. Medicine in general is shifting to recognize the importance of work–life integration, including support of childbearing at all stages of the medical career. This is demonstrated in the increasing pregnancy rates seen during residency, which have increased almost threefold since the 1980s [48, 59].

Improving female physicians' childbearing experience and their pregnancy outcomes could be achieved by creating an environment that is supportive of family planning and provides adequate maternity leave. Medical societies are now endorsing accommodations for physician wellbeing and have provided recommendations to employers and training programs. The American Association of Pediatrics (AAP) advocates that all training programs have a written policy for parental leave and recommends a minimum of 6–8 weeks of paid leave after the birth or adoption of a child [49]. Similarly, the American College of Obstetricians and Gynecologists (ACOG) recommends all medical schools, residency, and fellowship program should provide at least 6 weeks of paid parental leave as part of standard benefits. Additionally, ACOG recommends that programs and medical specialty boards allow resident physicians to be board eligible even if they take more than 6 weeks of leave [60]. Empowering women with options for pursuing desired training while following an opportune reproductive path is paramount in mitigating the burnout associated with family planning [61].

Vignette: A 35-year-old first-time mother and new attending returns to work as an obstetrician after 12 weeks of maternity leave. She successfully breastfed during maternity leave and has set a goal of exclusively breastfeeding her baby for 1 year. When she returns from matternity leave, she is placed on call for labor and delivery. She has four very busy call days and does not find time to pump appropriately. She breastfeeds her baby 1–2 times during the day, but given her inability to find time to pump during her busy call days, her milk supply drops and she stops breastfeeding when her infant is 6 months old – far short of her stated goal of breastfeeding to 1 year. This causes her to feel intense guilt and frustration.

Breastfeeding

In the postpartum period, the female body undergoes significant hormonal changes [62, 63], in part related to lactation. Prolactin levels increase during the end of pregnancy to help develop mammary tissue in preparation for milk production [62]. Once newborns latch, the prolactin level increases. While prolactin is increasing, there is a fall of estrogen and progesterone to aid in milk production. An increase in gonadotropin-releasing hormone (GnRH) results in elevated LH and FSH which suppresses ovulation and menstruation. Oxytocin levels increase as an infant suckles resulting in breast milk let down as a result of contraction of the myoepithelial cells around the alveoli [62]. These intricate and substantial hormonal fluctuations contribute to physiologic consequences and may influence mood and other symptoms. For example, increased prolactin levels in nursing mothers have been linked to lower anxiety [63].

Oxytocin's physiological effects include promoting uterine contraction and reducing postpartum uterine bleeding. It also boosts a state of calm and reduces stress in the mother, while enhancing feelings of affection between the newborn and mother that promotes bonding. In order to stay in tune with an infant's needs, milk production is reduced by a feedback inhibitor of lactation. This protects breasts from deleterious effects of engorgement such as clogged milk ducts and mastitis; however, it also results in decreased production if unable to remove milk in a timely manner whether through nursing or breast pumping [62].

Breast milk provides the nutrition an infant needs in the first 6 months of life, and breastfeeding plays an integral role in the neuroendocrinology of the mother–child interaction [62]. Because of this, the American Academy of Pediatrics (AAP) recommends exclusive breastfeeding for up to 6 months and continued breast-feeding in conjunction with solid foods until 1 year or longer [64]. The World Health Organization also supports exclusive breast-feeding for the first 6 months with continuation up to 2 years or beyond while introducing complementary foods [65]. Breast milk contains fats, carbohydrates, vitamins, minerals, water, as well as anti-infective properties [62, 66]. The anti-infective properties arise from immunoglobulins, white blood cells, and whey proteins, which kill bacteria, viruses, and fungi, and oligosaccharides, which prevent bacteria from attaching to mucosal surfaces. The nutritional properties and connection breastfeeding provides between mother and infant makes it an integral part of child rearing for many women [62]. Further, research finds that breastfeeding provides maternal protection against breast cancer, ovarian cancer, and endometrial cancer [67–69].

Reaching breastfeeding goals can be challenging for female physicians. A shorter maternity leave means that women must start pumping breast milk early to create a backup supply available once they are back at work. Infants of female physicians may be introduced to a bottle early on depending on how much maternity leave is taken. This may be challenging if the infant refuses the bottle, or then prefers the bottle over the breast. The infant's response to bottle-feeding may influence a mother's decision or ability to continue breastfeeding, making it difficult to reach breastfeeding recommendations outlined by the WHO and AAP [70].

In order to continue breastfeeding and provide infants with breast milk, women must commit to pumping throughout the work day. Busy clinical schedules and lack of suitable locations to pump create challenges for physician mothers. Disruption of a pumping routine can negatively impact a woman's milk production. In many specialities, it can be nearly impossible to structure clinical work around a breast pumping schedule. Beyond the challenges of scheduling times to pump, female physicians may perceive judgment by colleagues when they are excused to pump and may feel they are missing valuable patient or educational experiences. These challenges in sum may lead to early breastfeeding cessation. Additional cited barriers for female physicians include 80 hour work weeks during training, stress associated with the burdens of clinical, research and educational production, night shifts, anxiety related to increased need to control, analyze, and measure infant feeding, and suboptimal medical education related to breastfeeding [71]. In organizations where compensation is dependent on number of patients seen, pumping can effect a woman's compensation. Not surprisingly, motherhood, especially for those who choose to breastfeed, is noted to be one of the principal causes of the gender pay gap [72]. In dual physician households, women shoulder more household responsibilities including child rearing than men; on average, women with children work less hours outside the home per week than male counterparts with children [73, 74].

Physician mothers are classified as a high-risk group for not meeting organizational and personal breastfeeding goals [71]. One study found that while 56% of female physicians intended to breastfeed for 1 year, only 34% met this goal [75]. Another study showed that over one third of physician mothers did not meet their goal to breastfeed to 12 months [76]. Meeting breastfeeding goals illustrates the complicated trade-offs female physicians navigate between home and work responsibilities. Falling short on breastfeeding goals can lead to feelings of guilt and dissatisfaction; while at the same time missing integral educational, patient, and work experiences results in disruption of career development [77]. When physician mothers reach their personal breastfeeding goals, they are more likely to support and counsel other physician moms and colleagues, as well as their patients about breastfeeding [71].

Aiding women with their breastfeeding goals would undoubtedly help mitigate the stressors faced by female physicians. Fortunately, federal laws have made it so that hospitals and clinics must have dedicated space available for lactation spaces and time for breast milk expression [78]. Additionally, many provide hospital grade pumps with phones and computers nearby. However, while lactation spaces are required, hospital grade pumps and an adequate workspace (i.e. including a computer or telephone) are not. Hospital grade pumps allow for an average of 15.5 min per pumping session versus 24 min with a portable pump [79]. Hospitals and clinics can help mitigate female physician burnout resulting from breastfeeding by providing hospital-grade pumps and adequate lactation room facilities to allow for increased efficiency and productivity during work hours. Other suggestions for improving the breastfeeding experience for female physicians include:

- Not having to make up missed work due to pregnancy or maternity leave
- Providing longer maternity leave
- Allowing sufficient time for pumping
- Increasing the level of support for breastfeeding efforts at work [76]

Lastly, social support and authentic connection is a critical aspect to achieving better outcomes for female physician mothers [80]. Social media groups may provide support for breastfeeding physician moms. Participating in support groups and improving breastfeeding education to both females and males would help to normalize and bring to the forefront the benefit of supporting breastfeeding for all involved. It is also important to provide support to women who make the decision, or who, for various reasons have to, discontinue breastfeeding before meeting WHO and AAP recommending durations. Self-compassion is also critical. Breastfeeding can be challenging for all women. Emphasis on choosing the plan that makes most sense for the infant and physician mother as a whole should be the focus.

Vignette: A 48-year-old female anesthesiologist started to notice significant issues with her sleep, waking up multiple times at night secondary to night sweats, resulting in fatigue that interfered with work. She was prescribed zolpidem, but her symptoms continued to worsen. It became clear that the symptoms began the same time she started to notice changes to her menstrual cycle with less frequent menses and intensified with the cessation of menses 12 months prior. Shortly after being prescribed transdermal estradiol and oral progesterone, her vasomotor symptoms were nearly completely gone and she noted improved energy and sleep.

Menopause

Menopause is defined retrospectively on a clinical basis 12 months after the last menstrual cycle. In the United States, the average age of menopause is 51. Women often begin to develop symptoms of menopause during perimenopause, a few years before menopause, when the ovarian hormones begin to fluctuate greatly [81]. The first sign of perimenopause typically is a change in the menstrual cycle. Menopausal symptoms include hot flashes, night sweats, joint pain, sleep disturbance, changes to cognition and mood, vaginal dryness, or other sexual health problems [82]. These symptoms are sometimes debilitating and can negatively impact a woman's quality of life. Additionally, untreated women may have higher healthcare resource utilization and more indirect work productivity loss, compared to controls [83]. As many as 75% of women will experience bothersome vasomotor symptoms (VMS) during menopause, and the average duration of menopausal symptoms can be as long as 7.4 years and longer for some [84]. Up to 42% of women aged 60–65 may still report VMS. Therefore, it is important to consider treatment for menopause.

Prior to the Women's Health Initiative (WHI) in the 1990s, women were being prescribed menopausal hormone therapy (HT) for symptoms, and also to prevent certain chronic diseases such as cardiovascular disease. In fact, observational and basic science studies showed that HT reduced coronary heart disease and all-cause mortality by nearly half [85, 86]. The WHI set out to evaluate the cardiovascular outcomes of HT. In 2002, the estrogen (conjugated equine estrogen) + progestin (medroxyprogesterone acetate) arm was closed early due to increased risk of cardiovascular disease and breast cancer [87]. This information drastically changed practice and has had ripple effects in menopause medicine.

Subanalysis of the WHI as well as subsequent random control data demonstrates that the risks identified in the WHI are for women who initiate HT more than 10 years from their last menstrual cycle or after age 60 [88–91]. Subsequently, guidelines have issued support of the use of HT early in menopause for symptomatic women [81, 89]. Many nonhormonal therapies, most off label, have been identified as effective for treating the vasomotor symptoms of menopause in women who choose not to use HT or have contraindications, such as selective serotonin reuptake inhibitors (SSRI), serotonin and norepinephrine reuptake inhibitors (SNRI), gabapentinoids, clinical hypothesis, and cognitive behavioral therapy [92]. Additionally, it has become clear that women who go through menopause early (surgically or otherwise) should be on HT at least until the average age of menopause to prevent long-term health consequences, such as osteoporosis, cardiovascular disease, and dementia, regardless of the presence of vasomotor symptoms [27]. Despite this updated and robust information, many women are not being treated, likely for many reasons including lack of comprehensive menopause training [93, 94].

No specific studies have evaluated the impact of perimenopause or menopause specifically on female physicians. However, menopause generally coincides with the most productive time in a female physician's career. By her 50s, most women are finished with childbearing and children are often old enough to allow more time to dedicate to herself and career if she chooses. The potential for menopausal symptoms to impact career productivity, along with well-established quality of life improvements, is a reason to consider therapy for menopausal symptoms. For women without absolute contraindications (e.g., hormone responsive breast cancer, underlying clotting disorder) and significant vasomotor symptoms, HT is a reasonable option to consider.

Conclusion

Female physicians face challenges unique to women during their careers. Hormonal fluctuations throughout a woman's life span, from menarche through menopause, can contribute to temporary and long-term physiologic consequences. Women in medicine must integrate the challenges of their profession while planning and executing their reproductive life plan. Addressing symptoms related to hormonal fluctuations, including pharmacologic and nonpharmacologic therapies, can be considered. Additionally, institutional support of female physicians by providing adequate maternity leave, breastfeeding, and pumping resources, as well as support and wellbeing programs, can help mitigate distress and burnout often faced by female physicians.

Take home points

– The impact of fluctuating sex steroids, especially during puberty, menses, pregnancy, and menopause, can lead to many physiologic changes in a woman's life. This has the potential to impact the female physician career and should be addressed.
– There are many menstrual-related symptoms and disorders. These can be addressed by treatment with SSRIs (for PMS/PMDD) or combined hormonal contraceptives in appropriately selected women.
– Reproductive life planning for female physicians is impacted by their education trajectory and unique work demands. Many times this leads to attempting pregnancy later in life, which can

lead to infertility and more health consequences to the woman and her fetus. In turn, interrupting reproductive life planning affects female physician's satisfaction with their career paths.

– Improving services for female physicians during training and throughout their careers, including improved maternity leave and supporting breastfeeding, is recommended. Assisting women in achieving their breastfeeding goals benefit both mother and baby in innumerable ways.

– Most women experience menopause symptoms which can last up to 7.4 years. Considering treatment with HT is an option, especially for those less than age 60 or within 10 years of menopause. Treatment can significantly improve symptoms of menopause as well as quality of life.

References

1. Del Rio JP, Alliende MI, Molina N, Serrano FG, Molina S, Vigil P. Steroid hormones and their action in women's brains: the importance of hormonal balance. Front Public Health. 2018;6:141.
2. Truss M, Beato M. Steroid hormone receptors: interaction with deoxyribonucleic acid and transcription factors. Endocr Rev. 1993;14(4):459–79.
3. Miller VM, Duckles SP. Vascular actions of estrogens: functional implications. Pharmacol Rev. 2008;60(2):210–41.
4. Orshal JM, Khalil RA. Gender, sex hormones, and vascular tone. Am J Physiol Regul Integr Comp Physiol. 2004;286(2):R233–49.
5. Kling JM, Miller VM, Mulvagh SL. Hormonal transitions and the cardiovascular system in women. Heart Disease in Women. 2015;
6. Weissman MM, Bland RC, Canino GJ, et al. Cross-national epidemiology of major depression and bipolar disorder. JAMA. 1996;276(4):293–9.
7. Altemus M, Sarvaiya N, Neill EC. Sex differences in anxiety and depression clinical perspectives. Front Neuroendocrinol. 2014;35(3):320–30.
8. Hampson E. Estrogen-related variations in human spatial and articulatory-motor skills. Psychoneuroendocrinology. 1990;15(2):97–111.
9. Ryu A, Kim TH. Premenstrual syndrome: a mini review. Maturitas. 2015;82(4):436–40.
10. Johnson SR, McChesney C, Bean JA. Epidemiology of premenstrual symptoms in a nonclinical sample. I. Prevalence, natural history and help-seeking behavior. J Reprod Med. 1988;33(4):340–6.

11. Pope CJ, Oinonen K, Mazmanian D, Stone S. The hormonal sensitivity hypothesis: a review and new findings. Med Hypotheses. 2017;102:69–77.
12. Yonkers KA, O'Brien PM, Eriksson E. Premenstrual syndrome. Lancet. 2008;371(9619):1200–10.
13. Skovlund CW, Morch LS, Kessing LV, Lidegaard O. Association of hormonal contraception with depression. JAMA Psychiat. 2016;73(11):1154–62.
14. Yonkers KA, Simoni MK. Premenstrual disorders. Am J Obstet Gynecol. 2018;218(1):68–74.
15. Association AP. Diagnostic and statistical manual of mental disorders. 5th ed. Arlington: American Psychiatric Association; 2013.
16. Hofmeister S, Bodden S. Premenstrual syndrome and premenstrual dysphoric disorder. Am Fam Physician. 2016;94(3):236–40.
17. Marjoribanks J, Brown J, O'Brien PM, Wyatt K. Selective serotonin reuptake inhibitors for premenstrual syndrome. Cochrane Database Syst Rev. 2013;6:CD001396.
18. Brace M, McCauley E. Oestrogens and psychological well-being. Ann Med. 1997;29(4):283–90.
19. Skovlund CW, Morch LS, Kessing LV, Lange T, Lidegaard O. Association of hormonal contraception with suicide attempts and suicides. Am J Psychiatry. 2018;175(4):336–42.
20. Faubion SS, Kuhle CL, Shuster LT, Rocca WA. Long-term health consequences of premature or early menopause and considerations for management. Climacteric. 2015;18(4):483–91.
21. Crosignani PG, Testa G, Vegetti W, Parazzini F. Ovarian activity during regular oral contraceptive use. Contraception. 1996;54(5):271–3.
22. Grossman BN. Managing adverse effects of hormonal contraceptives. Am Fam Physician. 2010;82(12):1499–506.
23. Colquitt CW, Martin TS. Contraceptive methods. J Pharm Pract. 2017;30(1):130–5.
24. Oriel KA, Schrager S. Abnormal uterine bleeding. Am Fam Physician. 1999;60(5):1371–80; discussion 1381–1372.
25. Gierisch JM, Coeytaux RR, Urrutia RP, et al. Oral contraceptive use and risk of breast, cervical, colorectal, and endometrial cancers: a systematic review. Cancer Epidemiol Biomark Prev. 2013;22(11):1931–43.
26. Collaborative Group on Epidemiological Studies on Endometrial Cancer. Endometrial cancer and oral contraceptives: an individual participant meta-analysis of 27 276 women with endometrial cancer from 36 epidemiological studies. Lancet Oncol. 2015;16(9):1061–70.
27. IARC Working Group on the Evaluation of Carcinogenic Risks to Humans. Pharmaceuticals. combined estrogen-progestogen contraceptives exit disclaimer. IARC Monogr Eval Carcinogen Risks Hum. 2012;100A:283–311.

28. Havrilesky LJ, Moorman PG, Lowery WJ, et al. Oral contraceptive pills as primary prevention for ovarian cancer: a systematic review and meta-analysis. Obstet Gynecol. 2013;122(1):139–47.
29. Wentzensen N, Poole EM, Trabert B, et al. Ovarian cancer risk factors by histologic subtype: an analysis from the Ovarian Cancer Cohort Consortium. J Clin Oncol. 2016;34(24):2888–98.
30. White ND. Hormonal contraception and breast cancer risk. Am J Lifestyle Med. 2018;12(3):224–6.
31. Wu JP, Moniz MH, Ursu AN. Long-acting reversible contraception-highly efficacious, safe, and underutilized. JAMA. 2018;320(4):397–8.
32. Summary chart of U.S. medical eligibility criteria for contraceptive use. https://www.cdc.gov/reproductivehealth/contraception/pdf/summary-chart-us-medical-eligibility-criteria_508tagged.pdf.
33. Caserta D, Ralli E, Matteucci E, Bordi G, Mallozzi M, Moscarini M. Combined oral contraceptives: health benefits beyond contraception. Panminerva Med. 2014;56(3):233–44.
34. Mendoza N, Sanchez-Borrego R. Classical and newly recognised non-contraceptive benefits of combined hormonal contraceptive use in women over 40. Maturitas. 2014;78(1):45–50.
35. Foxcroft KF, Callaway LK, Byrne NM, Webster J. Development and validation of a pregnancy symptoms inventory. BMC Pregnancy Childbirth. 2013;13:3.
36. Hendrick V, Altshuler LL, Suri R. Hormonal changes in the postpartum and implications for postpartum depression. Psychosomatics. 1998;39(2):93–101.
37. O'Keane V, Marsh MS. Depression during pregnancy. BMJ. 2007;334(7601):1003–5.
38. O'Hara MW, McCabe JE. Postpartum depression: current status and future directions. Annu Rev Clin Psychol. 2013;9:379–407.
39. Meltzer-Brody S, Colquhoun H, Riesenberg R, et al. Brexanolone injection in post-partum depression: two multicentre, double-blind, randomised, placebo-controlled, phase 3 trials. Lancet. 2018;392(10152):1058–70.
40. Takeuchi M, Rahman M, Ishiguro A, Nomura K. Long working hours and pregnancy complications: women physicians survey in Japan. BMC Pregnancy Childbirth. 2014;14:245.
41. Moe TG. Pregnancy in fellowship: building a career and family. J Am Coll Cardiol. 2014;64(7):734–6.
42. Wang YJ, Chiang SC, Chen TJ, Chou LF, Hwang SJ, Liu JY. Birth trends among female physicians in Taiwan: a nationwide survey from 1996 to 2013. Int J Environ Res Public Health. 2017;14(7). https://doi.org/10.3390/ijerph14070746.
43. Gyorffy Z, Dweik D, Girasek E. Reproductive health and burn-out among female physicians: nationwide, representative study from Hungary. BMC Womens Health. 2014;14:121.

44. Bering J, Pflibsen L, Eno C, Radhakrishnan P. Deferred personal life decisions of women physicians. J Womens Health (Larchmt). 2018;27(5):584–9.

45. Grant-Kels JM. Maternity leave for residents and young attendings. Int J Womens Dermatol. 2015;1(1):56.

46. Chatani Y, Nomura K, Ishiguro A, Jagsi R. Factors associated with attainment of specialty board qualifications and doctor of medical science degrees among Japanese female doctors. Acad Med. 2016;91(8):1173–80.

47. Lake R. How long is the average maternity leave? 2019. Retreived from https://www.thebalancecareers.com/how-long-is-the-average-maternity-leave-4590252.

48. Blair JE, Mayer AP, Caubet SL, Norby SM, O'Connor MI, Hayes SN. Pregnancy and parental leave during graduate medical education. Acad Med. 2016;91(7):972–8.

49. Section on Medical Students, Residents, and Fellowship Trainees; Committee on Early Childhood. Parental leave for residents and pediatric training programs. Pediatrics. 2013;131(2):387–90.

50. Lerner LB, Baltrushes RJ, Stolzmann KL, Garshick E. Satisfaction of women urologists with maternity leave and childbirth timing. J Urol. 2010;183(1):282–6.

51. Johnson K, Posner SF, Biermann J, et al. Recommendations to improve preconception health and health careDOUBLEHYPHENUnited States. A report of the CDC/ATSDR Preconception Care Work Group and the Select Panel on Preconception Care. MMWR Recomm Rep. 2006;55(RR-6):1–23.

52. Kransdorf LN, Raghu TS, Kling JM, et al. Reproductive life planning: a cross-sectional study of what college students know and believe. Matern Child Health J. 2016;20(6):1161–9.

53. Tyden T, Verbiest S, Van Achterberg T, Larsson M, Stern J. Using the reproductive life plan in contraceptive counselling. Ups J Med Sci. 2016;121(4):299–303.

54. Scully RE, Stagg AR, Melnitchouk N, Davids JS. Pregnancy outcomes in female physicians in procedural versus non-procedural specialties. Am J Surg. 2017;214(4):599–603.

55. Stentz NC, Griffith KA, Perkins E, Jones RD, Jagsi R. Fertility and childbearing among American female physicians. J Womens Health (Larchmt). 2016;25(10):1059–65.

56. Willett LL, Wellons MF, Hartig JR, et al. Do women residents delay childbearing due to perceived career threats? Acad Med. 2010;85(4):640–6.

57. Stein Z, Susser M. The risks of having children in later life. West J Med. 2000;173(5):295–6.

58. Schueller-Weidekamm C, Kautzky-Willer A. Challenges of work-life balance for women physicians/mothers working in leadership positions. Gend Med. 2012;9(4):244–50.

59. Mundschenk MB, Krauss EM, Poppler LH, et al. Resident perceptions on pregnancy during training: 2008 to 2015. Am J Surg. 2016;212(4):649–59.

60. American College of Obstetricians and Gynecologists. Paid parental leave. Statement of Policy. Washington, DC: American College of Obstetricians and Gynecologists; 2016.

61. Petek D, Gajsek T, Petek SM. Work-family balance by women GP specialist trainees in Slovenia: a qualitative study. BMC Med Educ. 2016;16:31.

62. Infant and young child feeding: model chapter for textbooks for medical students and allied health professionals. Geneva: World Health Organization; 2009. Session 1: The importance of infant and young child feeding and recommended practices and Session 2: The physiological basis of breastfeeding.

63. Asher I, Kaplan B, Modai I, Neri A, Valevski A, Weizman A. Mood and hormonal changes during late pregnancy and puerperium. Clin Exp Obstet Gynecol. 1995;22(4):321–5.

64. Eidelman AI. Breastfeeding and the use of human milk: an analysis of the American Academy of Pediatrics 2012 breastfeeding policy statement. Breastfeed Med. 2012;7(5):323–4.

65. The World Health Organization's infant feeding recommendation. Global strategy on infant and young child feeding. 2001. https://www.who.int/nutrition/topics/infantfeeding_recommendation/en/.

66. Dieterich CM, Felice JP, O'Sullivan E, Rasmussen KM. Breastfeeding and health outcomes for the mother-infant dyad. Pediatr Clin N Am. 2013;60(1):31–48.

67. Cramer DW. The epidemiology of endometrial and ovarian cancer. Hematol Oncol Clin North Am. 2012;26(1):1–12.

68. World Cancer Research Fund/American Institute for Cancer Research. Continuous Update Project Expert Report 2018. Diet, nutrition, physical activity and breast cancer. www.aicr.org/continuous-update-project/breast-cancer.html. 2018.

69. Anstey EH, Shoemaker ML, Barrera CM, O'Neil ME, Verma AB, Holman DM. Breastfeeding and breast cancer risk reduction: implications for black mothers. Am J Prev Med. 2017;53(3S1):S40–6.

70. Kassing D. Bottle-feeding as a tool to reinforce breastfeeding. J Hum Lact. 2002;18(1):56–60.

71. Jones LB, Mallin EA. Dr. MILK: support program for physician mothers. Breastfeed Med. 2013;8(3):330–2.

72. Greenfield R. Breast pumping at work makes the gender pay gap worse: working moms who breastfeed face long-term career consequences. Bloomberg. 2018;

73. Butkus R, Serchen J, Moyer DV, et al. Achieving gender equity in physician compensation and career advancement: a position paper of the American College of Physicians. Ann Intern Med. 2018;168(10):721–3.

74. Ly DP, Seabury SA, Jena AB. Hours worked among US dual physician couples with children, 2000 to 2015. JAMA Intern Med. 2017;177(10):1524–5.

75. Sattari M, Levine D, Bertram A, Serwint JR. Breastfeeding intentions of female physicians. Breastfeed Med. 2010;5(6):297–302.

76. Sattari M, Serwint JR, Neal D, Chen S, Levine DM. Work-place predictors of duration of breastfeeding among female physicians. J Pediatr. 2013;163(6):1612–7.

77. Riggins C, Rosenman MB, Szucs KA. Breastfeeding experiences among physicians. Breastfeed Med. 2012;7(3):151–4.

78. Labor USDo. Wage and hour division: frequently asked questions- break time for nursing mothers. https://www.dol.gov/agencies/whd/nursing-mothers.

79. Creo AL, Anderson HN, Homme JH. Productive pumping: a pilot study to help postpartum residents increase clinical time. J Grad Med Educ. 2018;10(2):223–5.

80. Luthar SS, Curlee A, Tye SJ, Engelman JC, Stonnington CM. Fostering resilience among mothers under stress: "authentic connections groups" for medical professionals. Womens Health Issues. 2017;27(3):382–90.

81. Harlow SDGM, Hall JE, Lobo R, Maki P, Rebar RW, Sherman S, Sluss PM, de Viliers TJ, STRAW + 10 Collaborative Group. Executive summary of the stages of reproductive aging workshop + 10: addressing the unfinished agenda of staging reproductive aging. J Clin Endocrinol Metab. 2012;97(4):1159.

82. The North American Menopause Society 2017 Hormone Therapy Position Statement Panel. The 2017 hormone therapy position statement of The North American Menopause Society. Menopause. 2018;25(11): 1362–87.

83. Sarrel P, Portman D, Lefebvre P, et al. Incremental direct and indirect costs of untreated vasomotor symptoms. Menopause. 2015;22(3):260–6.

84. Avis NE, Crawford SL, Greendale G, et al. Duration of menopausal vasomotor symptoms over the menopause transition. JAMA Intern Med. 2015;175(4):531–9.

85. Davidson MH, Maki KC, Marx P, et al. Effects of continuous estrogen and estrogen-progestin replacement regimens on cardiovascular risk markers in postmenopausal women. Arch Intern Med. 2000;160(21): 3315–25.

86. Grodstein F, Manson JE, Colditz GA, Willett WC, Speizer FE, Stampfer MJ. A prospective, observational study of postmenopausal hormone therapy and primary prevention of cardiovascular disease. Ann Intern Med 2000;133(12):933–41.

87. Rossouw JE, Anderson GL, Prentice RL, et al. Risks and benefits of estrogen plus progestin in healthy postmenopausal women: Principal results from the Women's Health Initiative randomized controlled trial. JAMA. 2002;288:321–33.

88. Santen RJ, Allred DC, Ardoin SP, et al. Postmenopausal hormone therapy: An Endocrine Society scientific statement. J Clin Endocrinol Metab. 2010;95:S1–S66.

89. de Villiers TJ, Gass MLS, Haines CJ, et al. Global consensus statement on menopausal hormone therapy. Climacteric. 2013;16:203–4.

90. Rossouw JE, Manson JE, Kaunitz AM, Anderson GL. Lessons learned from the Women's Health Initiative trials of menopausal hormone therapy. Obstet Gynecol. 2013;121:172–6.

91. Manson JE, Chlebowski TR, Stefanick ML, et al. Menopausal hormone therapy and health outcomes during the intervention and extended post-stopping phases of the Women's Health Initiative randomized trials. JAMA. 2013;228:1423–7.

92. Nonhormonal management of menopause-associated vasomotor symptoms: 2015 position statement of The North American Menopause Society. Menopause. 2015;22(11):1155–74.

93. Kling JM, MacLaughlin KL, Schnatz PF, et al. Menopause management knowledge in postgraduate family medicine, internal medicine, and obstetrics and gynecology residents: a cross sectional survey. Mayo Clin Proc. 2019;94(2):242–53.

94. Stuenkel CA, Davis SR, Gompel A, et al. Treatment of symptoms of the menopause: an Endocrine Society clinical practice guideline. J Clin Endocrinol Metab. 2015;100:3975–4011.

Part III
Empowering the Next Generation of Women Physicians

Synthesizing Solutions across the Lifespan: Early Career Solutions

15

Sallie G. DeGolia and Margaret May

Early in the process of co-writing this chapter, we made several (what turned out to be Sisyphean) attempts to meet up. Despite working at affiliated hospitals less than two miles apart and regularly converging in the same building at least once a week, we appeared unable to connect in person. Our attempts were thwarted by the usual suspects: sudden project deadlines, a gauntlet of conference calls and meetings, suicidal patients needing urgent attention (an occupational hazard of being psychiatrists), the illness of children requiring the use of precious sick leave, an imminent concern for a parent's heart condition leading to a trip to the emergency room—to say nothing of the general everyday complexity of our clinical, teaching, and administrative schedules.

Such a scenario is no surprise to today's women physicians. The early career years present unique risk factors for burnout, particularly for female physicians. This section focuses on the challenges and possible solutions relevant to this time period.

S. G. DeGolia (✉)
Department of Psychiatry and Behavioral Sciences, Stanford University, Stanford, CA, USA
e-mail: degolia@stanford.edu

M. May
Psychiatry & Behavioral Sciences, Palo Alto Veterans Affairs Health Care System, Palo Alto, CA, USA

© Springer Nature Switzerland AG 2020 481
C. M. Stonnington, J. A. Files (eds.), *Burnout in Women Physicians*,
https://doi.org/10.1007/978-3-030-44459-4_15

Challenges of the Early Career Phase

The early career phase is defined here as a timeframe spanning medical school, postgraduate training (internship, residency, and fellowship), and the first approximately 5 years of professional development. Transitioning out of the medical student role into residency and then out of the training role into one's first post-training position represent important inflection points during the early career phase. These transitions are typically associated with changes both in the structure of workplace obligations and in subjective experiences of professional identity. Because trainees are under particular evaluative scrutiny but lack accumulated clinical experience and may be reluctant to ask for help or demonstrate uncertainty, this timeframe is particularly associated with high risk to experience aspects of medical culture that invoke shame [14, 66, 71]. This is compounded by the reality of shifting subjective standards, tendencies to compare one's self to others, a fragile sense of belonging, and the experience of imposter syndrome which has been shown to be more relevant in women [97].

While the peri- versus post-training periods differ in notable ways, the early career phase is unified by a focus on establishing knowledge, clinical skills, and scope of practice and on developing a more confident, authoritative professional identity. On a practical level, the early career phase culminates in the establishment of a more stable occupational role after a protracted period of being in the student/learner role.

Women are likely to face four key areas of pressure or vulnerability in the early career phase which may impact their likelihood of experiencing burn-out:

- *Relationship and community building:* For most women, the early career phase coincides with a time period from the mid- to late-twenties through the mid- to late-30s during which the establishment of romantic partnerships, community belonging, and a new sense of family often occurs. For sociocultural as well as other reasons, women often have unique and demanding roles in such processes.
- *Reproduction and family:* Reproductive complexities may present themselves during this biological phase of life for

women. This includes the experience of unwanted pregnancies, desired pregnancies, difficulty achieving pregnancy, complications in pregnancy and childbirth, and alternate routes to starting families (such as adoption). Beyond pregnancy and childbirth, early family life presents strenuous demands on the infant's caretaker(s). Though adoption presents more opportunity for gender equality in terms of some burdens, women remain uniquely affected by all of these possibilities and experiences.

- *Expectations of productivity:* Traditional expectations around workplace productivity during the early career phase may not align with the above-mentioned tasks related to partnership, family, and community building which predominantly affect women. Needs around flexibility, work hours, sick leave, and other forms of institutional support are particularly important.

- *Gendered expectations during role changes:* Gendered expectations in the workplace that apply uniquely to the trainee period and early postgraduation career period must be confronted. During the trainee period, conformation to a subordinate trainee role may be reinforced particularly for women (and the opposite—criticism for stepping outside this role—may also occur) [41, 45, 74]. Yet the transition out of the trainee role demands occupying positions of authority and utilizing that authority effectively. Women may be at a disadvantage, for example, during various workplace negotiations (including contract negotiations) if they lack these skills to negotiate. Paradoxically, women who display such skills may also be penalized [8, 50]. Moving into attending-level roles requires greater use of authority and leadership.

Early Career Solutions

To date, there is a paucity of randomized controlled trials testing interventions to prevent, mitigate, or ameliorate burnout, which makes it difficult to propose evidence-based solutions or generalize findings. It is clear at this stage that wellness solutions are not "one size fits all" [103].

We use Stanford School of Medicine's wellness framework [7] to group challenges and solutions into three major domains that are conceptualized as impacting wellness: *Culture, Efficiency of Practice, and Resiliency.* Each domain is explored with an opening vignette, followed by corresponding early career challenges and individual and institutional solutions. Some solutions not only are specific to academic environments but may also be useful in mid- to large-sized group practices or other institutional settings. Most recommendations have been identified in the literature, with the addition of some solutions that have arisen from personal experience or anecdote. Importantly, though both levels of strategies are needed and have shown to reduce physician burnout, it remains unclear which interventions are most effective in specific populations and how individual and organizational solutions might be combined to achieve the most impact on physician wellness [101].

Culture of Wellness

It's 6:30 pm on a Thursday evening, usually dinnertime for all participants, but the only available time for three faculty women and their female supervisor to convene a weekly psychotherapy consultation group. The four women log on to a HIPAA-compliant platform for a 90-minute supervisory experience to engage in support, consultation and continuing education. During the session, one woman is seen through the online video lens with her infant crawling over her, desperately vying for her attention while her mother (the colleague) tries to attend to the case presentation. Another participant is seen crossing her living room where her school-aged children are seen studying as she lets the dog out, holding her laptop in front of her in order to continue contributing to the conversation. Near the end of the evening, the third faculty woman's husband interrupts to ask where something is in the kitchen. Two of the women eat dinner as they participate while the third nurses a child. The productive and lively discussion is concluded at 8 pm.

A *culture of wellness* is defined as "a set of normative values, attitudes, and behaviors that promote self-care, personal and professional growth, and compassion for colleagues, patients, and self" [85]. In the above vignette, assuming that these four colleagues felt non-coerced to perform some of their professional duties outside of normal work hours, the group has created a culture of wellness among themselves by acknowledging that this supervisory work can occur in a flexible manner (during off-hours, via an online platform) and can accommodate the family lives of those involved. This includes recognition that each member may make valuable contributions and attend meaningfully to the session, despite occasional interruptions or coinciding role performances. To the extent that the institution in which these physicians are embedded sanctions this activity (by making the online platform available and easy to use, allowing the participants to time-bank afterhours work activity, reflecting positively on the ingenuity of such arrangements, etc.), the institution is facilitating a culture of wellness.

Six critical spheres impacting women at early stages in their career development where individuals and institutions can promote a culture of wellness include (1) the culture of medicine at large, (2) flexible career policies, (3) mentorship, (4) leadership/faculty development, (5) enhanced connectedness, and (6) promotion of self-care. Potential solutions targeting each area are explored below.

The Medical Culture

The culture of medicine comprises formal and informal practices. Informally, women often report many small (and some large) experiences of gender discrimination from superiors, colleagues, staff, and patients [46]. Formally, various policies, procedures, and administrative structures have adversely impacted women and led not only to their slower career advancement but also ultimately to leaving academic careers at early states [15, 20, 21, 63, 80]. An important background force is that of unconscious bias impacting evaluation, recruitment, promotion, and possibly compensation practices [15, 20, 21, 63, 80]. This bias is compounded by sexual harassment [64] and gender discrimination [16, 46]. Compounding these issues at this stage in training is the fact that early career physicians are particularly vulnerable to making mistakes and/or feeling uncertain about their nascent skills and knowledge in the context of overwhelming responsibilities. Experiences of shame and imposter syndrome may be experienced by women in ways that intersect with gender roles and norms [13, 49].

Institutional Solutions

- Ensure new promotion and tenure policies that support women and minorities.
- Require zero-tolerance policies for sexual harassment and review the National Academy of Sciences' *Interventions for Prevention Sexual Harassment* [65]. Establish an Office of Diversity.
- Appoint a diverse hiring committee and change search procedures to identify and reduce bias and identify females.
- Seek alignment of rewards and incentives along culturally sensitive policies and missions.
- Appoint women to leadership positions to enhance recruitment, mentorship, and/or advancement of women.
- Improve data collection and management systems to track gender demographics of search committees and data on women and minority faculty in each department to identify barriers and solutions to women's career advancement.
- Review compensation data to identify any inequities and disparities.
- Track wellness among all faculty through regular anonymous wellness surveys to identify hot spots and develop interventions.
- Implement early and effective employee on-boarding orientations within departments to explore the relevant departmental policies, practices, and guiding cultural values. Include relevant organization charts and create a central online repository for standard operating procedures and other institutional policies,

best practices to address staff wellness, and where to inquire about workplace flexibility or current initiatives to improve efficiency of practice. Consider maximal utilization of the organization website to achieve these goals.

- Provide faculty development workshops associated with mentoring, clinical supervising, and teaching to address how to recognize shame in learners, more appropriately respond to medical errors or academic struggles, and help teachers recognize their role in potentially inflicting shame on others and prevent intentional shaming in the learning climate.

Flexible Career Policies

While women tend to prioritize a work-life balance [91], early career women experience more work-life conflicts than men [51]. These conflicts and the manner in which they are resolved have been shown to influence career decisions, career satisfaction, and burnout [20, 26, 27, 63]. One major solution to addressing this issue is the development of more family-friendly, flexible career policies as well as interventions that reduce barriers to accessing the use of such policies. Having the ability to adjust professional work effort allows women to tailor work hours to meet both personal and professional obligations. By allowing physicians to reduce their work hours, they are able to recover from burnout [84].

Flexible career policies are seen as important for recruitment, retention, and career satisfaction [61, 96]. Though faculty women tend to use these policies more than men, several barriers have prevented women, in particular, from using such policies [96]. Barriers have included lack of reliable information about program eligibility and benefits; workplace norms and cultures that stigmatize participation; influence of uninformed or unsupportive department leaders; and worries about burdening coworkers through participation, damaging collegial relationships, or unfavorably affecting workflow and grant funding. Furthermore, one academic center reported that use of family-friendly policies was significantly lower within the school of medicine compared to other schools within the academic center [96]. A study of resident use and perceptions of barriers of work-life policies also report that barriers affecting the use of work-life policies include policy awareness and perception of negative attitudes from leadership [104]. Not surprisingly, the potential impact on co-resident relationships was identified as among the most commonly identified barriers. Furthermore, those residents perceiving the highest barriers endorsed higher burnout. Conversely, those residents who perceived that leadership supported the use of such policies were more likely to be aware of and actually use work-life policies.

The American Association of Medical Colleges (AAMC) has identified a "good work-life policy" as one that includes (1) paid leave offered to both full and part-time faculty, (2) no required length of prior service in order to qualify for leave, (3) 12 weeks of paid leave (longest cited), (4) 6 months (longest cited) total leave (paid and unpaid), and (4) shared leave when both parents are on faculty [4]. However, even with strong policies, women have had difficulty identifying and/or accessing an institution's work-life policies, despite the fact the AAMC reported that over three-quarters of medical schools had policies allowing for the tenure clock to stop [4] and one-third had a policy allowing faculty to work less than full-time while remaining on a tenure-eligible track [12].

Underutilization of such policies is most commonly due to faculty not requesting their use. Reasons for this include (1) a lack of information and/or misinformation about the programs (faculty are either unaware of benefits or misinformed about their eligibility and how to access the benefits); (2) unsupportive workplace norms and cultures characterized by discouraging use of work-family benefits, a culture of overwork, pressure to publish and write grants, or fear of being perceived as not a "good faculty" member); (3) failure of the administration to plan for flexibility within interdependent teams (clinical, research, teaching) where a faculty member may feel obligated to fellow colleagues, in addition to the administration burdening faculty to plan for accommodations; and (4) lack of support of supervisors and managers [86].

Institutional Solutions

- Implement policies that allow flexible work arrangements for faculty.
  - Ensure that flexible policies are clear and easily accessible (e.g. include on department website, in new faculty/trainee orientations, and/or in faculty manuals).
  - Identify and address barriers to policy awareness and utilization.
  - Educate department chairs and key supervisors about the policies and ensure they facilitate participation and advocate for work-life integration.
  - Consider broadening leave policies to include leaves for family members with serious illness and catastrophic events (fire, divorce, custody disputes).
  - Make childcare leave and stop-the-clock policies as opt-out vs opt-in.
  - Track program utilization to ensure it is applied equitably.
  - Ensure that university leaders reinforce support of such policies.
- Consider programs that reduce on-the-job stress (e.g., emergency sick-child care programs, on-site child care, elder care, day care hours in line with physician schedules, remote access to EMR, telecommuting)
- Ensure that promotion and tenure are the same for all faculty regardless of leave use.
- Offer part-time tenure tracks for those institutions offering tenure.
- Develop a time-banking intervention to augment flexible career policies [30]. Faculty can "buy back" time spent on otherwise uncompensated or not adequately recognized activities that benefit teams and/or individual colleagues and are allowed to redeem credits for services that would free up time to meet other demands at work or home (e.g., housecleaning, laundry, meal delivery, car service, grant writing, manuscript editing, and speech coach).

- Align hospitals and school of medicine holidays to minimize child care issues.
- Schedule meetings within "official" work hours.
- Provide food services, laundry, dry cleaning, and other domestic conveniences on site to facilitate work-life integration.
- Clarify leadership/training program attitudes toward use of work-life policies.
- Consider solutions to build in greater flexibility to the workforce, such as hiring moonlighting physicians or shifting trainee rotation schedules to accommodate major life changes.

Individual Solutions

- Identify and understand your institution's flexible policies. Meet with your supervisor, human resources administrator, Office of Faculty, Diversity Office, or Office for Women.
- Be clear about your legal protections including the Pregnancy Discrimination Act of 1978 (protects women in pregnancy against discrimination based on pregnancy), Family and Medical Leave Act (FMLA) (unpaid or paid if earned or accrued, job-protected leave up to 12 weeks a year for eligible women), and the Fair Labor Standards Act (FLSA) (provides nursing mothers the right to express milk in the workplace for up to 1 year postpartum). For more information, review AAMC Toolkit [4]
- Negotiate your salary before you are hired! Remember, a man's starting salary tends to be higher than that of a woman's and taking leave or working part-time for more than 2 months can lead to smaller increases in salary [31]. Consider resources around negotiation skill-building prior to engaging in negotiation (for examples, see resources on www.leanin.org/education/negotiation).
- When flexible policies are not being appropriately followed by your institution, consult the faculty affairs dean, equity, diversity and inclusion dean, ombudsman, or other resource centers to help negotiate a solution.
- Consult the AAMC Toolkit [4] for further details of what and how to manage a leave of absence.

Mentorship

Mentorship has been shown to be helpful to the well-being of early career women and under-represented minority women mentees [1, 2, 98] and is a key strategy for faculty success [48]. Having a mentor and role models who are successful at integrating work and life may help foster academic advancement and prevent burnout [42, 69]. In fact, a lack of adequate mentorship and role models were some of the reasons for women's premature departure from academic medicine [20, 55]. Though these findings reflect an academic setting, they are likely to extrapolate to other settings in which professionals are embedded in an institution or other hierarchical occupational structure.

Despite the importance of mentorship, women compared to men have more difficulty finding mentors—particularly clinician educators [76]. This is notable given that women make up nearly 50% of current medical school classes with an increasing number of women entering early faculty positions. Still, women represent only 38% of academic medical center faculty [52, 63] and far fewer are in senior faculty or leadership positions [94].

Although mentoring comes in a variety of modalities (dyadic, peer, group, etc), a mentoring network can be particularly useful to women. DeCastro et al. [23] found that multiple mentors including peers and women helped mitigate challenges related to gender in mentoring and also provided varying skill sets to meet the diverse needs of female mentees. For example, negotiations required in the early career phase represent a point of vulnerability for women who have been shown in studies to be disadvantaged by gender bias, framing of negotiations, and lack of exposure to relevant skill building [8, 88]. Appraising employment contracts is a complex task that may fall outside a woman's expertise, and the process often involves negotiation around compensation, work hours, productivity expectations, terms of occupational flexibility, and amount of leave. Some institutions offer no negotiation around contract offerings, an experience which can echo the insubordination experienced in training. Mentorship can be invaluable to helping early career women navigate these complex issues.

One issue for women is whether it is important to have women mentors. Female mentors can be particularly useful given their differences in communication and language styles [72] and emphasis on support and collaboration over independence and competition [58]. They can serve as role models of success for mentees in areas such as workplace communication, boundary setting, negotiation, and work-life balance, particularly within the context of a male-dominated workplace environment [3, 23, 24]. However, mentoring across gender lines can produce excellent mentorship as well. Because of few underrepresented minorities in leadership including sexual and gender minority faculty, it is important for "allied" role models to serve as mentors [87]. After all, it is the *lack* of mentorship that has kept women from advancing—not who is doing the mentoring [23].

Institutional Solutions

- Develop an institutionally sponsored or organized mentorship program.
- Protect time for mentorship and/or provide credit for successful mentoring.
- Acknowledge and reward mentors.
- Train mentors, team leaders, and/or division chiefs in coaching skills and career development mentoring. Include topics with particular emphasis on unconscious bias; acknowledgment of complex challenges faced by early career women faculty including experiences of isolation, discrimination, and stereotyping; as well as information on how to access and use flexible career development policies to achieve personal and professional goals.
- Address barriers to mentoring.
- Facilitate support networks for early career women.
- Develop peer mentorship opportunities.

Individual Solutions

- Find a mentor. If no formal mentorship program is available, start meeting faculty. Go to social events hosted by your department and women's networking events in the institution, or attend national organizations where networking is encouraged. Set up informational meetings with interested faculty and ask about their interests. Consider identifying a scholarly project advisor or clinical supervisor with whom to work. This is a safe way to see if the advisor or supervisor shares your interests, values, and characteristics of a good mentor (consistent, listens actively, creates a safe environment where you can share your thoughts and feelings, able to strike a balance between autonomy and guidance, and treats you and your goals with respect) [44].
- Develop a personal mentor network. Identify and include peers and/or faculty within and outside your institution who have expertise in a number of diverse skills, given the range of one's career tasks (i.e., teaching, administration, and leadership). One mentor is often not enough! Ensure that at least one mentor is a woman and of high standing.
- Be proactive. Once a potential mentor(s) is identified, ask if they might have time to *regularly* mentor you. Take responsibility for the relationship: develop clear, specific goals and strategies to achieve goals, and set a meeting schedule and agenda. Engage in critical self-assessment, track your progress on goals, and ask for and integrate feedback. Use an Independent Development Plan (*see* Appendix 1) as a template to help self-reflect and guide mentoring discussions.
- Identify important topics to explore. Topics of particular interest to early career faculty might include how to access and effectively utilize flexible career policies and benefits; how to balance divergent commitments of clinical service, research, teaching, administration, and family; when to consider having a child and how to address this with administration and colleagues; how to manage sexual harassment, stereotype threats, and implicit bias; how to develop negotiation skills—particularly as they apply to compensation and resource acqui-

sition; and how to diplomatically say "no" when opportunities are not aligned with values or career goals. Other topics might include how to transition from training to practice, identifying core values that will enhance meaning and joy in your life, guidance around career choices, how to maintain a healthy lifestyle, and ways to think about promotion, scholarship, service involvement, and time management.

- Create peer mentorship groups. If not offered through the organization, find peers with whom you can meet on a regular basis to discuss issues that affect early career women or who share interest in specific research topics. You may want to bring in speakers to address particular relevant issues to the group. Such groups might also serve as writing groups where members can gain writing skills and publish while advancing their careers. Writing groups can commit to rotating first authorship and key tasks in article development to ensure that the entire group progresses academically.
- Consider sponsorship of group meetings through national organizations (i.e., AMWA).

Leadership and Faculty Development

Historically, women have been abandoning careers in academia at early career stages partly due to dissatisfaction based on few opportunities for professional development and difficulty networking because of a paucity of senior female mentors and poor access to those in positions of power [20]. As such, faculty development (FD) must focus not only on developing and practicing nascent skills of early faculty women starting out in their careers but also on skills of faculty in leadership positions who have significant impact on early career women. For women in non-academic settings, FD may be analogous to leadership development. Whether or not women desire to seek leadership roles, such skills may contribute to important role functions (e.g., greater sense of self-efficacy, institutional engagement, and experience of influence on workplace culture). Aside from leadership or other work-based skills, FD might also include ways to manage work-life challenges and promote well-being [10].

Leadership styles significantly impact the well-being of those they lead [83, 106]. As part of improving the skills of leaders, leaders need to understand that some early career faculty may base career success more on intrinsic factors such as a respect and passion for and recognition of work rather than on other conventional definitions of success including promotion, publications, and compensation [22]. By addressing those factors that are important for a women's meaningful career, leaders may be able to mitigate burnout and improve retention.

Unfortunately, since few women serve in leadership positions within schools of medicine [94], early career women have few female role models and senior mentors. Without an identifiable pathway to leadership, women's career opportunities may seem limited. As the number of women in leadership positions increases, a cultural transformation may lead to a more inclusive, collaborative, and less hierarchical environment [70], and, therefore, lessen burnout and enhance professional fulfillment.

Institutional Solutions

- Survey early career faculty regarding their FD needs and address barriers to engaging in FD.
- Task the Office of FD and/or Women and Diversity, and/or create a task force to review the current state of FD in the institution and make recommendations.
- Develop FD programs for early career women on key faculty skills (e.g., management, work-life balance, negotiation, career development, promotion/tenure, and wellness strategies) and workshops on transitioning from training to practice. When scheduling such programs, it is important to accommodate early physician's clinical demands and less-flexible schedules [36].
- Identify resources and funding for junior faculty to make use of faculty development opportunities and advertise them more effectively.
- Select leaders thoughtfully based on their ability to listen, engage, develop and lead physicians and assess them regularly [83].

- Implement leadership development programs for current leaders and/or workshops on leadership skills, communication, unconscious bias, and gender and diversity issues, including how to motivate early career women based on their values and meaning for success.
- Develop sponsorship programs to advocate and facilitate advancement of talented women [95].

Individual Solutions

- Identify and take advantage of FD offerings through your department, institution, and/or national organizations.
- Review benefits to determine whether there are funds to support going to FD opportunities outside the department/institution.
- Find out about leadership programs whether within your organization or external to your organization (AAMC, AMWA, AMA, specialty organizations).
- Ask your mentor to help you develop leadership and other important skills and/or advocate for your nomination to a leadership program.
- Seek positions on committees that help hone leadership and administrative skills and create visibility, as well as enhance regional or national reputations important for promotion. However, be careful to guard against those commitments that take up time without enhancing promotion. It is important to keep an eye on balancing service to oneself against service to the institution. Women may be more vulnerable to enlistment in "emotional labor" activities (for example, office caretaking or organizing office social activities) that are not as salient to promotion criteria.
- Seek out sponsors in positions of power to facilitate career development [6, 68].

Enhance Connectedness

Research has shown that support in the workplace can serve as a buffer against burnout [99]. Taylor et al. [93] proposed that women (among other species) respond to stress often through a "tend-and-befriend" approach instead of the often-described fight-or-flight response. As a biologically derived and adaptive response, "tending" or nurturing each other and "befriending" or creating social groups can serve to reduce stress. Facilitated engagement groups sponsored by a department or institution have been shown to enhance personal and professional growth and decrease stress and depression. A randomized, controlled study offering a protected-time, 12-weekly, 1-hr sessions mother's group mitigated burnout and distress for physician mothers and reduced cortisol levels, depression, and parenting stress [56]. Other strategies that have enhanced connectedness include wellness workshops [10], dinner events with early career faculty to explore wellness issues [102], social writing events [25], as well as reflection groups for medical students [33].

Institutional Solutions

- Offer facilitated early career female physician engagement groups with protected time.
- Sponsor informal social get-togethers with residents and families, such as happy hours and outdoor activities to promote healthy engagement among residents. Salles, Liebert, and Greco [77] described a surgery department that assigned one to two residents per year to serve as social event planners.
- Sponsor dinners among early career women faculty and other outside work activities to enhance informal engagements and build meaningful relationships between colleagues.
- Provide social writing groups where early career faculty can develop meaningful relationships among colleagues while developing important professional skills that contribute toward promotion.
- Implement wellness workshops for early and/or new faculty which might explore cost benefits of a successful academic career, challenges of maintaining a work-life integration, where to locate resources and develop strategies to maintain wellness, and how to map out a plan to reassess work-life balance at regular intervals.

- Implement a compassion cultivation program such as gratitude cards to be filled out by an individual for a valued colleague, or start meetings by asking each member to identify for what they have been grateful.
- Sponsor wellness workshops targeting early faculty women.

Individual Solutions

- Participate in available engagement groups for women—particularly around work-life integration, mother's group, or other early career women's issues.
- If such a group doesn't exist, consider starting one. Find a group of like-minded women who might be interested in forming a group. Meet during lunch hour or lobby for protected time.

Promote Self-Care

Higher rates of burnout, emotional exhaustion, self-blame [89], suicide [19], and inadequate sleep and excessive sleepiness [32] have been reported in female physicians. Female physicians are also more likely to report sickness presenteeism [38]. These all highlight the importance for institutions to support self-care and provide easy access to health services among this particular cohort. This is compounded by the fact that lack of time in one's schedule, stigma, denial of illness, and concerns of confidentiality result in barriers to seeking care [11, 18]. Institutional solutions need to not only decrease barriers but also support opportunities to seek self-care.

Institutional Solutions

- Review internal practices that might impede self-care seeking.
- Lobby to eliminate requirement to report mental health treatment if required by the state medical board [34].

- Provide self-assessment tools to compare to peers nationwide [28, 82] and web-based prevention tools (e.g., [37]).
- Encourage senior staff, including program directors and chiefs to model wellness.
- Disseminate information regarding wellness opportunities, including peer-assistance programs, so physicians are aware of them [78].
- Enhance accessibility to wellness programs and health care by offering more practical time slots and/or protected time, proximal locations.
- Implement systems to protect from overburdening residents who cover absences and to avoid low-morale consequences [17].
- Encourage importance of self-care when sick; discourage sick presenteeism [77].
- Provide trainee support groups and/or allow small group discussions to help trainees develop tools to manage stress [77].
- Provide structured wellness programs [29, 53, 79] and educate about risk factors and workplace stressors particularly associated with early women physicians; encourage healthy behaviors including an emphasis on positivity, maintaining balance, and promoting self-compassion to improve resilience and sleep quality.
- Provide healthy snacks and drinks for trainees.
- Provide a dedicated lactation room for postpartum colleagues and provide policies that allow for lactation breaks.
- Implement non-gender-associated, early career, evidence-based strategies including facilitating mental health treatment [40, 62]; incentivizing exercise and physical activity programs [100, 105], stress reduction [39, 60], mindfulness [35, 57, 73, 105], meditation [67], and coping skills programs [75]; and offering communication skills training [5, 9] and reflection groups for medical students [33].

Efficiency of Practice

A clinical instructor at a hospital affiliated with an academic center has worked for 3 years teaching students, supervising residents, and furthering various academic projects, at which point she begins to wonder when she can apply for promotion to assistant professor. After reaching out to a senior professor in the department leadership team for clarification on the appropriate timeline, she receives several vague replies related to some ambiguities in the process. The administrative assistant who coordinates appointments and promotions is new, adding to the slowdown. Finally, after several months, the original professor intercedes by email, making a clear declaration of support that the clinical instructor be allowed to apply for promotion now, as indicated by her scholarly activities and his support. Immediately after this email, the necessary materials are sent to the clinical instructor.

Efficiency of practice can be conceptualized as a ratio of "value-added clinical work accomplished" divided by time and energy spent [7]. Improving efficiency of practice usually boils down to maximizing the elements of clinical care that feel valuable and rewarding while minimizing the elements that feel inefficient, unnecessary to the central tasks of clinical caretaking, or clerical in nature. A common breakdown in efficiency of practice involves the growing burden of charting and management of tasks generated by the electronic health record (EHR), often leading to spillover of work outside normal working hours; a vignette portraying a woman physician completing chart tasks remotely after putting her children to bed paints a familiar scene. However, this opening vignette highlights several additional themes. First, efficiency of practice may refer not only to clinical work but also to any system that gets bogged down and impacts the wellness of physicians. In this vignette, the initial period of inquiry about advancement shows a breakdown of systems that could be better streamlined to anticipate the kinds of questions that early faculty may pose. It also demonstrates how an institutional leader can help facilitate efficiency of practice by interceding in a supportive and, importantly, *effective* manner. The delayed process has only created a demoralizing and aggravating experience to the vulnerable early faculty member seeking promotion. This illuminates the fact that enabling more efficient practice is also a way of conveying support and appreciation—on an individual level as well as an institutional one.

Efficiency of practice is attained not only through individual work practices but also through workplace systems including policies, technologies, and well thought-out staffing. As many of these inefficiencies vary according to specialty and local work environments, the challenges and solutions are largely local. We did not identify any studies targeting early career women and efficiency of care interventions per se; however, research clearly indicates that inefficient practice (e.g., necessitating hours spent at home on work-related tasks) increases odds of burnout [103]. Below we present some general individual and workplace solutions and highlight a few recommendations specific to the early career phase.

Institutional Solutions

- Integrate aspects of efficiency of practice into effective employee on-boarding orientations, including provision of organization charts, where to find standard operating procedures and other institutional policies, and information about current initiatives to improve efficiency of practice.
- Consider how the EHR can support the use of templates, and how best it is to distribute templates to trainees and new faculty.
- Enhance easy and fast access to IT support services and EHR support services. The latter is particularly important for the early career phase when the learning curve around the specific EHR used is steep.

- Consider a wide range of efficient practice ideas including use of scribes, use of technologies (such as dictation or voice-to-text), and number and quality of support staff to perform clerical tasks.
- Develop a mechanism where physicians come together, ideally within small work units, to identify local factors that, if modified, could improve system's issues. Through this participatory management and collaborative action planning, physicians feel engaged and empowered, working constructively with leaders to shape their own future [92]. Within a training program or academic department, this mechanism might be a committee or breakout session at the Annual Program Review targeting specific areas and brainstorming solutions for identified inefficiencies.

Individual Solutions

- Consider alternate avenues for crowdsourcing efficiency practices (both individual and institutional). For example, Facebook groups for women physicians may provide a shared national platform for deriving solutions to efficient practices and institutional support measures implemented throughout the country. (Regarding Facebook groups, there are also downsides to participating in such groups; confidentiality and professionalism concerns should be considered.)
- Seek out documentation templates from peers and superiors. Consider the role for documentation strategies involving dictation, voice-to-text technologies, or medical scribes.
- Consider how you might approach your supervisor or institution with requests about systems-practices, technologies, or support staff. Consider opportunities to bring these requests into negotiation.
- Ask around about EHR task management strategies with a particular eye toward understanding how to prioritize which tasks are most impactful regarding productivity measures, promotion, hospital accreditation, and patient outcomes. Women may be more likely to internalize a desire to "please" the institution via completion of these tasks, while the reality may be that few physicians are achieving them perfectly while still maintaining

good standing at their institution. Furthermore, cogent arguments about the inefficiency of certain tasks may be taken up by your leadership if you communicate with them about your clinical experience and rationale.

- As you transition from early to advanced trainee and early attending-type roles, begin to pay back/forward efforts to enhance the efficiency of practice for those working under you. Consider developing an orientation guide for trainees that explains practices specific to the institution or service rotation. Or provide high-quality documentation templates in order to model good documentation practices and make note writing more efficient for trainees.

Personal Resiliency

Six months after the birth of her first child, a second-year resident discovered that she was unexpectedly pregnant. The thought of having two infants during residency so close to together was emotionally overwhelming, yet the idea of ending the pregnancy was also laden. She decided to continue the pregnancy but struggled with fatigue and often fell asleep shortly after returning home. Following the birth, her milk production ceased early on (not uncommon in the setting of long work hours and difficulties arranging pumping), yet her child was doing well with the bottle, which allowed her partner to do the night feedings. During the day, the baby was in a hospital-affiliated daycare that had extended hours. Every morning of her inpatient rotations, the resident met up with a good friend and co-resident an hour earlier than usual to have breakfast together at a special café on campus. On mornings she was running late, this friend would bring her breakfast to the work room instead. The simple pleasures of a shared meal and supportive company buoyed her spirits during a stressful time. Several years later, she was able to reflect the support back in a similar manner during a time of her friend's need.

Personal resilience is defined as "the set of individual skills, behaviors, and attitudes that contribute to physical, emotional, and social well-being," thus enabling the prevention of burnout [7]. The opening vignette illustrates a scenario in which a supportive friend/ colleague has volunteered and been accepted into a critical helping role in establishing some self-care during a high-risk burnout period. It demonstrates the reality that meeting self-care needs takes support and teamwork and cannot be done alone sometimes. It also demonstrates that institutional solutions such as on-site daycare with extended hours and access to good, healthy food can facilitate greater self-care, but the decision around specific needs/wants (in this case, the routine of a special breakfast with a supportive friend) and the commitment to engage must ultimately be made by the individual.

Institutions that promote wellness programming and/or allow individuals to take advantage of activities that support personal resilience have contributed to a culture of wellness. However, the domain of *Personal Resiliency* focuses on those actions of the individual who engages in resiliency behaviors. These behaviors are particularly critical in a field in which self-denial of basic needs has been indoctrinated in training and when meeting those needs has at times been labeled selfish. It is also particularly important for women who are often called upon to care for others in our sociocultural systems, frequently shortchanging their ability to meet their own needs. Such expectations around other-caregiving at the detriment of self-care are likely to be reified in medical culture. Under *Culture of Wellness*, we identifed various institutional solutions that may facilitate personal resilience in early career women. Here we will focus on individual solutions associated with *Personal Resilience*.

Increase Connectedness

As mentioned under *Culture of Wellness*, being connected with others – whether colleagues, family and/or friends – is a crucial part of enhancing and maintaining personal resilience, particularly among women.

- Participate in available engagement groups for women, particularly peer-oriented groups which may address challenges of work-life integration, parenthood, or other early career women's issues. Check if your institution runs a program similar to Lean In (at Stanford, these were named "Voice and Influence" groups).
- If such a group doesn't exist, consider starting one. Find a group of like-minded women who might be interested in meeting together. Meet during lunch hour, for breakfast before work (lobby for protected time or time-banking). This type of group might also be developed outside of the work environment to include women peers who face similar challenges, even outside of the medical profession.
- Even in the absence of "formalized" groups, reach out to other women in your department or across the department to see if they are interested in having lunch. Formal mentorship is not the only reason to network and get together; generating informal connections with fellow women physicians is also rewarding.
- If getting together whether at work or outside of work presents a challenge, consider developing or joining a virtual journal or book club, connect through social media, or join a Facebook group which can bring women together.

Enhancing Self- Care and Compassion

In order to better manage the multiplicity of factors that impact early career women's wellness, engaging in personal self-care is critical. With the help of our institutions promoting easier access to needed services or providing a more supportive environment to facilitate our self- care (*see Culture of Wellness*), women will be more able to take advantage of such opportunities.

- Seek counseling and/or medical appointments as needed.
- Prioritize adequate sleep, healthy nutrition, and regular exercise [54]. Consider having walking meetings.

- Sign-up for support groups, mindfulness or meditation-based practices, time for reflection, and other evidence-based interventions that support wellness.
- Implement positive psychology exercises such as *3 Good Things* before going to bed by writing down three good things that happen to you during the day. This practice has shown to increase happiness and decrease depressive symptoms [81].
- Be thoughtful about which hobbies you want to prioritize and consider those that are maximally replenishing. Recognize that without intentional planning, these activities may erode. Approach time management like financial management: with intention, goals, and a positive attitude.
- Learn to set compassionate limits and boundaries with work-related tasks and activities. Decline requests (ideally by expressing gratitude and responding quickly) that are unmanageable or not in line with career goals. Though in the early career this can feel presumptuous at times, learning to say "no" and to avoid becoming over-committed is a central task that any leader or later-phase physician will emphasize as important.

Meaning in Work

Becoming a doctor is a respected career path leading to a position of societal authority. For these reasons, the decision to become a physician is often reinforced by those around us and perhaps only rarely questioned. But what does it mean to become a physician today and how has the career of a physician changed over the last 50 years as women have entered the workforce? The early career phase is an important stage to consider what this occupational role means to you, and what you desire out of a "career." Taking some time to deconstruct what meaning and functions we get out of our work lives will lead to more clarity in pursuing work goals. Consider the following:

- What roles do you want your work to play? These might include financial goals, the acquisition of power or influence, scientific inquiry-related goals, a sense of service, providing specific community caretaking, teaching, community outreach, having a voice and platform, connecting with individuals on a day-to-day basis, having a flexible job, experiencing engagement and excitement, experiencing intellectual stimulation, etc.

- What are your own core values? Consider completing a value card sort at important junctures [59] to align your work life with your broader values (*see* Table 15.1).
- Think of your career as a journey, not an arc. The metaphor of "rising to the top" is rarely as simple as that directionality presumes. When connecting with potential mentors, pay attention to the ways that their careers may have fortuitously veered in unforeseen directions, often related to connections that came about organically.
- Consider the roles that failures played in career trajectories. Consider writing a "failure resume" as a means to explore the generative and learning role that failure can play [90].
- Consider a wide range of settings and employment opportunities. As women have entered the medical workforce, the positions that doctors can occupy has broadened.
- Consider the ways that academic institutions have traditionally been organized and how tenure-track pathways have been shaped by an era in which men often had partners working at home. Challenge your institution to rethink how women might have a slightly different trajectory, and reflect on how to inhabit a strong and assertive vision for that trajectory. Research indicates that women demonstrate more productivity later in their careers [43, 47].

As institutions strengthen their culture of wellness and reduce the inefficiencies of practice for early career women, these women will be able to invest more time in personal resilience activities and will be better prepared to move through subsequent career and life stages with more meaning and joy.

Table 15.1 Card sort example *(arrange values according to the importance in your life)*

Least important	Not important	Neutral	Important	Very important
Working with data	Financial reward	Challenge	Autonomy	Change and variety
Fame	Taking risks	Helpfulness	Being innovative	Genuineness
Self-control	Predictability	Taking responsibility	Caring	Integrity
Virtue	Adventure	Efficiency	Being valued	Mastery
Solitude	Power	Detailed work	Achievement	Learning
Non-conformity	Independence	Acceptance	Career progression	Self-knowledge
	Attractiveness	Life of order	Safety	Solving problems
	Popularity	Stability	Authority	Family
	Spirituality	Comfort	Commitment	Compassion
	Duty	Intimacy	Tolerance	Collaborative work
		Fitness	Humor	Growth
		Fun	Physical/mental health	Honesty
		Humility	Purpose	Justice
		Creativity	Contribute knowledge	Passion

Adapted from Miller, C'de Baca, Matthews, Wilbourne 2001

Appendix 1

Individual Development Plan

Your name: _____ Today's date:_____

Distribution of areas of effort (definitions)

1. *Education (Teaching/Scholarly Activity)*—student/resident teaching, advising, CME/curriculum teaching/involvement, new course development

2. *Research/Scholarly Activity*—basic science/clinical research, presentations and publications, funding and grant support and application, copyrights and patents, editing, and peer review
3. *Patient Care (Clinical Activities)*—direct care, chart reviews, related clinical activities
4. *Leadership & Management Skills*—participation or leadership in governance of the unit, department, program, school, personnel management, recruitment
5. *Self-Development*—training activities (CME training, earning advanced degrees, preparing for certification/re-cert, participation in professional academic associations or societies, consulting)
6. *Service*—committee membership, community outreach, and service

List your current time distribution by area estimating percent of duties and approximation of hours

Area	Percent of total duties	No. of hrs/week	How would you like to change this time distribution—New % time:
Education			
Medical student			
Resident			
Graduate student			
CME/others			
Research/scholarly activity			
Patient care			
Administration			
Self-development			
Service/citizenship			
TOTAL			

How (if at all) would you like to change this time distribution? Consider the above six categories:

1. Things you're doing now that you want to quit
2. Things you've just been asked to do that you want to refuse to do
3. Things that you're doing that you want to continue
4. Things that you're not doing that you want to start
5. Strategies for improving the balance within the above four categories

Specific Goals in Areas of Effort

Aspects necessary to achieve goals

	Expected Outcome	Resources	Collaborators	Time commitment	Barriers
Education					
Short-term goal #1:					
Short-term goal #2:					
Long-term goal #1:					
Long-term goal #2:					
Research/Scholarly activities					
Short-term goal #1:					
Short-term goal #2:					
Long-term goal #1:					
Long-term goal #2:					
Patient care (clinical activities)					
Short-term goal #1:					
Short-term goal #2:					
Long-term goal #1:					

	Expected Outcome	Resources	Collaborators	Time commitment	Barriers
Long-term goal #2:					
Leadership & management skills					
Short-term goal #1:					
Short-term goal #2:					
Long-term goal #1:					
Long-term goal #2:					
Self development					
Short-term goal #1:					
Short-term goal #2:					
Long-term goal #1:					
Long-term goal #2:					
Service/Citizenship					
Short-term goal #1:					
Short-term goal #2:					
Long-term goal #1:					
Long-term goal #2:					

Consider:

- *Were there specific areas of the IDP that were difficult for you to complete? If yes, which areas and what was difficult? Consider need for more self- development in this area.*
- *Are you "on track" to achieve your goals?*

- *What resources are available to help you achieve your short- and long-term goals?*
- *Critically assess your own competencies relative to your goals—In what areas do you need to improve and enhance your continued development?*

Adapted by Sallie G. De Golia 2019

References

1. Adesoye T, Mangurian C, Choo EK, Girgis C, Sabry-Elnaggar H, Linos E. Physician Moms Group. Perceived discrimination experienced by physician mothers and desired workplace changes: a cross-sectional survey. JAMA Intern Med. 2017;177(7):1033–6.
2. Allen BJ. Difference matters: communicating social identity. 2nd ed. Waveland: Long Grove; 2011.
3. Angelique H, Kyle K, Taylor E. Mentors and muses: new strategies for academic success. Innov Higher Educ. 2002;26:195–209.
4. Association of American Medical Colleges. Caretaking in academic medicine: from pregnancy through early parenting. 2018. https://www.aamc.org/download/488852/data/toolkitcaretakinginacademicmedicine pregnancythroughearlyyears.pdf. Accessed 15 Dec 2018.
5. Bar-Sela G, Lulav-Grinwald D, Mitnik I. "Balint group" meetings for oncology residents as a tool to improve therapeutic communication skills and reduce burnout level. J Cancer Educ. 2012;27(4): 786–9.
6. Bates CK, Gottlieb AS. Moving the needle on gender equity: a call for personal and organizational action. J Gen Intern Med. 2019;34(3): 329–30.
7. Bohman B, Dyrbye L, Sinsky CA, Linzer M, Olson K, Babbott S, Murphy M, DeVries PP, Hamidi MS, Trockel M. Physician well-being: the reciprocity of practice efficiency, culture of wellness, and personal resilience. NEJM Catalyst. 2017. https://catalyst.nejm.org/physician-well-being-efficiency-wellness-resilience. Accessed 4 Mar 2019.
8. Bowles HR, Babcock L, Lai L. Social incentives for gender differences in the propensity to initiate negotiations: sometimes it does hurt to ask. Organ Behav Hum Decis Process. 2007;103(1):84–103.
9. Bragard I, Etienne AM, Merckaert I, et al. Efficacy of a communication and stress management training on medical residents' self-efficacy, stress to communicate, and burnout: a randomized controlled study. J Health Psychol. 2010;15(7):1075–81.

10. Brown GE, Bharwani A, Patel KD, Lemaire JB. An orientation to wellness for new faculty of medicine members: meeting a need in faculty development. Int J Med Educ. 2016;7:255–60.
11. Brooks E, Early SR, Gendel EH, Miller L, Gundersen DC. Helping the healer: population-informed workplace wellness recommendations for physician Well-being. Occup Med. 2018;68:279–81.
12. Bunton SA, Corrice AM. Evolving workplace flexibility for U.S. medical school tenure- track faculty. Acad Med. 2011;86:481–5.
13. Butkus R, Serchen J, Moyer DV, Bornstein SS, Hingle ST, Health and public policy committee of the American college of physicians. Achieving gender equity in physician compensation and career advancement: a position paper of the American college of physicians. Ann Intern Med. 2018;168(10):721–3.
14. Bynum WE, Artino AR, Uijtdehaage S, Webb AMB, Varpio L. Sentinel emotional events: the nature, triggers, and effects of shame experiences in medical students. Acad Med. 2019;94(1):85–93.
15. Carnes M, Bartels CM, Isaac C, Kaatz A, Kolehmainen C. Why is John more likely to become a department chair than Jennifer? Trans Am Clin Climatol Assoc. 2015;126:197–214.
16. Carr PL, Helitzer D, Freund K, Westring A, McGee R, Campbell PB, Wood CV, Villablanca A. Summary report from the research partnership on women in science careers. J Gen Intern Med. 2018; https://doi.org/10.1007/s11606-018-4547-y. Accessed 20 Dec 2018.
17. Caravella RA, Robinson LA, Wilets I, Weinberg M, Cabaniss DL, Cutler JL, et al. A qualitative study of factors affecting morale in psychiatry residency training. Acad Psychiatry. 2016;40(5):776–82.
18. Carroll A. Silence is the enemy of doctors who have depression. 2016. Available at: https://www.nytimes.com/2016/01/12/upshot/silence-is-the-enemy-for-doctors-who-have-depression.html. Accessed 26 Dec 2018.
19. Center C, Davis M, Detre T, et al. Confronting depression and suicide in physicians: a consensus statement. JAMA. 2003;289:3161–6.
20. Cochran A, Elder WB, Crandall M, Brasel K, Hauschild T, Neumayer L. Barriers to advancement in academic surgery: views of senior residents and early career faculty. Am J Surg. 2013;206(5):661–6.
21. Conrad P, Carr P, Knight S, Renfrew MR, Dunn MB, Pololi L. Hierarchy as a barrier to advancement for women in academic medicine. J Women's Health. 2010;19(4):799–805.
22. Cumbler E, Yirdaw E, Kneeland P, Pierce R, Rendon P, Herzke C, Jones CD. What is career success for academic hospitalists? A qualitative analysis of Early-career faculty perspectives. J Hosp Med. 2018;13(6):372–7.
23. DeCastro R, Griffith KA, Ubel PA, Stewart A, Jagsi R. Mentoring and the career satisfaction of male and female academic medical faculty. Acad Med. 2014;89(2):301–11.

24. Driscoll LG, Parkes KA, Tilley-Lubbs GA, Brill JM, Pitts Bannister VR. Navigating the lonely sea: peer mentoring and collaboration among aspiring women scholars. Mentoring Tutoring Partnership Learn. 2009;17:5–21.

25. Dunn LB, Mahgoub N, DeGolia SG. How to write, socially. In: Roberts LW, editor. Academic medicine handbook: a guide to achievement and fulfillment for academic faculty, 2nd edn. New York: Springer; 2020;255–60.

26. Dyrbye LN, Shanafelt TD, Balch C, Satele D, Freischlag J. Relationship between work-home conflicts and burnout among American surgeons: a comparison by sex. Arch Surg. 2011;146(2):211–7.

27. Dyrbye LN, Freischlag J, Kaups KA, et al. Work-home conflicts have a substantial impact on career decisions that affect the adequacy of the surgical workforce. Arch Surg. 2012;147(10):933–9.

28. Dyrbye LN, Varkey P, Boone SL, Satele DV, Sloan JA, Shanafelt TD. Physician Satisfaction and Burnout at Different Career Stages Mayo. Clin Proc. 2013;88(12):1358–67.

29. Eckleberry-Hunt J, Van Dyke A, Lick D, Tucciarone J. Changing the conversation from burnout to wellness: physician well-being in residency training programs. J Grad Med Educ. 2009;1(2):225–30.

30. Fassiotto M, Simard C, Sandborg C, Valantine H, Raymond J. An integrated career coaching and time-banking system promoting flexibility, wellness, and success: a pilot program at Stanford university school of medicine. Acad Med. 2018;93(6):881–7.

31. Freund KM, Raj A, Kaplan SE, Terrin N, Breeze JL, Urech TH, Carr PL. BInequities in academic compensation by gender: a follow-up to the National Faculty Survey cohort study. Acad Med. 2016;91(8):1068–73.

32. Gander P, Briar C, Garden A, Purnell H, Woodward A. A gender-based analysis of work patterns, fatigue, and work/life balance among physicians in postgraduate training. Acad Med. 2010;85(9):1526–36.

33. Gold JA, Bentzley JP, Franciscus AM, Forte C, DeGolia SG. An intervention in social connection: medical student reflection groups. Acad Psych. 2019; https://doi.org/10.1007/s40596-019-01058-2.

34. Gold KJ, Andrew LB, Goldman EB, Schwenk TL. "I would never want to have a mental health diagnosis on my record:" a survey of female physicians on mental health diagnosis, treatment and reporting. Gen Hosp Psychiatry. 2016;43:51–7.

35. Goldhagen BE, Kingsolver K, Stinnett SS, Rosdahl JA. Stress and burnout in residents: impact of mindfulness-based resilience training. Adv Med Educ Pract. 2015;6:525–32.

36. Grisso JA, Sammel MD, Rubensein AH, Speck RM, et al. A randomized controlled trial to improve the success of women assistant professors. J Women's Health. 2017;26(5):571–9.

37. Guille C, Zhao Z, Krystal J, et al. Web-based cognitive behavioral therapy intervention for the prevention of suicidal ideation in medical interns: a randomized clinical trial. JAMA Psychiat. 2015;72(12):1192–8.

38. Gustafsson Sendén M, Schenck-Gustafsson K, Fridner A. Gender differences in reasons for sickness presenteeism – a study among GPS in a Swedish health care organization. Ann Occup Environ Med. 2016; 28:50.
39. Gunasingam N, Burns K, Edwards J, Dinh M, Walton M. Reducing stress and burnout in junior doctors: the impact of debriefing sessions. Postgrad Med J. 2015;91:182–7.
40. Haskins J, Carson JG, Chang CH, Kirshnit C, Link DP, Navarra L, et al. The suicide prevention, depression awareness, and clinical engagement program for faculty and residents at the University of California, Davis Health System. [Research Support, Non-U.S. Gov't]. Acad Psychiatry. 2016;40(1):23–9.
41. Heilman ME, Okimoto TG. Why are women penalized for success at male tasks?: the implied communality deficit. J Appl Pscyhol. 2007;92(1):81–92.
42. Hoff T, Scott S. The gendered realities and talent management imperatives of women physicians. Health Care Manag Rev. 2016;41(3):189–99.
43. Holliday EB, Jagsi R, Wilson LD, Choi M, Thomas CR Jr, Fuller CD. Gender differences in publication productivity, academic position, career duration, and funding among U.S. academic radiation oncology faculty. Acad Med. 2014;89(5):767–73.
44. Humphrey HJ. Mentoring in academic medicine. Humphrey HJ, editor. Philadelphia: ACP Press; 2010.
45. Jago AG, Vroom VH. Sex differences in the incidence and evaluation of participative leader behavior. J Appl Psychol. 1982;67(6):776–83.
46. Jagsi R. Sexual harassment in medicine — #MeToo. N Engl J Med. 2018;378:209–11.
47. Jagsi R, Guancial EA, Worobey CC, et al. The "gender gap" in authorship of academic medical literature–a 35-year perspective. N Engl J Med. 2006;355(3):281–7.
48. Jotkowitz AB, Clarfield AM. Mentoring in internal medicine. Eur J Intern Med. 2006;17:399–401.
49. Kay K, Shipman C. The confidence gap [online]. The atlantic 2014: May 2014. Available at: theatlantic.com/magazine/archive/2014/05/the-confidence-gap/359815/. Accessed 16 July 2019.
50. Kray LL, Thompson L, Galinsky A. Battle of the sexes: stereotype confirmation and reactance in negotiations. J Pers Soc Psychol. 2001;80(6):942–58.
51. Langballe EM, Innstrand ST, Aasland OG, Falkum E. The predictive value of individual factors, work-related factors, and work–home interaction on burnout in female and male physicians: a longitudinal study. Stress Health. 2011;27:73–81.
52. Lautenberger DM, Dandar VM, Raezer CL, Sloane RA. The state of women in academic medicine: the pipeline and pathways to leadership 2013–2014. Washington, D.C.: AAMC Group on Women in Medicine

and Science; 2014. pp. 1–17. https://members.aamc.org/eweb/upload/The%20State%20of%20Women%20in%20Academic%20Medicine%202013-2014%20FINAL.pdf . Accessed 21 Dec 2018.

53. Lefebvre DC. Perspective: resident physician wellness: a new hope. [review]. Acad Med. 2012;87(5):598–602.

54. Lebensohn P, Dodds S, Benn R, Brooks AJ, Birch M, Cook P, et al. Resident wellness behaviors: relationship to stress, depression, and burnout. Fam Med. 2013;45(8):541–9.

55. Levine RB, Lin F, Kern DE, Wright SM, Carrese J. Stories from early-career women physicians who have left academic medicine: a qualitative study at a single institution. Acad Med. 2011;86:752–8.

56. Luthar SS, Curlee A, Tye SJ, Engelman JC, Stonnington CM. Fostering resilience among mothers under stress: "authentic connections groups" for medical professionals. Womens Health Issues. 2017;27(3):382–90.

57. Martins AE, Davenport MC, Del Valle MP, et al. Impact of a brief intervention on the burnout levels of pediatric residents. J Pediatr. 2011;87(6):493–8.

58. Mayer AP, Files JA, Ko MG, Blair JE. Academic advancement of women in medicine: do socialized gender differences have a role in mentoring? Mayo Clin Proc. 2008;83:204–7.

59. Miller WR, Baca JC, Matthews DB, Wilbourne PL. Personal values card sort. University of New Mexico; 2001. http://www.motivationalinterviewing.org/sites/default/files/valuescardsort_0.pdf. Accessed 16 July 2019.

60. Milstein JM, Raingruber BJ, Bennett SH, Kon AA, Winn CA, Paterniti DA. Burnout assessment in house officers: evaluation of an intervention to reduce stress. Med Teach. 2009;31:338–41.

61. McNall LA, Masuda AD, Nicklin JM. Flexible work arrangements, job satisfaction, and turnover intentions: the mediating role of work-to-family enrichment. J Psychol. 2010;144(1):61–81.

62. Moutier C, Norcross W, Jong P, Norman M, Kirby B, McGuire T, et al. The suicide prevention and depression awareness program at the University of California, San Diego School of Medicine. Acad Med. 2012;87(3):320–6.

63. National Academy of Sciences[a], National Academy of Engineering and Institute of Medicine Committee on Maximizing the Potential of Women in Academic Science and Engineering. Beyond bias and barriers: fulfilling the potential of women in Academic Science and Engineering. Washington, D.C.: National Academies Press; 2007. pp. 1–12. https://www.nap.edu/read/11741/chapter/1. Accessed 1 Dec 2018.

64. National Academies of Sciences[b], Engineering, and Medicine. Sexual harassment of women: climate, culture, and consequences in academic sciences, engineering, and medicine. Washington, D.C.: National Academies Press; 2018. https://doi.org/10.17226/24994. http://sites.nationalacademies.org/shstudy/index.htm. Accessed 29 Dec 2018.

65. National Academies of Sciences[c], Engineering, and Medicine. Interventions in preventing sexual harassment. 2018. https://www.nap.edu/resource/24994/Interventions%20for%20Preventing%20Sexual%20Harassment%20final.pdf . Accessed 29 Dec 2018.
66. Niemi PM, Vainiomaki PT. Medical students' distress- quality, continuity and gender differences during a six-year medical programme. Med Teach. 2006;28:136–41.
67. Ospina-Kammerer V, Figley CR. An evaluation of the Respiratory One Method (ROM) in reducing emotional exhaustion among family physician residents. Int J Emerg Ment Health. 2003;5(1):29–32.
68. Patton EW, Griffith KA, Jones RD, Stewart A, Ubel PA, Jagsi R. Differences in mentor-mentee sponsorship in male vs female recipients of National Institutes of Health Grants. JAMA Intern Med. 2017;177(4):580–2.
69. Perlman RL, Ross PT, Lypson ML. Understanding the medical marriage: physicians and their partners share strategies for success. Acad Med. 2015;90(1):63–8.
70. Pololi L, Conrad P, Knight S, Carr P. A study of the relational aspects of the culture of academic medicine. Acad Med. 2009;84:106–14.
71. Radcliffe C, Lester H. Perceived stress during undergraduate medical training: a qualitative study. Med Educ. 2003;37:32–8.
72. Robinson JD, Cannon DL. Mentoring in the academic medical setting: the gender gap. J Clin Psychol Med Settings. 2005;12:265–70.
73. Rosdahl JA, Kingsolver KO. Mindfulness training to increase resilience and decrease stress and burnout in ophthalmology residents: a pilot study. Invest Ophthalmol Vis Sci. 2014;55:5579.
74. Rudman LA, Glick P. Prescriptive gender stereotypes and backlash toward agentic women. J Social Issues. 2001;57(4):743–62.
75. Saadat H, Snow DL, Ottenheimer S, et al. Wellness program for anesthesiology residents: a randomized, controlled trial. Acta Anaesthesiol Scand. 2012;56(9):1130–8.
76. Sambunjak D, Straus SE, Marusic A. Mentoring in academic medicine: a systematic review. JAMA. 2006;296:1103–15.
77. Salles A, Liebert CA, Greco RS. Promoting balance in the lives of resident physicians: a call to action. JAMA Surg. 2015;150(7):607–8.
78. Schrijver I, Brady KJ, Trockel M. An exploration of key issues and potential solutions that impact physician wellbeing and professional fulfillment at an academic center. PeerJ. 2016;10(4):e1783. https://doi.org/10.7717/peerj.1783. eCollection 2016.
79. Schmitz GR, Clark M, Heron S, Sanson T, Kuhn G, Bourne C, Guth T, Cordover M, Coomes J. Strategies for coping with stress in emergency medicine: early education is vital. J Emerg Trauma Shock. 2012;5(1):64–9.
80. Sege R, Nykiel-Bub L, Selk S. Sex differences in institutional support for junior biomedical researchers. JAMA. 2015;314(11):1175–7.

81. Seligman MEP, Steen TA, Park N, Peterson C. Positive psychology progress: empirical validation of interventions. Am Psychol. 2005;60(5):410–21.

82. Shanafelt TD, Kaups KL, Nelson H, et al. An interactive individualized intervention to promote behavioral change to increase personal well-being in US surgeons. Ann Surg. 2014;259:82–8.

83. Shanafelt TD, Gorringe G, Menaker R, et al. Impact of organizational leadership on physician burnout and satisfaction. Mayo Clin Proc. 2015;90(4):432–40.

84. Shanafelt TD, Sinsky C, Dyrbye LN, West CP. Potential impact of burnout on the U.S. physician workforce. Mayo Clin Proc. 2016;91(11):1667–8.

85. Shanafelt T, Trockel M, Ripp J, Murphy ML, Sandborg C, Bohman B. Building a program on well-being: key design considerations to meet the unique needs of each organization. Acad Med. 2019;94(2):156–61.

86. Shauman K, Howell LP, Paterniti DA, Beckett LA, Villablanca AC. Barriers to career flexibility in academic medicine: a qualitative analysis of reasons for the underutilization of family-friendly policies, and implications for institutional change and department chair leadership. Acad Med. 2018;93(2):246–55.

87. Sitkin N, Pachankis JE. Specialty choice among sexual and gender minorities in medicine: the role of specialty prestige, perceived inclusion, and medical school climate. LGBT Health. 2016;3(6):451–60.

88. Small DA, Gelfand M, Babcock L, Gettman H. Who goes to the bargaining table? The influence of gender and framing on the initiation of negotiation. J Pers Social Psycho. 2007;93(4):600–13.

89. Spataro BM, Tilstra SA, Rubio DM, McNeil MA. The toxicity of self-blame: sex differences in burnout and coping in internal medicine trainees. J Women's Health. 2016;25(11):1147–52.

90. Stefan M. A CV of failures. Nature. 2010;468:467.

91. Strong EA, DeCastro R, Sambuco D, Stewart A, Ubel PA, Griffith KA, Jagsi R. Work-life balance in academic medicine: narratives of physician-researchers and their mentors. JGIM. 2013;28(12):1596–603.

92. Swensen S, Kabcenell A, Shanafelt T. Physician-organization collaboration reduces physician burnout and promotes engagement: the Mayo clinic experience. J Healthcare Manag. 2016;61(2):105–27.

93. Taylor SE, Klein LC, Lewis BP, et al. Biobehavioral responses to stress in females: tend-and-befriend, not fight-or-flight. Psychol Rev. 2000;107(3):411–29.

94. Travis EL. Academic medicine needs more women leaders. AAMC News-Diversity and Inclusion. January 16, 2018. https://news.aamc.org/diversity/article/academic-medicine-needs-more-women-leaders/. Accessed 27 Dec 2018.

95. Travis EL, Doty L, Helitzer DL. Sponsorship: a path to the academic medicine C-suite for women faculty? Acad Med. 2013;88(10):1414–7.

96. Villablanca AC, Beckett L, Nettiksimmons J, Howell LP. Career flexibility and family-friendly policies: an NIH-funded study to enhance women's careers in biomedical sciences. J Women's Health. 2011;20(10):1485–96.

97. Villwock JA, Sobin LB, Koester LA, Harris TM. Impostor syndrome and burnout among American medical students: a pilot study. Int J Med Educ. 2016;7:364–9.

98. Voytko ML, Barrett N, Courtney-Smith D, Golden SL, Hsu FC, Knovich MA, Crandall S. Positive value of a women's junior faculty mentoring program: a mentor-mentee analysis. J Women's Health. 2018;27(8): 1045–53.

99. Wallace JE, Lemaire JB. On physician well-being – you'll get by with a little help from your friends. Soc Sci Med. 2007;64:2565–77.

100. Watson DT, Long WJ, Yen D, et al. Health promotion program: a resident well-being study. Iowa Orthop J. 2009;29:83–7.

101. West CP, Dyrbye LN, Erwin PJ, Shanafelt TD. Interventions to prevent and reduce physician burnout: a systematic review and meta-analysis. Lancet. 2016;388:2272–81.

102. West CP, Dyrbye LN, Satele D, Shanafelt TD. A randomized controlled trial evaluating the effect of COMPASS (colleagues meeting to promote and sustain satisfaction) small group sessions on physician well-being, meaning, and job satisfaction. J Gen Intern Med. 2015;30:S89.

103. West CP, Dyrbye LN, Shanafelt TD. Physician burnout: contributors, consequences and solutions. J Intern Med. 2018;283:516–29.

104. Westercamp N, Wang RS, Fassiotto M. Resident perspectives on work-life policies and implications for burnout. Acad Psych. 2018;42:73–7.

105. Weight CJ, Sellon JL, Lessard-Anderson CR, et al. Physical activity, quality of life, and burnout among physician trainees: the effect of a team-based, incentivized exercise program. Mayo Clin Proc. 2013;88(12):1435–42.

106. Williams ES, Manwell LB, Konrad TR, Linzer M. The relationship of organizational culture, stress, satisfaction, and burnout with physician-reported error and suboptimal patient care: results from the MEMO study. Health Care Manag Rev. 2007;32(3):203–12.

Synthesizing Solutions Across the Lifespan: Mid-Career

16

Janis E. Blair

Mid-Career Physicians

To discuss and address the challenges and potential solutions for women in the mid-career stage, one must first define "mid-career." While there is no consensus of definition, the timing of the middle of a career is most often relative to the end of postgraduate medical training. This timing then becomes problematic when considering that the period of postgraduate training may range from a 2- to 3-year residency to those involving 1, 2, or even 3 multi-year, post- residency subspecialty fellowships. Some authors define middle career as 11–20 years out of training [1], while others define it even earlier (6–10 years post training [2]). Very little literature specifically addresses physicians in the latter group [1–4]. In reality, both could be describing the same general age group, due to the variability in length of training. For the sake of definition, this section will assume the mid-career female physician to be roughly 40–55 years of age, possibly with children who may range from grammar school aged to college aged (or perhaps even early in their own careers).

J. E. Blair (✉)
Division of Infectious Diseases, Mayo Clinic, Scottsdale, AZ, USA

Mayo Clinic College of Medicine and Science, Rochester, MN, USA
e-mail: Blair.Janis@mayo.edu

© Springer Nature Switzerland AG 2020   521
C. M. Stonnington, J. A. Files (eds.), *Burnout in Women Physicians*,
https://doi.org/10.1007/978-3-030-44459-4_16

In this stage of career, women may be dealing with numerous issues that contribute to burnout or depression, and categories include family, personal health, and career issues. One study demonstrated that the highest rate of burnout occurred in practicing physicians who had been in the workforce for 6–10 years; this time frame occurs near the beginning of the mid-career, where time spent in clinical practice, research education, or administration may be in conflict with requirements for promotions [2].

Studies have shown that the general practice style of women physicians differs from male physicians, in that women tend to provide more preventative care, counseling [5], and follow guidelines more often [6]. In addition, patients score women physicians higher in empathy and note that they speak with less technical jargon, using more egalitarian language than their male counterparts [7]. Female physicians have practice outcomes that show reduced mortality and readmission of hospitalized patients [5], better diabetes outcomes [8], and other advantages. Given all the benefits that women physicians offer to their patients and institutions, and the huge cost of turnover associated with burnout [9, 10], institutions must find better ways to support women physicians. Women themselves must be aware that their struggles are not unique and find ways to support one another and make time for self-care.

Family By way of carryover from early in a physician's career, work-home conflicts likely continue into the mid-career timeframe, but change in character as children grow/develop and begin to have educational and social (school activities, sports, clubs, etc.) obligations of their own. The turbulence of teenage children may be present. Prolonged primary attention of the spouse or partner on children rather than the couple may be taking place and can take a physical and emotional toll. The life changes associated with empty nesting may be a challenge during this period, and some mid-career women may even be raising or caring for grandchildren at this stage of life. Dual-career homes may continue to challenge couples.

During mid-career, physicians may also be addressing the health of their parents and aging loved ones, who may need additional medical care or a change in homes or supervision. Grieving the death of a parent is likely to occur as well.

Personal Health In this time period, many women physicians will be dealing with challenges in personal health. Perimenopause or menopause is often associated with numerous physical and emotional changes, and increases the risk of depressed mood, anxiety, and a decreased sense of well-being [11]. In addition, particular or unique medical illnesses/challenges may develop. In this middle career stage of life, with so many other responsibilities, some women may have neglected or sacrificed their own health and well-being over the course of years and may be facing poor levels of fitness, overweight, or obesity.

Career Middle career is a time of increased work load for both men and women working in the medical field. Studies of US physicians at various career stages show that mid-career physicians reported more hours worked, more overnight call, and a low sense of work-life balance and satisfaction with career choice; this is accompanied by high emotional exhaustion and burnout when compared with physicians in early or late career stages [1, 2]. Compared with their male colleagues, fewer women surgeons (any career stage) reported that their schedules allowed adequate time for optimal family and personal life [12], and they experienced more emotional exhaustion and burnout. Physicians in the mid-career stage were more likely than other stages to plan to leave medicine within the next 24 months for reasons other than retirement [1].

A woman physician's career trajectory may have slowed down compared with her male colleagues as result of child bearing and raising a family earlier in her career [12], and requirements for promotion may not have been met as a result of the time spent up to that point in clinical, educational, research, or administrative activities [2].

Finally, even in the face of workplace changes, practice buy-outs, supervisors who do not value physicians, or other suboptimal practice situations, physicians may stay in a particular practice longer than the ideal duration, viewing departure as a weakness rather than a positive change [3].

Potential Solutions

In the face of these potentially untenable and overwhelming circumstances, the mid-career physician is at very high risk for burnout. "By not paying attention to our own deepest needs and nourishing those needs, we 'run out of gas' in our relationships and service to others, whether they be patients, family, or friends." [13] Potential solutions for burnout are abundant, but it is unlikely that one solution will address all struggles, and physicians will need a toolbox of strategies and solutions that work in any particular circumstance.

Personal Health and Well-Being

- *Make and keep appointments with your health care practitioner.* This may seem like an obvious recommendation, but too often personal health can take a backseat in the lives of busy people [14]. Having seen a primary medical practitioner within the previous 1 year, and being up to date with all age- and sex-appropriate health care and screening guidelines are all strongly correlated with high overall quality-of-life scores among surgeons [15].
- *Exercise regularly.* High quality-of-life scores are positively associated with compliance with Centers for Disease Control and Prevention (CDC) recommendations for aerobic exercise [15]. Key guidelines for adults include 150–300 min of moderate-intensity aerobic exercise per week, or 75–150 min of moderate-to vigorous-intensity exercise. In addition, muscle-strengthening activities (of moderate or greater intensity) should be performed at least twice weekly [16].
- *Schedule and prioritize a regular sleep routine.* As a group, physicians sleep less than the general population [17]. Women in perimenopause or menopause may have chronic difficulty sleeping. Chronic partial sleep deprivation is associated with functional impairment [18], and poor sleep can affect personal

health. For adults up to 60 years of age, the CDC recommends 7 hours of sleep on a regular basis [19, 20].

- *Plan and implement optimal nutrition* [3, 4, 21]. The CDC recommends healthy eating patterns within appropriate calorie levels to achieve and maintain healthy body weight, support adequate nutrition, and reduce the risk of chronic diseases [22]. Such a nutrition plan includes a variety of nutrient-dense foods across and within all food groups. It limits added sugars, saturated fats, and sodium. Planning and packing meals and snacks from home saves money and provides control over ingredients that are consumed.

- *Cultivate important relationships.* Spending time with family, spouse, children, extended family, friends, and colleagues is an important strategy in the resilience and wellness of physicians [4, 21, 23, 24]. Working married women have noted that one of the most important relationships that determine career satisfaction is a supportive spouse [24]. Turn off the television, computer, electronic medical record, and telephone and be present.

- *Cultivate religious or spiritual activity* [4, 21, 25]. In the Women Physicians' Health Study, those with deep faith connections and convictions were more likely to desire to be a physician again if given the chance to do so. The authors hypothesized that powerful philosophical convictions were not swayed by the problems that troubled other physicians [26].

- *Adopt a healthy philosophical outlook*, such as being positive or focusing on success [4, 21].

- *Recognize signs of depression* and seek counseling if able [3]. Although some have argued that burnout is a depressive syndrome, others have countered that burnout is job related and situational, driven by the work environment. Depression is a more context-free symptom complex that can be triggered by burnout and/or, if occurring independent of burnout, increased likelihood of work-related burnout [27].

- *Plan regular times of solitude*. This allows for time to reflect on goals, achievements, values, and direction, and to figure out whether changes in activities are needed [23].

Personal Well-Being at Work

- *Adopt a broad range of wellness strategies, both at home and at work.* One study on the well-being of surgeons indicated that, rather than a single strategy to achieve wellness, a repertoire of practices were necessary to achieve high levels of personal well-being [15].
- *Eat lunch.* While doing this, do not attend to emails, return telephone calls, or chart, but try to eat with someone else [28] in order to help nurture supportive relationships.
- *Insist on some control over work schedule.* Lack of control over one's work schedule is strongly associated with burnout [29–31], and efforts to improve control have successfully reduced burnout [31].
- *Set limits on work* [4]. Establish boundaries and be able to say "no" to extra tasks, patients, committee assignments, or other requests in order to move toward balance [23]. The Physician Work Life Study of more than 2300 physicians in primary and specialty care found not only that women were more burned out than their male colleagues, but also that the risk of burnout increased by 12–15% for every additional 5 hours worked beyond a 40-hour work week [32].
- *Find meaning in work.* A study of surgeons in 2010 demonstrated several factors that were associated with the lowest levels of burnout and highest quality of life; these factors included finding meaning in work, maintaining a focus on what is important in life, sustaining a positive outlook, and incorporating a balanced work/life philosophy [15]. Other studies have endorsed the need to find meaning in work [4], having and working toward professional goals [33], and the need to increase the aspects of work that are most meaningful to the individual [34]. Additional sources of meaning include teamwork, autonomy, scholarly activity, and medicine as a calling [2]. Interestingly, patient and clinical care, factors that often cause burnout, may also contribute heavily to a sense of meaning [2].
- *Have a mentor* [4]. Mentors help mentees identify professional goals, optimize their career fit, identify and manage specific stressors [33], and maintain accountability. If a single mentor does

not fulfill all needs, consider multiple mentors to address particular issues. Where mentors do not exist, consider a coach [35].

- *Cultivate a circle of supportive colleagues* who listen and support through stressful situations. Such interactions are associated with decreased emotional exhaustion [36]. Although avoidance and denial are common coping strategies, these strategies have been shown to be associated with higher levels of emotional exhaustion [36]. Understand that to receive such support, one also must provide it to others.
- *Use humor and laugh with others.* Humor and laughter are common coping strategies for physicians [36] and are advocated by physicians as a way to avoid burnout [37].
- *Take the time to regularly affirm* and support colleagues and coworkers. Be generous and gracious [24].
- *Take your vacation days* and use compensation time and unscheduled times to get away from the office and the computer. Increased use of such wellness promotion strategies are related to lower burnout and higher quality of life [36].
- *Conduct yourself with respectful, professional behavior.* This is completely within the control of professionals regardless of their circumstances. Professional, respectful behavior promotes trust and is positively correlated with workplace satisfaction and decreased burnout [38]. Give and expect the same from others.
- *Consider a possible change in career*, either within or outside the current place of practice. This could entail moving a practice to another setting or institution [3, 39], but could alternatively involve staying in the same location, but replacing some clinical activity with activities such as administration, teaching, leadership, consulting, or political activity [39, 40]. In one study, physicians who spent >80% of their time in patient care had higher rates of burnout [2].

Help from Leadership and Institutions

Health care organizations have an enormous impact on the well-being or burnout of their physician workforce in numerous ways, including influence on workload and job demands, providing resources for the job, promoting culture and values, providing meaning in work, allowing personal control and flexibility, practice support, supporting social networks, and supporting work-life balance [10]. Institutions are increasingly recognizing the business case for creating programs and an empowered and well-resourced infrastructure to meaningfully support clinician well-being [41]. Listed below is a non-comprehensive list of ways that leadership and institutions can work to address burnout.

- Physician leaders and administrators should acknowledge the problem of physician burnout and be prepared to measure and implement strategies for its reduction on an ongoing basis [9, 10, 42].
- Physician leaders and supervisors may benefit from leadership training to inspire and engage physician staff with the goal of preventing burnout and skepticism [43].
- Institutions should provide adequate administrative support systems [4].
- Institutions should support schedule flexibility as an important variable to women physician satisfaction [44, 45].
- Women physicians should be provided opportunities to advance their careers [44]. This may involve provision of mentors, and time for research or skill development at the individual level. At the level of the institution, committees that promote, recognize, and honor work and accomplishments should ensure that qualified women are adequately represented among nominees [46].
- Institutions should offer reduced-hour schedules to physicians who want to enhance their work-life balance. However, part-time opportunities may be associated with low-challenge work, and in such situations, the intent to quit is high [47]. Reduced-hour physicians should be supported with strong supervisor/administrative support, challenging and stimulating work, and opportunities for promotion [47]. Women in reduced-hour jobs should understand and pursue the credentials needed to gain promotion and inform supervisors of their desire to be considered for promotion.

- Institutions should compensate fairly between men and women. In the American Board of Emergency Medicine longitudinal survey [40], compensation fairness was more important to personal satisfaction than the actual salary itself.
- Institutions should cultivate a community of support. This could be achieved by a number of strategies.
    - Provide formal space for physician peer interactions (physician lounge or dining room) [10].
    - Provide support and time for participation in innovative activities such as an "Authentic Connections Group [48]," "Facilitated Small Group sessions [49]," or other groups [38] to foster social connectedness [42], resilience, engagement, empowerment, and reduced stress in the workplace.
- Physicians should promote policies that support zero tolerance for abusive behavior in the workplace [24].
- The clerical burden on physicians' use of the electronic health record (EHR) is one of the major drivers of physician dissatisfaction [50, 51]. Institutions must improve the EHR to minimize "clicks" and improve the EHR-user experience. The American Medical Association has published multiple modules toward this end, the AMA Steps Forward program. Granular suggestions and ideas are offered under the following general umbrellas 1. Aligning leadership and clinician EHR users; 2. optimizing software and hardware solutions; 3. reducing the burden of EHR documentation and order entry; 4. optimizing team skills and teamwork; 5. optimizing flow of information; and 6. leveraging EHR use data.
- Institutions should show support for "resilience champions (physicians with an interest in fostering resilience and who can serve as a resource for other physicians) within each department at hospitals or academic medical centers." [3]
- Institutions should facilitate and fund organizational science [10].
- Institutions and physician leaders should show support for work-life integration by providing the following:

- Annual reviews with a focus on developing and supporting work-life integration in addition to concerns regarding productivity and academic advancement [3].
- Provision of benefits such as on-site daycare, back-up childcare, in-house nanny recruitment/referral services, and assistance with elderly to help alleviate family stressors and decrease distress and burnout [28, 45, 52].

Bibliography

1. Dyrbye LN, Varkey P, Boone SL, Satele DV, Sloan JA, Shanafelt TD. Physician satisfaction and burnout at different career stages. Mayo Clin Proc. 2013;88(12):1358–67.
2. Anandarajah AP, Quill TE, Privitera MR. Adopting the quadruple aim: The University of Rochester Medical Center experience: moving from physician burnout to physician resilience. Am J Med. 2018;131(8):979–86.
3. Worley LL, Stonnington CM. Self-care, resilience, and work-life balance. New York: Springer International; 2017.
4. Spickard A Jr, Gabbe SG, Christensen JF. Mid-career burnout in generalist and specialist physicians. JAMA. 2002;288(12):1447–50.
5. Tsugawa Y, Jena AB, Figueroa JF, Orav EJ, Blumenthal DM, Jha AK. Comparison of hospital mortality and readmission rates for medicare patients treated by male vs female physicians. JAMA Intern Med. 2017;177(2):206–13.
6. Rochon PA, Gruneir A, Bell CM, Savage R, Gill SS, Wu W, et al. Comparison of prescribing practices for older adults treated by female versus male physicians: a retrospective cohort study. PLoS One. 2018;13(10):e0205524.
7. Howick J, Steinkopf L, Ulyte A, Roberts N, Meissner K. How empathic is your healthcare practitioner? A systematic review and meta-analysis of patient surveys. BMC Med Educ. 2017;17(1):136.
8. Berthold HK, Gouni-Berthold I, Bestehorn KP, Bohm M, Krone W. Physician gender is associated with the quality of type 2 diabetes care. J Intern Med. 2008;264(4):340–50.
9. Shanafelt T, Goh J, Sinsky C. The business case for investing in physician well-being. JAMA Intern Med. 2017;177(12):1826–32.
10. Shanafelt TD, Noseworthy JH. Executive leadership and physician well-being: nine organizational strategies to promote engagement and reduce burnout. Mayo Clin Proc. 2017;92(1):129–46.
11. Shifren JL, Gass ML. The north american menopause society recommendations for clinical care of midlife women. Menopause. 2014;21(10):1038–62.

12. Dyrbye LN, Shanafelt TD, Balch CM, Satele D, Sloan J, Freischlag J. Relationship between work-home conflicts and burnout among american surgeons: a comparison by sex. Arch Surg. 2011;146(2):211–7.
13. Christensen JB. Spirituality in everyday life. West J Med. 2001; 174(1):75–6.
14. Blair JE, Files JA. In search of balance: medicine, motherhood, and madness. J Am Med Womens Assoc (1972). 2003;58(4):212–6.
15. Shanafelt TD, Oreskovich MR, Dyrbye LN, Satele DV, Hanks JB, Sloan JA, et al. Avoiding burnout: the personal health habits and wellness practices of us surgeons. Ann Surg. 2012;255(4):625–33.
16. Physical activity guidelines for Americans. Department of Health and Human Services, USA. Available at: https://health.gov/paguidelines/second-edition/pdf/PAG_ExecutiveSummary.pdf. Accessed 12 Jan 2019.
17. Most physicians sleep fewer hours than needed for peak performance, report says. Available at: www.sciencedaily.com/releases/2008/03/080304075723.htm.
18. Schulman DA. When it comes to sleep health, do you practice what you preach? Vol 2019. 2013.
19. Watson NF, Badr MS, Belenky G, Bliwise DL, Buxton OM, Buysse D, et al. Recommended amount of sleep for a healthy adult: a joint consensus statement of the american academy of sleep medicine and sleep research society. Sleep. 2015;38(6):843–4.
20. Are you getting enough sleep? Available at: https://www.cdc.gov/features/sleep/index.html.
21. Weiner EL, Swain GR, Wolf B, Gottlieb M. A qualitative study of physicians' own wellness-promotion practices. West J Med. 2001; 174(1):19–23.
22. CDC. Follow healthy eating patterns across the lifespan.
23. Williams B. Woman in medicine: making it work. Tenn Med. 2007;100(9):29–30.
24. Sotile WM, Sotile MO. The key to excellence: successful executives keep the flame alive at work and home! J Oncol Manag. 1999;8(3):21–6.
25. Blair JE, Files JA. In search of balance: medicine, motherhood, and madness. J Am Med Wom Assoc. 2003;58(4):212–6.
26. Frank E, McMurray JE, Linzer M, Elon L. Career satisfaction of us women physicians: results from the women physicians' health study. Society of general internal medicine career satisfaction study group. Arch Intern Med. 1999;159(13):1417–26.
27. Melnick ER, Powsner SM, Shanafelt TD. In reply-defining physician burnout, and differentiating between burnout and depression. Mayo Clin Proc. 2017;92(9):1456–8.
28. Humikowski CA. Beyond burnout. JAMA. 2018;320(4):343–4.
29. Moore LR, Ziegler C, Hessler A, Singhal D, LaFaver K. Burnout and career satisfaction in women neurologists in the United States. J Womens Health (Larchmt). 2019;28(4):515–25.

30. Olson K, Sinsky C, Rinne ST, Long T, Vender R, Mukherjee S, et al. Cross-sectional survey of workplace stressors associated with physician burnout measured by the mini-z and the maslach burnout inventory. Stress Health. 2019;35(2):157–75.

31. Dunn PM, Arnetz BB, Christensen JF, Homer L. Meeting the imperative to improve physician well-being: assessment of an innovative program. J Gen Intern Med. 2007;22(11):1544–52.

32. McMurray JE, Linzer M, Konrad TR, Douglas J, Shugerman R, Nelson K. The work lives of women physicians results from the physician work life study. The sgim career satisfaction study group. J Gen Intern Med. 2000;15(6):372–80.

33. Shanafelt T, Chung H, White H, Lyckholm LJ. Shaping your career to maximize personal satisfaction in the practice of oncology. J Clin Oncol. 2006;24(24):4020–6.

34. Shanafelt TD, West CP, Sloan JA, Novotny PJ, Poland GA, Menaker R, et al. Career fit and burnout among academic faculty. Arch Intern Med. 2009;169(10):990–5.

35. Bickel J. Looking for mentor replacement therapy? A coach may be the answer. J Am Med Womens Assoc (1972). 2003;58(4):210–1.

36. Lemaire JB, Wallace JE. Not all coping strategies are created equal: a mixed methods study exploring physicians' self reported coping strategies. BMC Health Serv Res. 2010;10:208.

37. Swetz KM, Harrington SE, Matsuyama RK, Shanafelt TD, Lyckholm LJ. Strategies for avoiding burnout in hospice and palliative medicine: peer advice for physicians on achieving longevity and fulfillment. J Palliat Med. 2009;12(9):773–7.

38. Shapiro DE, Duquette C, Abbott LM, Babineau T, Pearl A, Haidet P. Beyond burnout: a physician wellness hierarchy designed to prioritize interventions at the systems level. Am J Med. 2019;132(5):556–63.

39. Keyes LE. Underpaid women, stressed out men, satisfied emergency physicians. Ann Emerg Med. 2008;51(6):729–31.

40. Cydulka RK, Korte R. Career satisfaction in emergency medicine: the ABEM longitudinal study of emergency physicians. Ann Emerg Med. 2008;51(6):714–22.e1.

41. Shanafelt T, Trockel M, Ripp J, Murphy ML, Sandborg C, Bohman B. Building a program on well-being: key design considerations to meet the unique needs of each organization. Acad Med. 2019;94(2):156–61.

42. Swensen S, Kabcenell A, Shanafelt T. Physician-organization collaboration reduces physician burnout and promotes engagement: the mayo clinic experience. J Healthc Manag. 2016;61(2):105–27.

43. Shanafelt TD, Gorringe G, Menaker R, Storz KA, Reeves D, Buskirk SJ, et al. Impact of organizational leadership on physician burnout and satisfaction. Mayo Clin Proc. 2015;90(4):432–40.

44. Clem KJ, Promes SB, Glickman SW, Shah A, Finkel MA, Pietrobon R, et al. Factors enhancing career satisfaction among female emergency physicians. Ann Emerg Med. 2008;51(6):723–28.e8.
45. Mobilos S, Chan M, Brown JB. Women in medicine: the challenge of finding balance. Can Fam Physician. 2008;54(9):1285–86.e5.
46. Kuhn GJ, Abbuhl SB, Clem KJ. Recommendations from the Society for Academic Emergency Medicine (SAEM) task force on women in Academic Emergency Medicine. Acad Emerg Med. 2008;15(8):762–7.
47. Hartwell JK. Psychological contracts: a new strategy for retaining reduced-hour physicians. J Med Pract Manage. 2010;25(5):285–97.
48. Luthar SS, Curlee A, Tye SJ, Engelman JC, Stonnington CM. Fostering resilience among mothers under stress: "authentic connections groups" for medical professionals. Womens Health Issues. 2017;27(3):382–90.
49. West CP, Dyrbye LN, Rabatin JT, Call TG, Davidson JH, Multari A, et al. Intervention to promote physician well-being, job satisfaction, and professionalism: a randomized clinical trial. JAMA Intern Med. 2014;174(4):527–33.
50. Sinsky C, Colligan L, Li L, Prgomet M, Reynolds S, Goeders L, et al. Allocation of physician time in ambulatory practice: a time and motion study in 4 specialties. Ann Intern Med. 2016;165(11):753–60.
51. Sinsky CA, Dyrbye LN, West CP, Satele D, Tutty M, Shanafelt TD. Professional satisfaction and the career plans of us physicians. Mayo Clin Proc. 2017;92(11):1625–35.
52. Baptiste D, Fecher AM, Dolejs SC, Yoder J, Schmidt CM, Couch ME, et al. Gender differences in academic surgery, work-life balance, and satisfaction. J Surg Res. 2017;218:99–107.

Late Career Solutions. Transitional Zone – Retire or Retread

17

Suzanne M. Connolly

Scenario

Dr. B. is a 59-year-old internist working full-time in a group practice. She was diagnosed with cancer for which she underwent surgery and has recently returned to her clinical practice. New teaching responsibilities for medical students and residents in addition to adjustment to a new electronic medical record system have increased her workload considerably. Her older husband, a retired teacher, is to undergo hip replacement in a few months and she has elderly parents she assists. Although she has an adult son, he and his young family live abroad and cannot help with family needs. She is overwhelmed; she is emotionally exhausted, stressed, and does not feel she can accomplish all at hand. She is seriously considering her options.

Dr. B. is not unlike many senior career women who have responsibilities for family members and multiple stressors in the workplace. Early retirement may be a viable option, but careful considerations of the ramifications of this decision and exploration of alternative strategies to address her work–life situation are imperative. Options she might consider include part-time work,

S. M. Connolly (✉)
Department of Dermatology, Mayo Graduate School of Medicine,
Scottsdale, AZ, USA

© Springer Nature Switzerland AG 2020 535
C. M. Stonnington, J. A. Files (eds.), *Burnout in Women Physicians*,
https://doi.org/10.1007/978-3-030-44459-4_17

re-balancing her clinical and educational responsibilities if possible in her group practice, and investigating temporary solutions such as whether she is eligible for family medical leave.

As Dr. B. contemplates her decision, she must consider a number of factors. Is she happy with her clinical practice? Does she enjoy patient care and the camaraderie of the group practice? Does she look forward to the prospect of working with young people entering the profession of medicine? Should she more seriously consider her health as a factor in her decision given her recent diagnosis of cancer? Would retirement allow her the ability to better care for her parents? Is she physically able to care for them or should she explore services available to them? What is her financial status: can she afford to retire? If she participates in a pension plan, does retirement earlier than planned or reduction in hours of work negatively impact her distribution? Does she have interests other than medicine? What type of lifestyle does she envision in her retirement years? Does she have the means to support it?

Retirement presents a transitional zone, a proverbial yin and yang, that is, the receptive and active principles seen in all forms of change. When do physicians retire? Why do some retire early and some delay retirement? What considerations might facilitate continuing to practice or choose retirement? Are there factors that influence female physicians differently than their male counterparts when deciding how and when to retire?

When Do Physicians Retire?

This is a question addressed in a systematic review of 65 English-language studies which were mostly cross-sectional in design, methodologically strong, and with results deemed credible [1]. Retirement was defined as "fully retired"; primary care and specialty physicians were included. Most studies originated in the United States with others based in Australia, Canada, Finland, Israel, the Netherlands, New Zealand, and the United Kingdom. The average age for expected and actual retirement of physicians reported was 60 years and 69 years, respectively; retirement occurred later than planned. Studies analyzed were published from

1976 to March, 2016; thus, the socioeconomic and healthcare delivery environment varied greatly over the span of these decades.

In a more recent survey of late-career physicians defined as age 50 years and older in primary care or various specialties conducted by Hanover Research on behalf of CompHealth, an American healthcare staffing company found that respondents intended to retire at an average age of 66 years [2]. In a study based on data from the American Medical Association (AMA) Physician Masterfile which included 77,987 physicians age 55–80 years and with retirement defined as leaving clinical practice, the median retirement age of all physicians who left clinical activity from 2010 to 2014 was 64.9 years [3]. Retirement age was similar across primary care specialties. Female primary care physicians had a median age at retirement that was about 1 year earlier than males (0.5 year for female family physicians and 1.3 years for female general internists). If retirement was defined as retirement from any type of professional medical activity, median retirement age across all primary care specialties occurred about 1 year later for both males and females. Thus, physicians tend to retire in their mid- to late-60s. To put this in perspective, the average retirement age of the general employed population in the United States is 63 years; thus, as of 2014, physicians tend to work longer than the average American.

Why Do Some Physicians Retire Earlier Than Expected?

This data was collated in the systematic review of physician retirement planning noted above. The list of reasons is unsurprisingly long given the span of years included in the report. Low job satisfaction, medical-legal issues, and health and financial concerns were common factors. Loss of autonomy, low morale, dissatisfaction with regulations, frustration with colleagues, feeling undervalued, and frank loss of interest in work were aspects of low job satisfaction notated. Excessive workloads and burnout were frequently cited reasons for early retirement, *especially within the last decade*. Lack of satisfaction with the regulation of medicine and bureaucracy and management viewed as oppressive gave rise to medical-legal issues. Poor health, cognitive decline, difficulty with sleeping, and psychological stress were other factors noted in more recent years. Some retired early to preserve health. Some viewed increasing costs of maintaining a practice including malpractice insurance fees and lower reimbursements as factors against continuing to practice; others had pension security.

In the CompHealth survey reported in 2017, doctors were not as satisfied with their careers as they had been; 59% of physicians noted their satisfaction had decreased since they began to practice. But they still had high overall career satisfaction: 82% were satisfied or completely satisfied with their careers. Concerns about staying competitive in the changing healthcare environment (38%), declining personal health (37%), providing quality patient care (26%), mastering technology (23%), and failing health of spouse/ partner were concerns about working past 65 years of age in this survey.

In a large national cohort survey of all United Kingdom-trained medical graduates of 1974 and of 1977, factors influencing the decision to retire or to continue to practice were collated [4]. The median age of the 1974 graduates was 64 years (men: 64 years; women: 63 years) and for the 1977 graduates 61 years (men: 61 years; women: 60 years). Forty-four percent of all respondents were retired (38% of men; 56% of women), 26% had retired but returned to practice (29% of men; 20% of women), and 29% continued to work in medicine (32% of men; 23% of women). For those retired, the reasons cited in decreasing order of importance were desire for more time for leisure or pursuit of other interests, increased pressure of practice (43%), retirement of spouse, family reasons, financial reasons (poor reimbursements, financial security), and on-call work. More men than women cited on-call work hours as a factor. Those retirees from the younger 1977 cohort were significantly more likely to retire due to pressure of work, reduced job satisfaction, or financial reasons, suggesting these factors are more relevant to earlier retirement. Of those retired, they did so earlier than planned due to changes in the work environment (14%) or due to personal circumstances (13.7%).

According to a recent large survey of pediatricians conducted by the American Academy of Pediatrics, 27% of those still working would retire if it were affordable [5]. Increased regulation in medicine, decreased clinical autonomy, and insufficient reimbursements were rated by >50%of respondents as the most important factors. For those pediatricians who had retired, nearly 27% rated the effort to keep up with clinical advances and changes in practice as important factors in deciding to retire.

Possible cognitive decline has become a factor receiving greater emphasis in recent years as a greater number of senior physicians continue to practice [6]. There has been an aging of the medical workforce with a 374% increase in the number of actively practicing physicians over the age of 65 years in the United States from 1975 to 2015. In 2015, 23% of practicing physicians were 65 years or older. For some professionals such as air pilots, air traffic controllers and firefighters, periodic testing is required or there is a mandatory retirement age. While there are not uniform requirements for physicians, some hospitals and institutions have introduced mandatory age-based assessments. Another assessment of competency is maintenance of certification requirements which have increasingly been implemented in the medical profession and have become another factor in early retirement considerations.

The situation of Dr. B. is not unusual. Common factors that favor an early retirement include personal health, family concerns, and the burden of practice including aspects of delivery of care. Data also confirms that retirement at age 59 years is earlier than average; her health and family concerns along with practice demands are well-recognized factors impacting this consideration.

Why Physicians Retire Later Than Planned

This is often due to career satisfaction, a desire to be active and focus on the social and stimulating intellectual aspects of the medical profession, a sense of responsibility to patients, ongoing financial obligations, and/or lack of interests outside of medicine [1]. In a survey of late-career physicians in the United States, age 50 years or older, the top three reasons for working beyond the age of 65 years were enjoyment of the practice of medicine, enjoyment of the social aspects of working and the desire to maintain current lifestyle [2]. Institutions can play a role in promoting physician satisfaction and practicing medicine for a longer period. Flexibility in work hours, emphasis on career development, and awareness of the value of some degree of personal autonomy over work are examples of ways the workplace can promote satisfaction and a longer period of time in practice [1].

Some cannot imagine life without medical practice. A loss of identity and/ or sense of purpose with retirement from a demanding profession for which years of training were required are not an uncommon concern of many; little time may have been taken to develop or maintain interests outside of medicine. In a small but highly detailed study of academic Canadian physicians, manifestations of threats to personal identity included apprehensions about self-esteem after retirement, a loss of a sense of belonging, concerns about clinical competency, and continuity of patient care [7]. Women physicians and other professional women may have a more difficult time than men adjusting to retirement. They are more likely to have a sense of loss with retirement compared to a sense of relief shared by non-professional women workers. And while the latter are more likely to base retirement decisions on family issues and responsibilities, professional women are more likely to base the decision on pension eligibility and health concerns [8].

Thus, among potential reasons for later retirement are the following:

- Career satisfaction
- Sense of responsibility for patients
- Lack of interests outside of medicine
- Concerns about loss of identity with leaving professional practice
- Lack of financial ability to maintain desired lifestyle or pension eligibility

Pattern of Retirement

This is an important consideration, not only for the physician but also for the institution or group in which he/she practices. It impacts patients too. Institutional flexibility has been noted to be a positive driver of retaining physicians and facilitating retirement planning [1]. There is benefit to the institution to know retirement plans and, thus, better meet appropriate staffing demands. In a population-based retrospective cohort study of all physicians over 50 years of age in British Columbia, Canada, four retirement patterns for physicians were identified by payment data analysis: slow decline in practice activity by 10% to <25%, rapid decline by 25% to 90%, maintenance of practice with little change in activity until full retirement, or an increase in practice activity by 10% or more until retirement [9]. About 40% reduced their practice activity by at least 10% in the 3 years preceding retirement. Women physicians retired earlier as did those practicing in rural areas. Research is needed on why women physicians retire earlier [10]. In a study of pattern of retirement of academic physicians age 65 years or older, four potential retirement trajectories were identified: abrupt, progressive reduction in practice activity, some reduction such as half-time followed by abrupt retirement, and continued activity until serious illness or death [11].

Physicians prefer gradual retirement. In a small but highly detailed study, 89.5% of physicians surveyed preferred to retire gradually [12]. Flexible and fewer work hours, part-time employment, job-sharing, and decreased time on-call are among the possible options of gradually cutting back on clinical practice [1, 12, 13]. Sharing care between an incoming new physician and a late-career physician wanting to reduce hours can afford a smooth transition for the physicians, greater patient satisfaction, and also ease the impact of retirement on other members of a group practice. These approaches can be viewed as ways of keeping physicians in the workforce and improving work satisfaction. In some specialties greater part-time work before full retirement was noted among women compared to men [14, 15].There are caveats with part-time work: compensation might not be comparable to full-time work if pay is considered on an hourly basis of compensation; an individual may actually put in full-time effort and hours, yet be compensated an a part-time basis; the characteristics of one's clinical practice might be impacted, such as limiting type of patient to be evaluated or procedures performed; one might be perceived as less dedicated; opportunities to engage in special projects may be viewed by others as an inconvenience [16]. Additionally, the aim is to reduce hours of work and care needs to be taken that the same number of patients are not scheduled in a reduced time frame! Impact on pension plan is a key consideration. Contemplation of any reduction in number of hours worked at any time in one's career must be coupled with careful review of the impact on future pension distributions. One guide for part-time employment has been developed by the American College of Physicians [17].

Another consideration is full retirement followed by continued professional clinical activity in a *locum tenens* position or, for some specialties, telemedicine. Medical consulting such as for law firms, pharmaceutical industry, medical device company, insurance companies, or other entities are among other options for those retirees who wish to continue to participate in medicine professionally but without clinical patient activity [18].

In summary, most physicians prefer gradual retirement which permits a growth into the next phase of life.

- Reduction in work hours might be accomplished by flexible and fewer hours of work, job-sharing, or decreasing on-call demands.
- Creative institutional flexibility in considering gradual retirement options can be a positive force.
- Any reduction in hours of work must be preceded by careful review of the impact on current and future financial status including pension distributions.
- Any contractual agreements between the physician and institution or group require careful review.
- There are many options after retirement for continued participation in medicine professionally that do not include direct patient care.
- For Dr. B. in the scenario, there is a sense of urgency as she contemplates her next step. She regrets that she has not spent time exploring these issues and strategically considering her late career options.

Planning

This is the key to successful retirement. The word "*retire*" connotes withdrawal, an exit, or departure, all rather negative descriptors. To this author "*retread*" is a more optimistic term to apply to this phase of life where freedom of personal and/or professional reinvention and continued growth can occur. There are what the author terms the *Five F's of Retirement Planning*: *F*itness, *F*amily, *F*riends, and *F*un, all of which cultivate a sense of personal well-being, and *F*inances. The goal should be transition "to" another phase in life not only "from" medicine. Ideally, retirement planning – so called " exit strategies" – should receive as much enthusiastic attention as career planning and preferably early on in one's career. It is better not to be like "the dog chasing the car," that is, all in for the chase but not knowing what to do when it's caught [19]. The success of this transition zone has a great deal to do with thoughtful, early planning and knowing one's self. The plan should be adaptable to withstand unexpected situations such as some of those experienced by Dr. B. in the scenario, but flexible enough to permit ability to embrace new opportunities that might arise and offer further zest to life. This can be a time of reinvention: "I am the master of my fate/ I am the captain of my soul" [20].

A myriad of meaningful activities are possible after retirement that can include volunteer work inside or outside of medicine [21]. Many rewarding opportunities might be considered, such as mentoring, teaching, writing, donating time to free medical clinics locally or abroad, or speaking to the community about public health issues. Local medical societies, national and subspecialty medical associations, medical schools, and training programs as well as community non-medical volunteer networks such as the Corporation for National and Community Service (https://nationalservice.gov), family, and friends can all be resources to access. There is meaning in life after full-time clinical practice. Healthcare organizations and medical societies have an opportunity to educate late-career senior physicians about the possibilities.

Six significant practical insights about retirement were recently shared by survey technique of 1200 retired American physicians [22]. They underscore the need to take the time to truly consider options, to know one's goals, wants, and needs. The first emphasis was the benefit of a gradual transition to retirement such that time could be taken to cultivate life outside of medicine, a so-called "growing into retirement" phase of 1–2 years, as has been outlined above. Defining and planning meaningful activities was stressed. Assessing goals before retirement and considering strategies to achieve them, taking care of one's health, and making a commitment to enjoy retirement were other important insights shared by these retirees. The last two insights related to financial wellness: financial planning and priority spending. Financial planning with one's spouse/ partner and a financial advisor was considered of utmost importance and, ideally, initiated early in one's career. Re-assessment of wills, insurances, power of attorney, estate plan, and advanced directives should be done. The last insight shared by this group was the importance of prioritizing spending to live within one's means. A clever way of thinking of finances over the years of retirement might be to consider three phases of this chapter: go go, go slow, no go!

The importance of early financial planning cannot be over emphasized as it can impact not only the timing of retirement but also the possibilities of what retirement will look like [23, 24]. Conversely, poor financial planning is a barrier to retirement [1, 12]. Planning for retirement should occur over one's medical career [23–27]. Early considerations ideally include establishing a team of advisors including a financial expert, attorney, and accountant; obtaining life and disability insurances and considering insurance for long term care, too; and creating a will, developing advanced directives and establishing power of attorney. Mid-career actions might include paying off debts, maximizing retirement contributions, monitoring investments, re-assessing insurance needs, updating wills, and developing an estate plan. At age 50 years and older, updating financial goals, reviewing annual budgets especially expenses, and reviewing pension plans and other potential sources on income need to be the focus. Review of wills, advanced directives, and power of attorney should be done at every phase as with any major life transition such as having children. Insurance, especially health insurance, must be considered carefully, particularly if retirement occurs before the age of Medicare eligibility in the United States.

Barriers to retirement planning can include poor personal financial management including simply a lack of personal interest, rigid institutional policies that favor full retirement over gradual, and a professional culture that favors work over other aspects of life [1, 28]. Facilitators of physician retirement include financial planning resources offered to physicians at multiple times throughout their careers, opportunities for gradual transition toward retirement, and the introduction of the concept of career mentorship by supporting collaborations between younger and older physicians [12]. There is an opportunity for organizations to provide easily accessible support [29]. Areas of support could include retirement planning, basic income tax services, college planning for children, short- or long-term disability planning, or other areas of financial counseling such as life insurance, long-term care insurance, basic estate planning. But also organizations can provide support for professional issues such as burnout, time management, and work-life integration, as well as for personal issues such as those facing Dr. B. in the scenario above. Professional medical associations such as the American Medical Association, the American College of Physicians, and many specialty societies also offer guidance, resources, and support.

If a physician decides to retire, any contractual agreements must be carefully reviewed. Any employment contracts with a group should be assessed, especially with respect to advanced notification of retirement [27]. In a group practice, responsibility for patient records and patient transition would be assumed by the group. For those in private practice, state requirements for record storage, retention, and accessibility need to be reviewed and arrangements made for this as well as smooth transition of patients to other providers. Requirements of malpractice carriers and state medical licensure need to be reviewed thoroughly.

With her recent surgery for cancer, Dr. B. has reviewed her will and advanced directives, but she did not review her long-term financial plan including her group's pension plan in which she has participated, details of her contractual arrangement with her group, nor her insurance policies. She regrets not having taken full advantage of financial counseling services offered by her group early on in her career; she let demands of the practice and of her family supersede time spent on long-term planning. Only now does she fully appreciate how important planning throughout her career should have been. Her inclination is to retire from full-time practice, but she is uncertain what impact early retirement will have on her future. Planning in advance for the expected and unexpected would have placed her in the "driver's seat" instead of circumstances driving her.

In summary, a retirement plan should

- Begin early in one's career and be re-assessed throughout the span of a career
- Be based on realistic goals with thoughtful strategies to achieve them
- Be flexible enough to adapt to unexpected circumstances
- Be developed by a team with expertise in finance, law, insurance, and accounting
- Be financially sound with attention to a realistic budget
- Be attentive to contractual arrangements with the workplace and to whether the employer supports late career transitions to retirement
- Take advantage of any planning services offered by the employer
- Embrace a healthy lifestyle and a commitment to enjoy this phase of life and late career
- Be open to new opportunities

Healthcare institutions would be wise to offer comprehensive retirement planning that includes but is not limited to financial planning and is triggered at key times throughout the course of a physician's career. Such programs could prevent sudden unexpected departures, decrease burnout, and increase fulfillment by tapping the wisdom of senior physicians. These early-, mid-, and late-career discussions either within one's specialty department, HR, or other office geared toward support of the clinicians could include:

- Assistance with financial planning, wills, advanced directives, and adequate insurance health and malpractice coverage
- Surveys of "what is important to me" to clarify interests inside and outside of medicine
- Strategies for gradually scaling back over time and increasing attention to other pursuits or family focused activities
- Wellness coaching
- Opportunities to be mentored by retired or late-career physicians
- Opportunities for mentoring students, trainees, and early career physicians
- Opportunities to refine and tailor one's practice over time to take advantage of an individual's expertise and interests

How Physicians Adjust to Retirement

This has been the subject of a systematic review of peer-reviewed English-language literature published with quantitative and/or qualitative analysis [30]. Generally, retirement was viewed as positive. Financial security, good health, engagement in meaningful activities, and improvement in quality of time spent with family including spouse and relatives correlated with adjusting well to retirement. Having a plan enhanced adjustment. Poor health of a spouse had a negative impact and correlated with depression in the retiree; some retirees suffer depression with leaving active medical practice [31].

AMA Insurance has reported on the financial preparedness of retired physicians in the United States and retirement satisfaction [32]. The survey included 1202 physicians representing the broad spectrum of medical and surgical specialties; 13% were female and 85% of respondents were married. Twelve percent had retired at less than 60 years of age; 14% retired at age 75 years or greater. Eighty percent of respondents were either satisfied or very satisfied with retirement, while 9% were either dissatisfied or very dissatisfied with retirement. Eleven percent of respondents were neutral. Most retired physicians were leading full, active lives with over 80% spending time with friends and family, as well as leisure activities (76%) and travel (60%). A significant percent (41%) engaged in volunteer work, taught (16%), worked part-time (17%), consulted (15%), or started a new business (4%). No details were given about the amount of time devoted to past profession.

The top 5 factors that impacted satisfaction in this survey were age at retirement, financial knowledge and status, initiation of savings early in career, and use of a financial planner. Those who retired under age 60 years were more likely dissatisfied or very dissatisfied; those who retired between the ages of 60 and 65 years were most satisfied. Nearly 30% of those who retired before the age of 60 years viewed their financial status as behind where they would like to be. Seventy-one percent of the respondents who judged themselves financially savvy and understood their personal finances were more satisfied with retirement compared to those who rated themselves as not very knowledgeable. Nearly 3 out of 4 retired physicians worked with a professional financial advisor and they were more likely to be satisfied with their retirement than those who did not. Forty-seven percent of those who did not use a financial advisor preferred to handle their own finances.

Satisfaction in retirement also depends on being confident that financial fitness extends throughout retirement, and this confidence depends on a number of facets including at what age one retires, health, and longevity. Overall, in the AMA Insurance survey, respondents were confident that their retirement funds would last. Living within one's means, wise investment decisions, generous savings, and having a financial advisor who shared that view bolstered confidence. Conversely, market volatility and less savings lowered confidence that retirement funds would last. Major health issues, unexpected costs that rapidly reduced savings, supporting other family members, or having spent too much early in retirement years reduced confidence.

Returning to Dr. B. in the scenario, if she had made retirement readiness a part of her overall career planning, she could deliberate more confidently on a broader range of options leading to a satisfying retirement – even at age 59 years. Greater satisfaction in retirement is more likely achieved if the following factors are considered:

- Be enthusiastic about retirement planning and begin it early in the course of a career; be attentive, reassess, and adjust the plan over time.
- Be knowledgeable about finances, work with a professional financial advisor, and save early.
- Be aware of contractual arrangements and insurance coverages – including that for health.
- Be open to opportunities along the course of a career trajectory; in particular, be aware of potential possibilities permitting a gradual retirement that do not impact pension distribution.
- Be engaged in meaningful activities; know your interests and what gives you satisfaction.
- Be healthy!

Gaps and Opportunities

The limited data currently available indicates that there is substantial overlap but also key differences between male and female physicians in terms of when and why they retire, the patterns of retirement, reasons for retirement, and how they adjust to retirement. As greater numbers of women approach retirement age, there is an opportunity and a need to investigate in detail all aspects of their retirement including planning and to develop more tools to support this phase of career and life. Among opportunities are the following:

- Study ongoing demographic trends among male and female physicians including age at retirement, pattern of retirement, reasons for retirement, perceived key stressors that might have impacted time of retirement, and details of degree of financial planning undertaken and when it was initiated. Such data can inform future workforce needs and needs of female physicians in particular.

- There is no data to the author's knowledge of minority female physicians and aspects of their retirement.
- Develop educational tools about retirement that are geared to female physicians.
- Gather data about activities undertaken by female physicians in retirement, in particular volunteerism, care for family members or friends, and professional versus non-professional activities.
- Assess satisfaction of retired female physicians and factors that positively or negatively impact it.

References

1. Silver MP, Hamilton AD, Biswas A, Warrick NI. A systematic review of physician retirement planning. Hum Resour Health. 2016;14(1):67.
2. CompHealth. Survey report – Physician views on retirement. 2017. Available from: https://comphealth.com/resources/wp-content/uploads/2017/07/CPHY20200_PhysicianViewsOnRetirementReport_rw_v1.pdf.
3. Petterson SM, Rayburn WF, Liaw WR. When do primary care physicians retire? Implications for workforce projections. Ann Fam Med. 2016;14(4):344–9.
4. Smith F, Lachish S, Goldacre MJ, Lambert TW. Factors influencing the decisions of senior UK doctors to retire or remain in medicine: national surveys of the UK-trained medical graduates of 1974 and 1977. BMJ Open. 2017;7(9):e017650.
5. Rimsza ME, Ruch-Ross H, Simon HK, Pendergass TW, Mulvey HJ. Factors influencing pediatrician retirement: a survey of American Academy of Pediatrics Chapter Members. J Pediatr. 2017;188:275–9.
6. Dellinger EP, Pellegrini CA, Gallagher TH. The aging physician and the medical profession: a review. JAMA Surg. 2017;152(10):967–71.
7. Onyura B, Bohnen J, Wasylenki D, Jarvis A, Giblon B, Hyland R, et al. Reimagining the self at late-career transitions: how identity threat influences academic physicians' retirement considerations. Acad Med. 2015;90(6):794–801.
8. Price CA. Retirement for women: the impact of employment. J Women Aging. 2002;14(3–4):41–57.
9. Hedden L, Lavergne MR, McGrail KM, Law MR, Cheng L, Ahuja MA, et al. Patterns of physician retirement and pre-retirement activity: a population-based cohort study. CMAJ. 2017;189(49):E1517–e23.
10. Silver MP. Physician retirement: gender, geography, flexibility and pensions. CMAJ. 2017;189(49):E1507–e8.

11. Moss AJ, Greenberg H, Dwyer EM, Klein H, Ryan D, Francis C, et al. Senior academic physicians and retirement considerations. Prog Cardiovasc Dis. 2013;55(6):611–5.
12. Pannor Silver M, Easty LK. Planning for retirement from medicine: a mixed-methods study. CMAJ Open. 2017;5(1):E123–e9.
13. Silver MP. Critical reflection on physician retirement. Can Fam Physician. 2016;62(10):783–4.
14. Orkin FK, McGinnis SL, Forte GJ, Peterson MD, Schubert A, Katz JD, et al. United States anesthesiologists over 50: retirement decision making and workforce implications. Anesthesiology. 2012;117(5):953–63.
15. Merline AC, Cull WL, Mulvey HJ, Katcher AL. Patterns of work and retirement among pediatricians aged >or=50 years. Pediatrics. 2010;125(1):158–64.
16. Moawad H. Why working part time may not be a good idea. 2016. Available from: https://www.mdmag.com/physicians-money-digest/con-tributor/heidi-moawad-md/2016/12/why-working-part-time-may-not-be-a-good-idea.
17. American College of Physicians. Part Time Employment for Physicians 2017. 2017. Available from: https://www.acponline.org/system/files/documents/running_practice/practice_management/human_resources/part_time.pdf.
18. Blau JM, Paprocki RJ, Baum N. Road to retirement part III: other options for retiring physicians. J Med Pract Manage. 2015;31(2):78–81.
19. Larson DL. Preparing for retirement: reflections on mistakes made and lessons learned. Aesthet Surg J. 2015;35(2):225–7.
20. Bartlett J. Familiar quotations. Rarebooksclub Com. Boston, USA; Little, Brown and Company, 2012.
21. Singer D. Moving forward: retirement opportunities for senior physicians. Rhode Island Med J (2013). 2017;100(9):26–8.
22. Farouk A. 6 Key physician retirement insights From doctors already there 2018. Available from: https://www.ama-assn.org/practice-management/career-development/6-key-physician-retirement-insights-doctors-already-there.
23. Blau JM, Paprocki RJ, Baum N. Road to retirement: not necessarily the road less traveled – part I. J Med Pract Manage. 2015;30(6):373–6.
24. Blau JM, Paprocki RJ, Baum N. Road to retirement: part II – advice on advisors. J Med Pract Manage. 2015;31(1):26–8.
25. Clemons MJ, Vandermeer LA, Gunstone I, Jacobs C, Kaizer L, Paterson AH. Lost in transition? Thoughts on retirement – "will you still need me, will you still feed me, when i'm sixty-four?". Oncologist. 2013;18(11):1235–8.
26. Heyl AR. The transition from career to retirement: focus on well-being and financial considerations. J Am Med Women's Assoc (1972). 2004;59(4):235–7.
27. American Medical Association. 4 Must-Dos before physicians retire. Available from: https://www.ama-assn.org/practice-management/career-development/4-must-dos-physicians-retire.

28. Silver MP, Williams SA. Reluctance to retire: a qualitative study on work identity, intergenerational conflict, and retirement in academic medicine. Gerontologist. 2018;58(2):320–30.
29. Shanafelt TD, Lightner DJ, Conley CR, Petrou SP, Richardson JW, Schroeder PJ, et al. An organization model to assist individual physicians, scientists, and senior health care administrators with personal and professional needs. Mayo Clin Proc. 2017;92(11):1688–96.
30. Silver MP, Hamilton AD, Biswas A, Williams SA. Life after medicine: a systematic review of studies of Physicians' adjustment to retirement. Arch Commun Med Public Health. 2015;1(1):026–32.
31. Lees E, Liss SE, Cohen IM, Kvale JN, Ostwald SK. Emotional impact of retirement on physicians. Tex Med. 2001;97(9):66–71.
32. Moy P, Hegwood JM. 2018 Report on U.S. physicians' financial preparedness: retired physicians segment. AMA Insurance; 2018. Available from: https://www.amainsure.com/physicians-in-focus/2018-report-retired-physicians-financial-preparedness.html.

Changing the Culture and Managing Imposter Syndrome

18

Chee-Chee Stucky

The face of burnout is unquestionably ugly. And the effects of burnout aren't just confined to the hospital. Burnout infiltrates every part of our lives, including our families, our friends, and our physical and mental health. Many drivers of burnout, including lack of work-life balance and emotional exhaustion, disproportionately affect women [1]. It's time to address this issue. Unfortunately, attempting to eradicate each risk factor one by one would be like playing a game of Whac-A-Mole. This is because many of the drivers originate from a deeper force: the overall culture of medicine. It is a complex culture founded by self-sacrificing physicians who worked countless hours, denying themselves personal comfort to ensure excellent care for their patients. For decades this philosophy was the standard, but the turn of the century brought about work-hour restrictions and a shift of expectation toward well-being, particularly for physicians in training. Although these regulations reduced the number of weekly hours worked by residents, many institutions struggled with inadequate staffing which often shifted the work load to the attending physicians [2, 3]. As a result, the persisting culture of medicine still includes a "suck-it-up" mentality, which looks down on work-life balance and physician well-being, particularly when it comes to

C. C. Stucky (✉)
Department of General Surgery, Mayo Clinic,
Phoenix, AZ, USA
e-mail: Stucky.chee-chee@mayo.edu

© Springer Nature Switzerland AG 2020
C. M. Stonnington, J. A. Files (eds.), *Burnout in Women Physicians*,
https://doi.org/10.1007/978-3-030-44459-4_18

women, who traditionally believe we must work harder and longer to prove we are worthy of the title "doctor" [4]. This culture places women physicians at a significant disadvantage with inequalities in salary, career advancement, leadership opportunities, and performance standards. It is a setup for burnout [1]. And in my experience, those who express interest in rebuilding our culture to make it more sustainable are often met with disapproval. So why are we in medicine so reluctant to improve our environment? Shouldn't we want to make a culture that allows the next generation of physicians to look forward to going to work each day? If we don't make the change soon, we can only expect more burned out doctors.

While some have already accepted the onerous task of initiating culture change by altering practice and institution policies as well as researching best approaches to implementing change, a widely accepted process is yet to be established [5–7]. This may be a result of resistance to change, lack of awareness of the need for change, or lack of appreciation of the benefit that cultural change would bring, particularly for the next generation of physicians. Ultimately, there is no single modification that will result in a revitalized culture conducive to preventing physician burnout. The solution to the problem of a disillusioned culture will be multifactorial: starting specifically with transforming our individual approach to our colleagues, empowering the influencers, rebuilding the institution of medicine, and changing the way we look at ourselves.

Start with the Individual

With all of the amazing advancements of modern medicine, it would seem that the culture would progress at the same pace, to become one that is non-discriminating, forward thinking, and interested in the preservation of a bright future. Yet, among the generations within medicine, there are hold-outs. Published articles, national presentations, and social media are full of stories like that of Dr. Esther Choo, an emergency room physician in Oregon. After delivering twin babies, Dr. Choo struggled with the stress of returning to her medical career and research while caring for newborns at home. When she sought out encouragement from her professional *female* mentor, Dr. Choo received hostility instead [8]. Sadly, this story prompted innumerable replies from women in science of similar experiences with mentors stating "I had to go through it, so should you." Why is this a standard response by both men and women? First, let us acknowledge the fact that these dogmatic physicians undoubtedly had to struggle through a long period of education, followed by training and likely stretches of financial discomfort, only to have extreme stress and demands placed on him or her once past all of the training and education. We should all be incredibly thankful to these medical pioneers, especially the women who made it through such difficult times, because they paved the way for the next generation of physicians to start having a voice. But, unfortunately, what often happens when the next generation tries to implement their voice is that these same pioneers seemingly resent the fact that the more vocal physicians will theoretically not have endured the same struggles as they did. It is almost as though the expectation is that all physicians, no matter the generation, have to go through a rite of passage that includes poor work-life balance, discrimination, and isolated, extreme physical and emotional distress in order to prove our dedication to medicine. This way of thinking needs to be eradicated. We should be approaching the next generation from a different perspective. For instance, like so many other parents, my mother, an immigrant from Taiwan, worked tremendously long hours to help provide food and shelter for our family. She did so with the dream of having more opportunity for her children than she had herself. What if we as individuals had that same desire to make the opportunities better and more available for the next generation of physicians? What would that look like?

The first thing we would do is make a deliberate effort to eliminate microaggression from our conversation. Whether conscious or unconscious, microaggression is a behavior that ultimately insults a marginalized group of people. The halls of any teaching hospital have likely heard an attending physician comment on how the millennial residents need "nap time." This joke is in reference to changes in resident duty hours, specifically mandated limits on call shifts and hours and days worked. It is a small dig suggesting that residents are not working as hard as the earlier generations of physicians who never had work-hour restrictions. And there are other, more subtle microaggressions that are specifically directed toward women. For instance, have you ever noticed women doctors are addressed differently than men? Female residents are often told to have the nurses call them by their first names so they will not seem arrogant or unapproachable, but the same rule does not apply to the male residents [9]. Additionally, Dr. Files and colleagues demonstrated that male physicians introducing male physician speakers at Internal Medicine Grand Rounds used the professional title of "Dr." 72.4% of the time while female physicians introduced by men were afforded the use of their professional title only 49.2% of the time (p = 0.007) [10]. This simple difference seems innocent but actually demonstrates a lack of respect for the women physicians, their education and their position. Ultimately, these forms of individual microaggression thwart institutional effort toward well-being and equality. Changing our culture means individuals must stop making slighting comments passed off as jokes and start using edifying and respectful words in everyday conversations. Eliminating microaggression means we also must be willing to apologize when we misspeak. This is particularly important in the wake of the #MeToo movement in which individual male physicians across the nation have made comments like "Oh, can we even shake hands anymore?" implying that they no longer want to work with female colleagues for fear of being falsely accused of harassment [11]. Those who are thoughtful of their words and the impact they have on the opposite gender know that harassment is not actually a misperception of jokes. Implementing a tone of mutual respect for colleagues despite gender is the foundation of a culture conducive to women's academic success in medicine [12].

Each individual must also have a desire to change. Instead of upholding and clinging to the practices of the "good old days" we must ask ourselves, "How can we make things better?" It requires a personal effort to educate ourselves on the implicit gender bias that results in barriers for the advancement of women in medicine. This not only requires an individual to recognize divisive speech but also to have the self-confidence to carry out the amplification of others. Those who practice "amplification" use a technique first described by the *Washington Post* during the Obama administration in which female West Wing aides would restate important ideas of others and give recognition to the individual responsible for the idea [13]. Integrating this technique into our medical culture would build inclusivity and promote a role in decision making for junior women faculty whose voice might not otherwise be heard. Those who are successful in practicing this technique have often surrendered their own recognition for the advancement of their colleagues. It is this type of behavior that changes a culture.

Enable the Influencer

I recently met with one of our department's most senior woman surgeons. When we sat down to discuss her experience in the male-dominated world of surgery, I fully expected to hear horror stories of mistreatment particularly early in her career. This would have been around the time when surgeons were at their peak of pride for working long hours and spreading rumors of 100% divorce rates during their residencies. However, I was quite surprised to find out that this surgeon had a good experience as a woman in surgery early in her career. She did not note any feelings of being held back at the starting line. She affirmed that she was treated with respect and as a colleague even when just starting out as the only woman in a small group of male surgeons. It wasn't until mid-career that she began feeling the effects of gender discrimination. When asked what she thought the reason for her early career success was, she answered without hesitation: the chair of the department. He was an internationally-known surgeon who had a desire to build a world-renowned department of surgery. This particular chairman was unbiased when he recognized talent. He supported those who worked under him and was welcoming of all types of people. In essence, he set the cultural tone of the department, that of inclusivity and collegiality. And in this culture, the junior female surgeon thrived. Recent efforts to change the culture of medicine recommend a "top-down" approach, which places significant responsibility on the leader of the group – often the hospital CEO or department chairperson [5, 6, 14, 15]. In countries such as Sweden and Australia, action plans established by university vice-chancellors encourage the recruitment of women physicians for academic positions to redress gender inequities. While these are important steps, mandating leaders to proceed in this manner falls short of establishing a culture conducive to women's academic success. One might assume that if reluctant leaders are forced to implement mandated changes, the new culture is founded on unaddressed, inherent bias that will collapse at first opportunity. Since men are predominantly in leadership positions at academic hospitals, it is easy to place the blame on them for the lack of progress in our culture. However, as described in our earlier example, the chair of surgery and other male leaders have successfully cultivated environments where both women and men are nurtured. The way these leaders have been successful is by demonstrating sincere support of their faculty without prompting. To establish an enduring culture change that is inclusive and collegial, our leaders will deliberately seek out ways to promote equality for women in the intangibles: access to resources and office space, participation in formal and informal meetings, and adequate coverage for maternity leave. Boyle et al. have shown that men functioning as ambassadors of change have a positive impact on the job satisfaction of women in medicine [16].

Make no mistake, men are not to be entirely blamed for the lack of advocacy for women in medicine. Women in leadership have a major responsibility to promote their peers. In fact, we in the medical community have believed so strongly that women physician leaders will be the answer to the problems with our culture that for years, we have been pushing for more women in medicine. The Theory of Critical Mass has been applied to academic medicine, which suggests that once a proportion (>30%–35%) of faculty are women, their impact on culture change will be evident. Now that our entering medical school classes are consistently populated with 50% women students, we have finally achieved a critical mass of women faculty in academic health centers [17]. However, what researchers have found is that the evidence for an influential role of women as catalysts for change has yet to materialize. There are likely several reasons for this, one of which is a phenomenon labeled "Queen Bee Syndrome," and a point of discussion internationally. The traditional belief is that women mentors are not only less likely to promote their fellow women, but intentionally keep them at a lower level. The motives are thought to be multifactorial. These include everything from an evolutionary basis where women are used to competing with other women for survival and mating to women purposely acting like men to avoid appearing like the "other" women [17–19]. Regardless of the underlying motives of Queen Bee Syndrome, the cry for cultural change in medicine has brought about an awareness of this problem and a call for women to support each other through their academic careers.

So how do we remedy the fact that a critical mass of women in academic medicine has not substantially improved medical culture? Several studies suggest that the answer to our problem is by enabling "critical actors" or influencers to initiate cultural change. This means that we identify individuals – not critical masses – who are inspired to improve our culture and give them the resources and support to implement changes. Successful influencers are not only positioned as department chairs or medical school deans. They drive change in numerous ways including leadership within national societies and organizations, publishing research demonstrating gender inequities within our medical culture and speaking up through the media. On a smaller scale, that might include four young women surgeons meeting for lunch every few months to provide encouragement to each other, or female radiologists leading tumor boards overwhelmingly made up of male physicians, or hospital internists offering to take the final shifts of a female colleague at her gestational term. The inspiring voice of these influencers will result in a culture where women physicians feel empowered to ask for help and will find support in each other and their leaders in not only times of burnout but in our everyday practice.

Transform the Institution

The medical world still has a long way to go in addressing inequalities. Even the mandatory female quotas enforced by institutions were not successful in developing career satisfaction in junior women faculty. Why? Because gender parity is not the same as gender equality. Career satisfaction, and subsequently a reduction in burnout, results when women are valued for their contributions to medicine and research and respected for their knowledge and education. The intangible concepts of value and respect are not achieved by merely ensuring an equal ratio of women to men in the workforce. These core principles are established when medical institutions "sustainably promote gender equality in academic medicine." [5] This means institutions must eliminate the long-standing culture of discrimination, starting with salary gaps.

We have well-documented evidence that women physicians consistently have lower salaries and are less likely to be promoted in academic rank or leadership than their male colleagues of equal qualification [20–24]. Many explanations have been used to justify this fact including women are more likely to work part time, women more frequently work in underserved communities where the reimbursement is lower, and women are not as productive in research as their male counterparts. Yet, numerous studies have shown that when adjusting for covariates such as these, women physicians still earn up to 25% less than men [25]. Similarly, studies have shown that despite the required presence of gender-equitable policies within academic institutions, women still experience inadequate institutional support for advancement [7]. In 2018, the American Association of Medical Colleges reported 13% of all medical school faculty women held the title of full Professor, compared to 29% of men [26]. Others have noted that the time to promotion is statistically longer for women physicians than men [24]. In other words, by compensating women at a lower level than men and withholding their promotions, institutions are reinforcing a culture which validates disrespect toward women and perpetuation of bias. Institutions ready to transform the culture of medicine must do so by launching transparent salaries and setting overt a priori objectives for promotion across the establishment.

Does this mean that women working part time should be given equal salary and equal opportunity for promotion as those working full time? Time and again we hear the rationale that women physicians have "chosen to take a back seat" in their careers due to family priorities. This mindset notoriously suggests that women have less career motivations, less career confidence, and less ambition to take on leadership positions. However, if you were to ask one of our junior Endocrinologists what her work schedule is like now that she has reduced her full-time effort to 80%, she would tell you that she continues to see the same number of patients and produces the same amount and quality of research that she was doing at 100% effort. How did she do this? By cutting back hours at work, she gained flexibility allowing her to better manage both the demands of home and work. Thus, she is now working more efficiently in fewer allotted hours but for less income. The dedication demonstrated by this Endocrinologist would suggest that she continues to find fulfillment in her career and is equally motivated to help her patients as any other full-time employee. There is no reason that someone like this should be compensated at a lower rate or be passed over for promotion just because her position is considered a part-time effort. But this is a book about burnout—and one way to produce burnout is to be overworked. So, perhaps we should not base all compensation and promotion on productivity measures. In fact, recent studies show that women physicians are more successful than male colleagues when implementing preventive health measures [27]. They also have statistically lower readmission and 30-day mortality rates compared to male colleagues as Tsugawa et al. reported in *JAMA Internal Medicine* [28]. The data are clear that women physicians are overwhelmingly motivated, and therefore now is the time to be innovative when determining compensation goals and intentional in efforts to develop a diverse group of leaders. In fact, groups like the University of California, San Diego; Emory University; the University of Alabama at

Birmingham and several European institutions have implemented novel strategies that promote gender equality at a sustainable level [29]. These plans include quality-based rather than quantity-based salary, flexible work-hours and equal benefits for part-time employees. They also include mentorship across a team of multiple senior faculty, early participation of junior faculty in curriculum-based career development programs, and well-defined parameters of academic excellence that take into account longstanding disparities for those medical professionals at risk of experiencing inherent bias [5, 29]. For a cultural transformation to be successful, academic medical institutions must establish a new framework that looks past the bottom line and nurtures passion for the practice of medicine.

Managing Imposter Syndrome

Clearly, changing the culture of medicine to protect women physicians from burnout is going to take participation by everyone: including ourselves. Sometimes, we are our own biggest barrier to change. We speak up for equality in compensation, leadership opportunities, and recognition for high quality work, but deep down inside, we tell ourselves that our jobs well done came out of luck or hard work and in reality we're not worthy of success. This phenomenon is called Imposter Syndrome and plagues women around the world and throughout all facets of medicine [30, 31]. We may underestimate or downplay our abilities resulting in our over preparation or procrastination for tasks, which once accomplished seems undeserved. Ultimately, we convince ourselves that if we accept opportunities for advancement, we will eventually be discovered as a fraud. In reality, studies have demonstrated that women perform at the same level as their male counterparts despite the fact that they consistently underestimate their own ability [32].

There are many potential reasons for Imposter Syndrome and it is not a phenomenon isolated to women [30]. However, in this particular culture, we must recognize Imposter Syndrome as a barrier to change. If we want to see the medical culture revolutionize into one of mutual respect and value, we have to believe that we are deserving of such a culture and overcome Imposter Syndrome, transforming our thoughts and behaviors into those of women physicians who believe they are deserving of respect and value. Drs. Armstrong and Shulman have listed personal strategies to manage imposter syndrome [30]. These include acknowledging its existence, admitting imperfection but eliminating self-criticism, acting confident, and finding self-worth in personal strengths and values. Trying to tackle Imposter Syndrome in isolation is extremely difficult, so we must willingly ask for help from each other, support our colleagues, be willing to be vulnerable, and mentor those in earlier stages of change. We say it is time for a new culture, now we must believe it ourselves.

References

1. McMurray JE, Linzer M, Konrad TR, Douglas J, Shugerman R, Nelson K. The work lives of women physicians results from the physician work life study. The SGIM Career Satisfaction Study Group. J Gen Intern Med. 2000;15(6):372–80.
2. Coverdill JE, Finlay W, Adrales GL, Mellinger JD, Anderson KD, Bonnell BW, et al. Duty-hour restrictions and the work of surgical faculty: results of a multi-institutional study. Acad Med. 2006;81(1):50–6.
3. Bolster L, Rourke L. The effect of restricting residents' duty hours on patient safety, resident well-being, and resident education: an updated systematic review. J Grad Med Educ. 2015;7(3):349–63.
4. Shollen SL, Bland CJ, Finstad DA, Taylor AL. Organizational climate and family life: how these factors affect the status of women faculty at one medical school. Acad Med. 2009;84(1):87–94.
5. Hasebrook J, Hahnenkamp K, Buhre WFFA, de Korte-de Boer D, Hamaekers AEW, Metelmann B, et al. Medicine goes female: protocol for improving career options of females and working conditions for researching physicians in clinical medical research by organizational transformation and participatory design. JMIR Res Protoc. 2017;6(8):e152.
6. Expert Group on Structural Change. Structural change in research institutions: enhancing excellence, gender equality and efficiency in research and innovation. Report of the Expert Group on Structural Change. Brussels: European Commission; 2016.
7. Helitzer DL, Newbill SL, Cardinali G, Morahan PS, Chang S, Magrane D. Narratives of participants in National Career Development Programs for Women in Academic Medicine: identifying the opportunities for strategic investment. J Womens Health (Larchmt). 2016;25(4):360–70.

8. Choo EK. Twitter. In: @choo_ek, editor. 29 May 2019.

9. Gomer BT. Area physician changes first name to "Doctor". https://gomerblog.com/2018/11/area-female-physician-changes-first-name-to-doctor/.

10. Files JA, Mayer AP, Ko MG, Friedrich P, Jenkins M, Bryan MJ, et al. Speaker introductions at internal medicine grand rounds: forms of address reveal gender bias. J Womens Health (Larchmt). 2017;26(5):413–9.

11. Firth S. Could the 'Pence effect' undo #MeToo? Fears that men in healthcare will simply avoid women, to the latter's detriment. MedPage Today. 2019. https://www.medpagetoday.com/publichealthpolicy/generalprofessionalissues/78432.

12. Westring AF, Speck RM, Dupuis Sammel M, Scott P, Conant EF, Tuton LW, et al. Culture matters: the pivotal role of culture for women's careers in academic medicine. Acad Med. 2014;89(4):658–63.

13. Eilperin J. White House women want to be in the room where it happens. Washington Post; 2016.

14. Chesterman C. Not-tokens: reaching a "critical mass" of senior women managers. Empl. Relat. 2006;28(6):540–52.

15. Bickel J, Wara D, Atkinson BF, Cohen LS, Dunn M, Hostler S, et al. Increasing women's leadership in academic medicine: report of the AAMC Project Implementation Committee. Acad Med. 2002;77(10):1043–61.

16. Boyle PJ, Smith LK, Cooper NJ, Williams KS, O'Connor H. Gender balance: women are funded more fairly in social science. Nature. 2015;525(7568):181–3.

17. Helitzer DL, Newbill SL, Cardinali G, Morahan PS, Chang S, Magrane D. Changing the culture of academic medicine: critical mass or critical actors? J Womens Health (Larchmt). 2017;26(5):540–8.

18. Team RC. Queen bees: do women hinder the progress of other women? Reality Check. BBC. 2018. https://www.bbc.com/news/uk-41165076.

19. Ellemers N, van den Heuvel H, de Gilder D, Maass A, Bonvini A. The underrepresentation of women in science: differential commitment or the queen bee syndrome? Br J Soc Psychol. 2004;43(Pt 3):315–38.

20. Wiler JL, Rounds K, McGowan B, Baird J. Continuation of gender disparities in pay among Academic Emergency Medicine Physicians. Acad Emerg Med. 2019;26(3):286–92.

21. Mainardi GM, Cassenote AJF, Guilloux AGA, Miotto BA, Scheffer MC. What explains wage differences between male and female Brazilian physicians? A cross-sectional nationwide study. BMJ Open. 2019;9(4):e023811.

22. Jagsi R, Griffith KA, Stewart A, Sambuco D, DeCastro R, Ubel PA. Gender differences in the salaries of physician researchers. JAMA. 2012;307(22):2410–7.

23. Jena AB, Olenski AR, Blumenthal DM. Sex differences in physician salary in US Public Medical Schools. JAMA Intern Med. 2016;176(9):1294–304.

24. Zhuge Y, Kaufman J, Simeone DM, Chen H, Velazquez OC. Is there still a glass ceiling for women in academic surgery? Ann Surg. 2011;253(4):637–43.
25. Ly DP, Seabury SA, Jena AB. Differences in incomes of physicians in the United States by race and sex: observational study. BMJ. 2016;353:i2923.
26. AAMC Faculty Roster. Table 9: U.S. Medical School Faculty by Sex and Rank, 2018. 2019. Available from: https://www.aamc.org/download/495040/data/18table9.pdf.
27. Reid RO, Friedberg MW, Adams JL, McGlynn EA, Mehrotra A. Associations between physician characteristics and quality of care. Arch Intern Med. 2010;170(16):1442–9.
28. Tsugawa Y, Jena AB, Figueroa JF, Orav EJ, Blumenthal DM, Jha AK. Comparison of hospital mortality and readmission rates for medicare patients treated by male vs female physicians. JAMA Intern Med. 2017;177(2):206–13.
29. Chapman AB, Guay-Woodford LM. Nurturing passion in a time of academic climate change: the modern-day challenge of junior faculty development. Clin J Am Soc Nephrol. 2008;3(6):1878–83.
30. Armstrong MJ, Shulman LM. Tackling the imposter phenomenon to advance women in neurology. Neurol Clin Pract. 2019;9(2):155–9.
31. Butkus R, Serchen J, Moyer DV, Bornstein SS, Hingle ST, Physicians HaPPCotACo. Achieving gender equity in physician compensation and career advancement: a position paper of the American College of Physicians. Ann Intern Med. 2018;168(10):721–3.
32. Kay K, Shipman C. The confidence gap [online]. 2014. https://www.theatlantic.com/magazine/archive/2014/05/the-confidence-gap/359815/.

Changing the System

19

Stephanie Kivi and Lisa Hardesty

Introduction

Despite widespread knowledge that the current practice of health care is injuring physicians worldwide, very little has been done on a systems level to mitigate its spread. Responsibility for this trend is shared across a variety of domains, from governmental systems to large health-care employers, to the numerous small clinics scattered across the national landscape. Women physicians carry a growing and disproportionate burden of burnout, outpacing men with an estimated 20–60% increased odds of suffering from this preventable condition [87]. A variety of ideas have been shared in the literature to combat this epidemic, but the solution to an individual's burnout will not likely to be found in any one suggestion. The cure may be as complex as the female physician herself. Solutions that impact the drivers of burnout may be found among the layers of ideas found within this chapter

S. Kivi (✉)
Department of Family Medicine, Mayo Clinic Health System,
New Prague, MN, USA
e-mail: Kivi.Stephanie@mayo.edu

L. Hardesty
Department of Psychiatry and Psychology, Mayo Clinic Health System,
North Mankato, MN, USA
e-mail: Hardesty.Lisa@mayo.edu

© Springer Nature Switzerland AG 2020   567
C. M. Stonnington, J. A. Files (eds.), *Burnout in Women Physicians*,
https://doi.org/10.1007/978-3-030-44459-4_19

and will likely stem from a compilation of work pulled from several directions within the system; each owned and rolled out by different owners.

Burnout

How do we as a nation take care of the people who care for us? Is it not in our best interest to ensure that the people that we entrust with our lives are healthy?

How do we as employers expect a physician to work 80 hours a week without balancing their personal commitment with a system-wide effort to support that work? Is it not in our best interest to ensure an efficient workforce, showing respect for their personal engagement while enhancing our system-wide metrics?

How do we as educated women, with our perfectionistic tendencies, high levels of empathy, and dual jobs roles, at work and at home, take care of ourselves? Isn't it in our best interest to ensure that we are balanced and healthy, living long and strong?

Burnout was described as early as 1928 by S Dana Hubbard, the director of the Bureau of Public Health Education for New York City, when he noted that physicians took their own lives more than twice as often as other educated men. He recommended almost 100 years ago that "our scheme of medical practice, as it relates to hours and relief, (should) be revised" [31]. Unfortunately despite that century-old observation, research until recently has been in short supply and riddled with cross-sectional studies of short duration, diversity across specialties limiting transference, low N's, and inferred suggestions [87]. If burnout stemmed from a singular source, the issue would have been resolved; but no one entity is responsible for the diversity of causes. Complex problems such as governmental regulations, financial pressures, societal expectations of the patient populations drawn to a female physician, and the historical medical hierarchy created by men for men, most of whom had support at home and could focus on work [44], are examples of causes with seemingly immovable solutions. There are also less complex local issues, such as required patient volumes, call burden, and workflows created by Electronic Health

Records (EHRs) that could be seemingly managed at a team level but aren't routinely or easily addressed. Social factors further complicate things, as we continue to see a change within the patient/ physician dynamic, once a relationship known to combat the effects of burnout, now it carries the potential to undermine that value. As patients' increasing see health care as a business, their trust in clinicians and the health-care system erodes [6], while at the same time, we are seeing frustration among clinicians when patient's decisions differ from their professional recommendations [2]. That said, there is growing recognition within health-care organizations that they must act to thoughtfully address systemic drivers of burnout, and research studies on the topic are rapidly accumulating. By delving into the existing science and listening to the physicians, we can develop sound guidelines and innovations to move us toward a culture of health care that dares to care for our care givers.

Sex Differences That Impact Burnout

First it is important to point out that we need to read the current literature with an understanding that medical research has for many years been male dominated. Likewise, research on burnout has largely lacked female-specific causes and solutions, despite the known typical differences between men and women. Thus, in order to better understand some of the key systemic drivers of burnout, we need to recognize those disparities and only reach conclusions after keeping these factors in mind. Briefly, and not fully inclusive of what makes the genders unique, research suggests that when compared to men, women physicians/surgeons:

- Demonstrate higher levels of emotive empathy with patients [30], which puts them at higher risk for compassion fatigue when stressed [24]. In 1989 Carol Williams stated, "It is hypothesized that high emotional empathy may predispose helping professionals to emotional exhaustion and that emotional exhaustion, if not mediated by personal accomplishment, may lead to the development of depersonalization [89]."

- Have patient panels that are dominated by female patients, many of whom have complex psychosocial needs and require a more time-consuming type of communication.
- Lack exposure to female role models in leadership.
- Work in care teams where, despite being the "top of the pyramid," they may struggle with being verbally challenged, or be criticized more harshly, and interrupted more often by their female clinic support staff, thus having to navigate their work relationships differently than male physicians [30].
- Are historically taught to cope with stress by internalizing or ruminating. They are also more likely to use the maladaptive coping mechanism of self-blame, a tendency characterized by criticizing or blaming oneself for things that have happened [73]. "The internal ones, those self-perpetuating internal wars that so many women wage with themselves, can be just as damaging, if not more so (than external pressures). Perfectionism, guilt, over commitment, reluctance to delegate, and not setting realistic limits are all examples of internally generated stressors common among these high achievers." [13]
- More often feel unsafe in reoccurring situations at work.
- More often hold primary responsibility for their children and the management of their households [21] and feel a social pressure to do so.
- More often are in a dual career household [21].
- Historically tend to be in primary care, a field with high levels of burnout that has changed dramatically over time, that is, with its wide diversity of patient concerns intermixed with an increased complexity of patients, increased demands for non-face-to-face work, and increased demands for higher volumes due to declining reimbursement for primary care services, all complicated with cumbersome EHRs that not only have increased clerical tasks but have blurred that fine line of work/life balance. Primary care also sits at the front line, holding the lion's share of the growing list of quality metrics and the changing societal views on health care.

Of course, male physicians also struggle with burnout, but when looking at large factors that burn men and women out equally, such as EHRs designed for business offices and the burden of constant change and metrics that don't align with their personal values, women physicians may perceive those stressors differently than men do. Not better or worse, and even if all things are equal in a work environment, it is our experience that women tend to respond, relate, and live a different experience.

Overview of Five Categories of Work

Although not experts on burnout in the female physician, Dr. Hardesty and I work together on a team locally coordinating efforts to combat burnout. Like many of you, we've been reading and searching for practical solutions. Through listening to what physicians across the country are saying and what the experts offer as suggestions, we have chosen to break the work down into five basic categories. These categories are not suggestive of the causes of burnout but rather areas of work intended to offer insight into how a system, or an individual working in a system, might develop tactics in support of traditional organizational goals while improving the professional well-being of the physician (Fig. 19.1).

Our five focus categories include the following:

- Efficiency: How do you help a woman with work-life integration in an era where round the clock technology allows work to follow her without geographical boundaries and there is the expectation for immediate responsiveness? When under constant pressure to perform, an individual not used to taking short cuts starts to take them and may slip from emotional exhaustion into a deeper part of burnout defined by depersonalization. When there is a constant loss of efficiency partnered with increasing demands for her attention, are we surprised if there is an erosion of her personal integrity? Offloading a physician whenever possible, especially a woman who has historically done whatever it takes, is imperative to avoid this slide into burnout. This section includes some thoughts around the use of the Electronic Health Record (EHR), workflows, both indirect and direct care support, and nonclinical efficiency. Maslach et al. suggest that burnout is driven by "imbalances

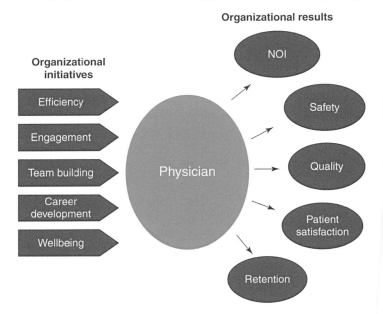

Fig. 19.1 Five categories of organizational initiatives showing direct relationships between the support of the physician and the drive for organizational results

between demands and resources" and efficiency is where we make up some of that ground. She states the risk of burnout further increases when "the workplace does not recognize the human side of work," a delicate balance complicated by work overload, lack of control, insufficient reward, unfairness, breakdown of community, and value conflict [43]. For every hour spent on patient interaction, the physician has an added 1–2 hours finishing the progress notes, ordering labs, prescribing medications, and reviewing results [90]. Simply put, systems that effectively reduce the burden of these clerical tasks for physicians will improve efficiency and reduce physician burnout.

• Engagement: How does an institution align with and retain a physician, constitutionally, socially, and emotionally? This includes aligning values, respecting the fine line between work and life, and being the voice of the physician and the patient. To combat burnout there is an organizational requirement for leadership engagement, which involves active listening, acting in response to what is heard, empowerment of staff, and aligning the why of every decision to a mission statement which is grounded in shared values.

- Team Building: How do we build a community, decrease the isolation of the female physician, and celebrate the commitment of the care giver? We have somehow isolated physicians within a sorority of peers. It is critical we prevent the dissolution of the team that occurs when no one has the space to give while ensuring that members of our teams have a place to turn.
- Career Development: How do we encourage our educated female physician and show her that there is a way to integrate her career and life, enhance her natural skill of leadership and curiosity, teach her to be assertive, and give her the support to promote herself beyond her own expectations? As members of one of the most rewarding and respected societies, we need to buck the trend of decreasing career satisfaction in medicine over the past 30 years [54].
- Well-Being: How do we ensure that our team is resilient and grateful? How innovative would we be to have a team that feels free to care fully about patients without consequence of burnout and feels free to fully engage at home without the consequence and feelings surrounding neglect of work? When one enters medical school, there is an assumption that there will be some personal sacrifices, loss of sleep, the occasional missed family event, stress due to involvement in high stakes situations; but not many physicians are ready for their career to evolve into depression, drug abuse, or suicidal thoughts. Women can engage in maladaptive coping strategies, overcommit, and be self-critical, perfectionistic, and overly idealistic. The organizational system must therefore value personal resilience, structured support groups, and physical health.

One caveat to keep in mind is that burnout is currently a hot topic, and in the time since we started researching the issue for this chapter, there have been several new studies reported and we are aware of several large ongoing research projects. This chapter is really meant as a guide, using the background of prior research with extrapolation of ideas, combined with some common sense. Because of the diversity inherent within the branches of medicine, and the fact that not all specialties practice the same, not all health systems use their teams in the same fashion, and all women are unique, our intention was to build a template that will be a starting point to help navigate the complexities within individual health-care systems or within an individual physician needing direction. For instance, a woman with an established career and grown children may be more interested in career advancement and her physical health than a young primary care physician, just starting her family, who needs support with call and workflow efficiency. As in all things, we are learning as we go and despite the fact that we are scientists and find comfort in statistics and facts that are proven beyond inference, we must embrace the uncertainty created by the lack of data. If the shoe fits (and we think it is pretty), we should wear it.

Also of note, the other chapters of this book have specific solutions embedded within them that address the topics identified within those pages. Some of those solutions may be included in the following pages, but we would encourage you to look to those authors for more specialized solutions.

Efficiency

The state or quality of being efficient, or able to accomplish something with the least waste of time and effort. (Siri 2020)

Throughout our long history, physicians have efficiently cared for patients as part of a care team. In many ways the team and its members remain the same, but the team roles played by each and the functional relationship between them have changed dramatically over the last decade. This change is primarily due to payer requirements and the subsequent health system response. Metrics and finances have required an organizational attempt to create efficiencies for itself by optimizing task alignment within its workforce, while minimizing cost and overhead. Not so long ago a physician was surrounded by team members, working side by side, assisting in the care of the patient, either directly or behind the scenes. By assisting at the physician's side or as experts in their fields, team members allowed physicians to do what they were trained to do, that is, practice both the art and science of medicine. Now with physician-based order entry, the continuous evolution of documentation requirements, and a necessary understanding of the complexities of coding and billing, physicians often feel the brunt of a system built to make the business office efficient at the expense of the patient interaction.

No discussion on efficiency in clinical practice can develop without first addressing the topic of the EHR. Embraced by the government in 2009 as a solution to escalating cost, quality, and safety concerns, its use, in many forms, is widespread. With its complexity, security, and inevitable updates, it has transformed how physicians interact with their patients, their partners, their staff, and their families at home. Designed for efficiencies beyond the face-to-face patient interaction, it can undermine the personal relationships between physicians and patients and what was a well-established way of "connecting to purpose," a connection defined later in this chapter as a solution to burnout. Since its inception, the EHR system, which is designed to solve multiple issues, has been decried as a leading cause of burnout. The system has been plagued with issues related to usability, interoperability, ergonomics, and cybersecurity, which impacts computer station timeout times and has a related requirement for multiple log-ins for noncommunicating internal systems that are accessed by a rotation of passwords of increasing complexity. We should also mention poorly designed workflows, "in-basket dumping," and documentation that evolved from voice to manual input, all inherent in a system that moved from something totally human to one based on a partnership between a human and a technological advancement. Even though physicians are spending 44% of their time computer-facing [4], they are producing less usable clinical notes. Despite being nearly four times as long as notes completed by physicians in other developed countries using the same EHR, the US clinical notes are difficult to navigate when searching for relevant clinical information [18]. Approaches to optimize clinical efficiency have been shown to decrease burnout, while in contrast, the "simple" requirement of adding physician order entry into a system worsens it [62]. Although it brings high levels of efficiency to different aspects of the patient encounter, for many it is considered the antithesis of efficiency for the physician. Wasted time, redundancy, unnecessary obstacles, and inflexibility are things encountered daily within the EHR for a care giver, leading to what has been estimated to be a dissatisfaction rate of 70% among physician users of the same [25].

Once trained in these complex systems, physicians are often expected to be proficient, despite being trained by nonclinicians in brief training sessions and being faced with the frequent updates often found within this complex system driven to change by both internal and external factors. How do we ensure proficiency when training is time limited and change occurs rapidly? In the past, physicians could multitask with the support of staff as part of the patient care team. Now, nothing happens unless a physician dedicates time to data input, with team members awaiting instructions at secondary terminals; thus, their proficient use of the EHR is imperative to a high-functioning team.

There are several reasons use of the EHR has been repeatedly linked to physician burnout, but for our purposes we will look at the gender-specific concerns that have been identified. Studies suggest that female physician struggles are amplified within the EHR. Data collection demonstrates that female physicians generally conduct longer visits, create longer notes, and have more "patient contacts" (including face-to-face, portal, and in-basket) than men do in the same time frame. They are also more likely to address patient calls within 24 hours of receipt and spend significantly more time in the EHR during off work hours, with less office visits closed on the same day. Thoughts on why this occurs span several ideas. First, many female physicians have a patient-centric communication style, partly because of learned communication behaviors and partly because it is a patient expectation [25]. Society measures female communication by a different standard, and patients are no different. "Our stereotype of men holds that they are providers, decisive, and driven. Our stereo-type of women holds that they are caregivers, sensitive and com-munal. Because we characterize men and women in opposition to each other, professional achievement and all the traits associ-ate with it get put in the male column," leaving women to approach being decisive and firm from a less direct and more time-consuming angle [57]. This expectation creates an environ-ment where if the female physician simply addresses computer requirements during a patient encounter, she will leave a differ-ent impression on the patient than a male physician who does the same. She is thought of as inattentive or rushed, and he is thought of as efficient. By extension, staff interactions for female physicians are layered with these same expectations, cre-ating an increased time burden for day-to-day communications at work. Female physicians are often seen as more collaborative, which is a time-consuming way to manage a care team, and they are significantly more likely to be interrupted during their quiet work time. As stated previously, female physicians are often the primary care giver at home which can require them to manage their time immediately after direct patient care differently than men; to meet the needs of their families, they may need to leave as close to clinic closure as possible, requiring more work late nights or on weekends.

Certainly, there has been innovation within the EHR space and increasingly there has been focus on optimizing its use to decrease burnout. Atrius Health, in Massachusetts, embraced several dif-ferent efficiency techniques and reduced the total number of clicks within its system by approximately 60 million in the first year [84]. Some ideas at improving efficiency within this space are noted below:

1. The use of scribes is one area that has not only decreased levels of burnout but has also been shown to be cost effec-tive, increasing productivity and quality at the same time. During a typical day physicians spend about 50% of their time on EHR functions and less than 30% in face-to-face interactions with patients. This is considered a disturbing trend for physicians that chose a career traditionally defined

by relationships with patients. Scribes allow physicians to remain face-to-face with patients, allowing them to work at the highest level of their license, touch more patients with less administrative burden, and get home to their families at the end of the day with loose ends more often tied up [23].

2. Health systems with EHRs should ensure physician proficiency after training and provide ongoing training to maintain competency with updates. There is evidence of benefit when physicians train other physicians despite increased cost. Physicians understand workflows and the questions of other physicians better than nonclinical staff [59].

3. If assigned a task not traditionally physician owned, adequate education and competence should be assured. For example, coding and billing, in and of itself a complex task, historically completed by trained professionals, now is often assigned to the physician through their EHR pathway.

4. Understanding that health care is changing and more health care is managed outside of the face-to-face interaction, time should be built into templates to allow for order entry, in-basket management, and interactions with team members. Because physicians are required to input the data that the work of other team members is built off of, it is not unusual for a physician to be tasked with a wide variety of miscellaneous assignments throughout the course of their day. Physicians are moving in and out of patient charts before their work is complete to allow the extended team to tend to other parts of the patient encounter. This screen jumping creates a very inefficient personal workflow but allows other team members to do their work within an allotted shift, leaving the physician alone after work to clean up tasks only assigned to them. With the realization that not every physician, especially female physicians, interacts with their team and their patients within the EHR environment the same, we must understand that traditional metrics for volumes and RVU production may not be sustainable without time built into the work day to complete their work. Disruption of quiet work time should be at a minimum for physicians, especially as many work environments have moved toward common rooms and shared office spaces. Work disruptions

are frustrating and are known to lower quality and safe care [47]. There is data to suggest that it may take up to 25 minutes to resume productivity at previous levels after even a brief interruption [41], and we know that women physicians are more likely to be interrupted by staff than their male counterparts. Nicola and colleagues showed the benefit of decreasing disruptions on burnout levels in their study of radiologists [49].

5. Create a streamlined way (or multiple ways through alternate venues) for clinicians to give feedback into the system with their ideas for optimization and increased efficiency and encourage them to submit their ideas [5].

6. Data also suggest that regular feedback on physician specific EHR utilization is helpful. Not as a right or wrong suggestion, because not every practice will use the EHR the same, but to help physicians see where their routine use of the EHR product might vary and where they may gain some efficiencies and grow into the EHR space alongside their partners. There is also the suggestion noted above that face-to-face time with a physician superuser or physician informaticist to lead team improvements may have added value [59].

7. Redirect, whenever possible, electronic messages that physicians do not need to touch and assign documentation responsibilities to medical assistants and other team members where appropriate. Team assignments and hiring patterns should keep this in mind. Staff should be used across the clinic setting to the highest level of their licensure wherever possible to keep non-physician-related tasks off of a physician's plate and out of their in-basket. Within 6 months of its 2015 roll out of APEX, the University of Colorado health system saw burnout rates among providers plummet from 53% to 13% while at the same time increasing their vaccination rates and referrals for preventative services, such as colonoscopy and mammograms. The new Family Medicine care model focused on "ambulatory process excellence." In this model medical assistants gathered data, reconciled medications, set patient visit agendas, and addressed preventative care concerns during the rooming process, after which the provider met directly with the

patient and medical assistant. During the physician encounter the medical assistant documented the visit and finished out the visit with the patient after the clinician departed, providing appropriate patient education [90].

8. Use wide-screen monitors that reduce scrolling and clicks, and create a login process that uses biometrics to reduce time and typing, that not only opens the computer but all aspects and applications of the chart.

9. In 2020, there is an expectation for timely responses to patient portal inquiries. Allow time in the schedule for this very important patient care option, as it is a great patient satisfier and drives quality [33]. The mental energy required by a physician when responding to patient questions or concerns via the portal is no different than when they are sitting across from each other face-to-face. Patient encounters should be contained during the work day to avoid care fatigue.

10. Ensure appointment lengths are appropriate for patients with special needs. For instance, a recent study showed clinicians are spending an average of 13 minutes per patient completing prescription monitoring queries and other institutional requirements related to controlled substance prescribing [75].

Other important considerations for efficiency surround the idea of nonclinical practice efficiency. This area of consideration is comprised of a large and growing number of non-patient-related tasks, many of which are electronic. These are often required tasks peripheral but imperative to the work of being a physician, so they should be considered routinely as part of their work and supported with efficiencies by whoever distributes the requirements:

1. Email management techniques should be taught, while email volumes should be closely monitored for appropriateness and kept to a minimum.

2. Work meetings should be held whenever possible during the traditional work day to respect time meant for family or for personal space.

3. Administrative assistants should be deployed wherever possible – with electronic changes occurring everywhere, it is not

uncommon for physicians to spend time with data input while enrolling in a CME, renewing a license or submitting a vacation request. State and federal licensure bodies, accreditation services, specialty boards, and other professional organizations with electronic platforms all require manual submission of certification requirements, data, and payments. These additional data entry points are time consuming and have providers working beyond their normal hours and yet are required for employment.

4. Ensure required training modules for employment purposes (how does the fire extinguisher work again?) are accounted for during regular work hours.

5. This will be discussed later in this chapter, but physicians are often the care team leader, where they are by design, trained or not, overseeing staff. We should ensure that they have time for that purpose so that responsibility doesn't fall at odds with patient care or personal time. To some extent, by the nature of residency training, we are the best fit for the job; but some education and support for the leadership role is necessary, especially in light of the fact that care teams are increasingly inclusive of professionals outside the traditional doctor/nurse relationship. Care team leaders may need additional background and insight into ways social workers, pharmacists, care coordinators, and behavioral therapists can aid in patient panel management and how best to support them as individual caregivers.

6. For hospital-based practices and those with call burden, ensure access to healthy sleep patterns, access to healthy nutrition, and time off of work after direct patient care. When physicians are physically and emotionally fatigued from constant clinical exposure, burnout is more prevalent [1, 35, 68]. Micro-aggressions occur when fatigue has set in. That toxicity can spread throughout the care team, where we may see teamwork, safety, and patient experience suffer. There is a tremendous amount of science supporting the benefits of sleep, everything from increasing work efficiencies, patient safety, and physician productivity to decreasing one's risk for developing cancer. Sleep also makes us a better, kinder, and gentler people.

Employers should encourage and help facilitate regular exercise for all physicians, as this has been shown as beneficial for both general and psychological health, thereby decreasing the incidence of burnout by approximately 44% [69].

7. Any physician in clinical practice will tell you that retention of current staff greatly enhances team and personal efficiency. Related to this concept is the stress on the system that is caused by the increased sick leave associated with burnout or the growing phenomenon of physicians practicing at less than full-time status. Short staffing, rescheduling patients, and the added clinical burden required when covering another's patient panel are associated with physician turnover and burnout [29]. Every effort should be made to ensure retention of good staff, as it enhances retention of other staff and is cost effective. The financial cost of burnout is twofold, as it has been shown to decrease both the productivity of the burned-out physician and it causes staff turnover. All physicians suffering from burnout are likely to be less productive over time, but there is some data that females suffering from burnout have a disproportionate loss of RVU productivity. Female gynecological oncologists with burnout experienced a twofold increase in RVU productivity loss and decreased professional effort when compared to males with burnout over the same period of time, approximately 1.1 million compared to 490,000 [83]. In general the cost to an institution to replace a physician is thought to be somewhere between 250,000 and 1 million dollars annually, depending on specialty, geography, and practice type. This is due to lost revenue, a decrease in patient satisfaction and quality metrics, ramp up of new physicians, and recruitment expenses. Han and colleagues estimated the cost of turnover and loss of productivity due to burnout among US physicians to be upward of $4.6 billion annually [27]. Some health-care systems are using float services, that is, physicians employed to float to areas of need to allow time off or to help cover after a physician departs. This makes practical sense at several levels, as it maintains patient services and supports the physicians at work and during time away. It delicately balances the inflex-

ibility of advertised clinic hours and on-call demand with the needs of the physicians.

8. And of course, efficiency for the pregnant physician or the physician just back from maternity leave, especially those working part time, is a critical issue. For them, being respectful of their energy is paramount in the fight against burnout, because for them, work-life integration is imperative. Clinical work has a way of stretching out from one day to the next week, haunting time meant for family and self. Most mothers are naturally efficient and are able to multitask, but if they are also working outside the home, they *have* to embrace these things. It is in everyone's best interest to create workflows within the work day to further promote healthy work-life integration. Connect with them and explore their ideas on how to streamline workflows to best meet their need, consider alternative scheduling options or creative ideas such as time banking for the first few months after their return. Stanford piloted "time banking" to reward team members for activities that are rarely recognized, such as serving on committees. Faculty were allowed to "trade" time spent on these activities for in-home support, such as meal delivery or cleaning services. They saw greater use of this pilot by women faculty, who doubled their responses of "feeling supported" by the end of the initiative [90].

A generally accepted fact within health systems is that even though full time is considered 40 hours of face-to-face time, the true expectation is for a physician to be engaged in some type of work for 80 hours a week. That said, if a health system requires 80 hours a week of work, and the science says that our expectation should be for physicians to get a healthy 56 hours of sleep a week, that leaves a mere 32 hours a week for family and personal time, just over 4 hours a day. Not much time left over if one needs to shower and get a handle on laundry. It would be a far better use of our time to create efficiency within the work day, allowing physicians to maintain a full-time patient panel, develop healthy sleeping patterns, and have 72 hours of daylight a week to spend doing things that keep them whole.

Engagement

A pledge, an obligation or an agreement (Siri 2020)

Like the relationship between efficiency and the EHR, no discussion on engagement can occur without understanding its connection to institutional leadership. Engagement begins and ends with those who lead, whether it is a team of four, or a thousand. Simply put, their relationship is symbiotic; you can't excel in the arena of engagement without excelling as a leader. Theirs is a relationship built on a foundation of shared values, which requires mutual loyalty and trust interlaced with integrity and faith. In fact, our nation's history is filled with companies saved from the brink of collapse by a surge in leadership engagement and, conversely, corporate success stories brought to the brink of collapse by failures in leadership. Over the last three decades, our nation has seen a significant shift in medicine away from the small clinic to large multispecialty corporations and with that there has been growth in the administrative branch of medicine. Some estimate that employment of administrators is far outpacing that of the family physician. Often these administrators are trained in the philosophies, strategies, and tactics used in traditional American industry, where the product is something tactical and not the health and wellness of a human being. Cantlupe and colleagues, in 2017, studied data revealing a growth of health-care administrators upward of 3200% between 1975 and 2000 [12].

Leaders instill in their people a hope for success and a belief in themselves. Positive leaders empower people to accomplish their goals. (Unknown)

As in any large company, leadership drives results, and in the business of medicine, it is no different. The consolidation of health care into larger entities has many advantages, but administratively, medicine differs from traditional industry in at least three significant ways: leaders leading leaders, imprecise metrics, and regulations and directives from multiple masters.

Leaders leading leaders Physicians are leaders, even if not always trained specifically as such. As the most highly educated team member, they are expected to step up to lead in stressful situations with decisions and directions. Physicians are trained to make life and death decisions – literally, life and death decisions. Unlike business leaders, administrative leaders in health care are often leading team members who may have more education and carry more personal responsibility than the leader themselves.

Imprecise metrics With the recent growth in metrics for physicians, many physicians struggle with the quantities of and complexities inherent to metrics involving patient care. They often have to make the difficult decision to prioritize, focusing on some, while holding back work on others. Some of the metrics drive reimbursement, which adds weight to their importance for the institution. Metrics range from productivity to patient experience, volumes, safety measures, and to any number of patient-specific outcomes. Work on any one specific metric may be counterintuitive to the successful management of another. Over the last several years, physicians have been witness to a revolving array of metrics with seemingly a different goal each year. Physicians, who in general are used to being successful and at the top of their class, can lose morale and become discouraged by scores falling within a lower percentile ranking than they are accustomed to. Let's face it, we don't pick metrics we are already good at, so by nature of design, we measure things we are trying to change. Physician buy-in may be better if the metrics on the dashboards reflected their daily work, namely concrete things that can be accomplished within the confines of the patient interaction. Indeed, a patient or person with personal pressures, preferences and insurance coverage issues that affect their ability to follow recommendations lives on the flipside of that metric, such as the diabetic who can't afford their insulin or the patient with hypertension who is not ready to stop smoking. The physician is not measured on their time educating patients or researching social options that may help a patient move toward a healthier lifestyle; they are measured on whether that diabetic's labs are in line with the set goal or if the hypertensive patient chooses to abstain from the use of tobacco products. For individuals driven to be 100%, those types of patient nuances feel like personal failures.

Patient experience starts with the first phone encounter and ends with the billing statement, and contains multiple system contacts in between, many of which are areas a physician does not own but can be reflected in a personal assessment of an encounter.

Volumes are subject to everything from an individual scheduler to weather, to the types of patients that make up a physician's patient panel. It is common sense to think that female physicians see a higher number of female patients, many of whom we've already noted require more time in the daily schedule. This panel makeup can translate to lower volumes; despite the fact, the time commitment and the work load are the same.

Certainly an individual physician owns parts and pieces to these metrics, all of which are built around very important things, but the current imprecise and imperfect metrics are being used to measure a physician's value. That is a heavy weight for someone that has spent a lifetime working toward a career where their sole purpose is adding value to another person's life. The rapid expansion of metrics and the seemingly singular focus on them by payers drive many physicians to feel that health-care governance has veered away from historical core values surrounding patient care and thus are in part a cause for the rising burnout rates.

Multiple masters Rules in medicine flow out from decision makers to the physician's day-to-day practice by many different routes: 1. legislative mandates meant to ensure good care at the best price; 2. specialty boards with requirements meant to ensure physicians remain competent within their field; 3. insurance payers' rules regarding everything from what should be said in a dictation to what medications are covered to the revolving evaluations of an individual's performance, requirements which have health-care employers reinforcing those mandates with metrics of their own; 4. local hospitals' staff requirements associated with credentialing and call; 5. individual care teams that need support and direction; and finally, 6. the patient with specific needs of their own. It seems that most days the list of what is needed from a physician outweighs the list of support that is offered to a physician in return. The complex web of rules, both written and unwritten, by multiple masters, each with its own values and metrics, means that each set of rules touch an individual physician in various ways, such as online postings on the performance of individual physicians by payers to personal dashboards colored from red to green to a patient's submitted commentary on a provider's professionalism and abilities.

No physician would tell you that safety and outcomes aren't important, nor would they argue about the need to ensure a healthy bottom line, but there is science showing that by aligning the engagement of a physician, alongside those traditional metrics, we will ensure better outcomes across the entire dashboard. In 2015, Shanafelt and colleagues released a study showing the impact of leadership on burnout. They concluded there was a linear relationship between how empathic, engaged, and involved leaders were and the degree of burnout expressed by staff. On a 60-point leadership assessment scale, for every one point increase in leadership skill as assessed by physicians, there was a 3.3% decrease in their level of burnout [61].

To the individual physician the benefits of sleep, time away from work, work confined to work hours, exercise, and pure, unadulterated face-to-face time with patients are well documented throughout our chapter and this book but Quint Studer, in his book *Healing Physician Burnout*, suggests that the benefits are not just for the individual physician but also reflect positively on safety, patient experience, volumes, productivity, and attrition [76]. The business side of medicine is slowly beginning to realize that if we fix burnout, other metrics will improve by extension.

> *From a purely financial standpoint, preventing and treating physician burnout just makes good sense. A healthcare system's largest producer of revenue is the medical staff. Most professions make a special point to take great care of their revenue producers. Healthcare can be no different. In healthcare, physicians are way more than the people who create the documentation for billing. They are the lifeblood of health care; they are the healers.*
> (Quint) [76]

In large entities, change is often slow, and in medicine change is further stymied by the multitude of decision makers. Today's reimbursement trends make it difficult to embrace this philosophy of engagement and reducing burnout in order to improve safety, productivity, and outcomes. What administration wouldn't want their physician to each have a scribe and have templates heavy in non-face-to-face time for work designed to improve quality care, and never be on call more than 1:20? The need to keep the lights on is real, so we seem stuck here in the muddy waters of physicians working in a vacuum of expectations with insufficient support to make them successful. Our nation's high burnout numbers, along with the US cost of burnout, that whopping 4.6 billion dollars annually (Han et al., 20), indicate that where we currently sit is not sustainable.

For that reason there has been a philosophical shift at many structural levels from the Triple Aim to the Quadruple Aim [8], a push to add physician well-being to the institutional metrics, alongside quality, cost, and safety. Organizations as a whole will now be able to reflect and begin to develop a relationship between administration and clinicians that is mutually beneficial, supporting the need of patients and physicians, while successfully managing their assigned metrics.

Before we move on to solutions, let's touch on the idea of hope. Would you think it crazy to say that leaders across the health-care system have been given this huge gift of burned out physicians? If so, consider reading Rich Bluni's book, *Oh No... Not More of That Fluffy Stuff! The Power of Engagement* [7]. He suggested that in many ways burnout "is a sign of hope." He highlighted that physicians burn out because they want something better; they want to be great care givers, they want to be good team members, they want to provide efficient and effective care, they want to support their employers, they want to personally be seen as green across the dashboard, and they want to be great spouses and community members. They basically want to be engaged in the things that surround them on a daily basis. As leaders, we spend much of our energy and time working with and fretting about the physicians who don't buy in to those things, physicians who are disengaged or disruptive. Physicians like that don't get burned out, they come to work disengaged and leave work disengaged. Burned out physicians, on the other hand, leave work with things tied up in a nice bow as they quietly and personally struggle. How lucky we are as a nation to have women and men so willing to give of themselves for the greater good; these are the individuals we want representing our institutions, and all we have to do as leaders now is listen and act.

Health-care leaders more than likely already understand the value and importance of their physicians, but practically, what should an institution consider when trying to create a culture of physician engagement:

- Make sure their leaders are adequately prepared to lead, both for those born a "natural" leader and especially for those that are not. Training in the nuances of leadership is important. Leaders need a skill set and a knowledge base to actively listen, address issues, and be prepared to meet the structural, practical, and emotional needs of the physician and the practice. The specifics of leadership development are beyond the scope of this chapter, but books and conferences abound on the subject.
- Make sure their leaders actively listen. They will be challenged with questions by very smart people who are much closer to the work of patient care. By listening to understand they will be better able to explain the "why" or find solutions to achieve buy in. Individuals who feel respected by their immediate supervisors report scores 56% higher in measures of well-being, 89% higher in measures of joy in work, and are significantly more likely to be retained [52].
- Make sure to ask for input from frontline physicians when a change is first contemplated, because team workflows and issues surrounding patient care are extremely personal to physicians. When change is necessary they will have insight as to how best to make a change that will be both impactful to the institution and consistent with their personal goals.
- Roll out frequent Individual Feedback Sessions to make sure physicians know: 1. where the institution stands with its metrics, 2.data reflecting their team's performance within the insti-

tutions metrics, and 3. where they sit personally. Build a bidirectional feedback session by asking about their personal goals, their thoughts around institution metrics, roadblocks to successful implementation of both, and ideas on how to remove them. Leaders need to pay special attention to the needs of a female physician, often prone to self-trepidation and sensitive to negativity. People with high levels of empathy can fare poorly in a system based on negative feedback. Performance review sessions need to speak to specifics and not conjecture. A comment like "staff say you are demanding" requires specific examples. An understanding of how burnout accentuates maladaptive coping mechanisms should be a primary focus when navigating the red, yellow, and green of any physician review. A study out of Medscape in 2019 revealed that 30% of physicians identified the "lack of respect from administrators/ employers, colleagues and staff" as a contributor to burnout [45]. Reviews should strengthen relationships with the institutional culture and not undermine the development of trust.

- Make sure there is a clear understanding of the "why" before any new roll out. "Why" a metric is important or "why" change is occurring is imperative for front line staff if buy-in is desired.
- Make sure that there is always follow up, whether or not the answer is a yes or a no or a maybe. A large part of the physician's day is spent "following up" on things, and physicians will quickly lose respect for leaders that fail this simple step. Physicians are very conscious of the role they play in following up on their patient concerns; leaders should be equally so with the concern of their physicians.
- Make sure to understand what any change means to the day-to-day physician-patient interaction with regard to the inflexible EHR workflow, which is already tasking the physician with clerical burden. If possible streamline the EHR for optimization of the work before any new task is added. The phrases "just one more patient" or "just three more clicks" should be food for thought. Gain understanding on how that one more patient may equate to an additional 1.5 hours of work or how that three more clicks will be amplified across an entire patient panel. Help them be mindful about how much energy is really

expended before, during, and after any type of patient encounter – whether it be virtually through an in-basket inquiry or phone call or more directly from a face-to-face visit.

- Provide structured opportunity for the physician to give feedback on the leaders to ensure relationships are constructive, and improvements, where needed, are ongoing.
- Make sure communication is respectful and that leaders are prepared in advance for group meetings or one-to-one sessions, as time is a precious commodity.
- Ensure your *physician* leaders are also trained; they leave medical school expected to be leaders but with little training in that regard. Many business leaders have specific training throughout their educations and careers, and for all of the reasons stated earlier, physicians in leadership positions need that training and practice as well. Physician leaders also often lead their partners and need to balance personal relationships with institutional priorities, making training in this regard imperative to prevent social isolation.
- Make sure your institutional values and mission statements are reflected in your decisions and actions. Alignment between institutional and individual physician values needs to remain at the forefront of organizational priorities, as there is a buffering effect specific to women under stress when values are congruent. Not only are values the basis for mission statements, something that physician subscribe to and are "promised" at the time they are hired, but when values are misaligned personal burnout intensifies [36].
- Make sure institutional priorities are visible to all and that an effort to decrease burnout is one of those priorities. Burnout should not only be measured routinely with results clearly displayed on timely dashboards, but there should be visible leadership within the practice addressing physician well-being and everything that implies.
- Create a taskforce with representation of multiple disciplines, reinforced with physician staff for specific directives. Membership should include the "owners" of defined solutions or those accountable to the practice for identified initiatives (your chief informational officer, head of scheduling, etc.)

- Establish open connections between physicians and all levels of leadership. Physicians are at the top of their work pyramids and should have routine contact with their immediate leader but also the leaders that sit atop the leadership pyramid to enhance the philosophy of belonging.
- Be nimble, remove bureaucracy whenever possible, and be mindful that one size does not fit all. Large institutions find efficiency with consistency, but in health care different specialties and different providers find efficiency with personalization.
- For female physicians, ensure your institution practices bias-free decision making.
- Create an environment of respect for physicians, both among colleagues and from patients. Be intolerant of toxic behavior from staff and patients alike [68]. Female physicians tend to feel less valued by patients [24], so share negative feedback sparingly and focus on successes in patient experience.
- Be grateful for your physicians, and thank them when appropriate. Offerings of gratitude beyond financial have been shown to decrease burnout [16]. Embrace the fact that they have lives outside of the work environment. They are a reflection of you, so support them as their health and performance reflects your values.
- Be respectful of the care team environment and it's maturation over time. Changing staff without physician involvement alters the nuances that patients expect and physicians depend on. Women are problem solvers by nature [13], so whenever possible, retain physician input for practice changes. Autonomy is a distinct modifier of burnout and care teams are instrumental in connecting physicians to a shared sense of purpose
- Check in routinely with practices that have experienced attrition. These teams are especially vulnerable to burnout and further attrition.
- Always communicate difficult messages in person and not via email.
- Focus groups are beneficial for soliciting information in an open forum. They build camaraderie and have within them the potential to prevent the toxicity inherent in "meeting after the meeting."

- Embrace the 80/20 philosophy, which suggests that those individuals who spend greater than 20% of their work effort doing the things they find most meaningful showed the lowest rates of burnout [60]. This may mean that a physician has a clinical or nonclinical work assignment of their own design created to advance their clinical practice or that of the institution. As Roth and colleagues suggested [56], burnout increased when providers spent more of 80% of their time dedicated to clinical care. Ask a physician where they find personal value during their work day and support a process that allows focused work in that area.

- Consider whether or not your work space is family friendly. If possible, offer flexible scheduling or childcare. Respecting a family friendly environment goes beyond identifying a room for lactating mothers. Historically, women carry more of the childcare responsibilities than men. When comparing the United States to the European Union, where there is more access to workplace childcare and extended maternity leaves are common, support by employers and an understanding of the importance of childrearing have been shown to significantly decrease the risk for burnout [53]. Managers should be sensitive to work-life issues and show willingness to assist where able. Work-life stressors are well known to be a major cause of burnout, and organizations that attempt to promote flexibility within their work structure to allow physicians to attend to family needs when they occur appear to be effective in mitigating burnout [21].

- Ensure patient panels are weighted appropriately and clinic templates are built allowing for the uneven demands of a patient panel laden with female patients. On average, female patients have more psychosocial complexity, have different needs (gynecologic), and require a caring communication style. Gendered stereotypes and expectations with their hidden social rules for women are more difficult and time consuming to manage. Women physicians are seen as domineering more so than men if they disagree with a patient's request, so they often have to communicate in such a way that the decision appears to be mutual. The excess work of listening, counseling, and preventive care may add 5–10 minutes to a visit, and if a female physician completes eight female physicals a day while a male physician does eight male physicals a day, there may be a difference of an hour or two worth of work between the two [37]. The flip side of this communication requirement and style is twofold. Studies have recurrently shown that female physicians provide better quality of care when compared with their male counterparts, striving to maintain high standards at work with greater adherence to evidence based practices [82] and it aligns with society's changing relationship with health care. Patients are moving away from the historical paternalistic interaction with physicians toward a model that is based on shared decision making [46].

- Be a visible voice of change at a national level. Let your physicians know you have heard them by advocating beyond your institution. Partner with your physicians providing feedback to professional societies and organizations on redundancies to minimize time requirements.

Improving institutional engagement is an essential element to stemming the increase of burnout among physicians today. Full engagement will help move the health industry closer to achieving all four parts of the Quadruple Aim by focusing process improvements within the only section (the support and health of their physician staff) that has been proven to move the other three forward as well.

The single biggest way to impact an organization is to focus on leadership development. There is almost no limit to the potential of an organization that recruits good people, raises them up as leaders and continually develops them. John Maxwell

Team Building

Activities used to enhance social relations and define roles within teams (Siri, 2020)

As the delivery of health care shifts and technology shapes the landscape, one thing remains perfectly clear. The medicine of tomorrow requires even more deliberate approaches to developing and connecting medical professionals, particularly women. Building a community in the work environment is essential to reducing silos, improving patient care and allowing women to prosper in the current environment. Waiting for connection to occur in the workplace is not enough; therefore, intentionally creating strategies to improve team building and overall connectivity is a vital strategy in moving the culture forward. One program conducted at the Mayo Clinic found that building small groups with a focus on meaning and engagement resulted in changes in measurements of burnout and enhanced engagement [86]. Similarly, a study of women physician and advanced practice provider mothers randomized to attending facilitated group sessions versus having a freed clinical hour showed significantly greater improvement in measures of well-being, depression, and emotional exhaustion for those attending the support groups [38]. Considering team-based care, creating shared practice models and enhancing innovation have demonstrated promise [34, 48] and can be built upon and modified to fit organizational strategies and objectives. Additional ideas for improving team building and connections are noted below:

1. Promote team-based care and team-based strategies such as partnered documentation, delegation of certain aspects of patient care and refill protocols [39].
2. Consider journal clubs, social support groups, second victim groups, and emotional support groups for women as potentially beneficial resources.
3. Offer CME-focused activities geared toward encouraging women in medicine. For example, the GRIT Women in Healthcare Leadership Conference was started by the Department of Anesthesiology and Perioperative Medicine and the Division of General Internal Medicine at Mayo Clinic in 2018 to promote growth, resilience, inspiration, and tenacity. The program intentionally builds a community that fosters optimism and connection and team-based care.
4. Provide resources that promote communication and healthy dialogue to offset the potential isolation that can exist in medicine.

5. Promote social support both inside and outside of the work environment. Encouraging the utilization of formal and informal resources in the work environment, carving out time for social experiences, and allowing time and space to connect with others in the natural environment can help support physicians to remain engaged and focused on patient care.
6. Focus on reward and recognition outside of more traditional programming. For instance, identifying those individuals who foster a healthy culture and bring positivity to the work environment, or physicians who exemplify a healthy integration of home and work.
7. Enhance the nurse and physician and advanced practice provider relationships. Build teams that bring women and men together and promote concepts such as teamwork, partnerships, shared care models, and similar core concepts for the medicine of tomorrow. Ultimately, bringing these individuals together and offering multiple resources build the workforce needed to combat the ambiguity of medicine.

Career Development

Lifelong process of managing learning, work, leisure, and transitions in order to move toward a personally determined and evolving preferred future (Siri 2020)

Increasing leadership competencies and fostering growth and career development are especially relevant to women physicians given the unique challenges described in this book. The intentional growth and development of women physician leaders will be critical for diminishing physician burnout and increasing entry of women in historically male-dominated specialties. Traditional career paths are not always available for female physicians. Having an awareness of the gender gap allows organizations to identify gaps in promotions, programming, pay, or services. Pay equity is a certain way to reward and acknowledge the commitment and talents of female physicians. The ideal years for career building often coincide with childrearing years and have been referred to as "The Motherhood Penalty" [51]. Making sure to promote academic, pay, and career promotion during these years is vital to changing the culture over time.

Practice and promotion practices that are free of gender bias are more difficult to build than anticipated. Time away from work related to the birth of a baby or breastfeeding schedules, unexpected illnesses, or school-related activities may be mistaken as a lack of commitment or prioritization of work. Time at work is often a measure of commitment rather than "work accomplished" or "overall productivity." For instance, a female physician who was identified as positive and energetic and engaged was going through infertility treatment. She lost time at work related to the treatments and appointments. This female physician was overlooked for a leadership title despite her tenure and leadership experience. These kinds of scenarios occur repeatedly in health-care settings across the nation. Consideration of time away from practice is particularly germane to medical specialties that hold longer or more erratic schedules, for example, surgical specialties and emergency medicine [85], and equitable promotions are key.

Holding routine discussions of promotional and future goals with physicians are needed to identify the unique contributions and challenges facing each physician. Combining a learning culture with leadership opportunities open to all and offering variety of options for education, publishing, writing, and practice bring the equity needed to promote cultural changes. Interventions must impact the culture, people, and the practice. Some ideas at improving career development are noted below:

1. Hold frequent and direct conversations with leaders and teams to align work with skills and talents and abilities. Often we discuss "allowing each team member to operate at the height of her/her licensure." Use that same statement to identify strengths and unique gifts thereby "allowing each female physician to operate at the height of her own strengths and abilities." The literature is clear, aligning talents and strengths with the work will bring the optimal levels of engagement and

retention and productivity (Shanafelt and Noseworthy, 2019; [28, 64, 66]). Assuring job fit and promoting the 20% meaningful work will serve as a place to start.

2. Flexible work time models, offering child care on-site option, illness-related daycare options, part-time employment without losing seniority or leadership potential, and connecting work schedules with home schedules are all reasonable considerations for building a culture that protects and promotes women physicians [55].

3. Educational options can range from courses and coaching and mentoring, to day-long/week-long CME conferences or retreats focusing uniquely on issues related to female physicians in the workforce.

4. Same sex mentoring and coaching [20, 22, 58] are vital components to on-boarding and retention, yet often do not occur. Early career physicians, particularly women, can get overlooked in the emerging talent pipeline if they decide on a nontraditional or nonlinear path due to family commitments. Mentoring and sponsorship by either sex is thus critical to maintain and develop opportunities for career advancement and leadership.

5. Creating a pipeline of talent requires awareness of the talent pool coupled with people practices that are free of gender bias. An often overlooked component of equitable promotion practices is validating and assuring that physicians build relationships with current leadership. Promoting visibility and connection is necessary, especially if the female physicians are not at the current "table" of leadership. This may involve placing women physicians in key leadership roles, creating leadership roles that are shared by two or more physicians and directly connecting physicians with top leaders for roundtable and one-on-one discussions. Mentoring, training, flexible work hours, fitness reimbursements, and the ability to work remotely have been identified as potential options for both career development and enhancing engagement and optimizing energy [14].

6. Education, support, and services that support alternative lifestyle options can empower the development of one's full

potential and abilities. For example, the Office of Diversity and Inclusion at Mayo Clinic offers Mayo Employee Resource Groups open to all employees to "celebrate, support and encourage diversity among employees. Mayo Clinic provides financial and administrative support and resources to ensure each group's success" (Mayo Clinic Office of Diversity and Inclusion, 2019 Web Page). Groups of interest to female physicians include those focused on leadership opportunities, emerging leaders, lesbian/gay/bisexual/transgender/intersex, multicultural nursing, and family resource. Bringing together like-minded individuals and their allies, along with financial and administrative support, appear to be the most important components to assure success of the groups.

Well-Being

Diverse and interconnected dimensions of physical, mental, and social conditions that are positive, lead to growth, and go beyond the traditional definition of health. (Siri 2020)

Developing a culture that supports the overall well-being of physicians consists of many aspects, including connection at work, internal support resources, actively involved leadership, and promoting excellent mental health practices [77]. Identifying preferences allows an individualized approach to well-being and fostering self-care. Providing well-being resources in the more traditional areas is a good start. Encouraging and carving out time for gratitude, higher meaning, compassion, trained attention, forgiveness, and reflecting can optimize individual efforts [40, 70] Promoting a culture of psychological safety is vital. Finally, it is critical to measure engagement and burnout regularly and create action plans that optimize the resources available. The categories of social, physical, and emotional well-being are especially key for female physicians.

The relationship between engagement and burnout is not completely unidirectional, but engagement does increase the likelihood of retaining and developing female physicians. Engagement considerations as noted above can be utilized to improve retention and growth. Moreover, female physicians may speak up in ways that are nontraditional and perhaps not always welcomed at leadership tables. Assertiveness may be mistaken for aggressiveness. Education and training are necessary to construct the skills and receptivity necessary to bring all voices to the table. Any skills that increase fluency and expertise within the culture of departments and organizations can help foster an environment of well-being.

Strategies to make it easier for physician staff, particularly women, to speak up and remain engaged include:

- Offering Crucial Conversation [50] workshops to develop skills for optimal handling of difficult conversations.
- Assertiveness training [72] courses can be important to enhance an awareness of how and when to express self in a skilled manner.
- Emotional intelligence [32, 71] is a core aspect of self-awareness and management and can be modified and tailored to the population of female physicians.

Courses or trainings that address self-limiting beliefs and self-depreciating self-talk or even imposter syndrome can offset negative mindsets and mood. Finally, whenever possible, foster autonomy and decision making for physicians. Small allowances can go a long way to mitigating burnout and increasing engagement. Empowering physicians to make decisions, engaging them in decisions that impact patients, and allowing instances of autonomous decision-making foster the emotional climate that promotes well-being and emotional engagement [3].

Overcommitment and time management challenges are often a source of stress for women physicians and can get in the way of goals to enhance well-being. Improving purposeful prioritization and intentional time management is foundational to clearing the template and opening up the schedule for more focused work. The Steven Covey model of "The 7 Habits of Highly Effective People" [15] for physicians can provide a useful tool to identify what is most urgent and important, while identifying time wasters or derailers that lessen productivity and a sense of satisfaction. This model conveys that physicians often prioritize everything as "urgent"/"important" and therefore challenges individuals to strive to move as much as possible to "nonurgent"/"not important" to create activities that are meaningful and lasting and impactful. Focusing on work that is meaningful at least 20% of the time can engage physicians and lessen burnout (Shanafelt and Noseworthy 2019; [66, 67]). Following the foundational work, physicians will have more time and opportunity to create interventions throughout the day that stay aligned with a purposeful plan. For instance, one physician structured her day so that she lessened overall interruptions by meeting with her nurse three times per day only. This reduced nonessential discussions and opened up more time for patient focused care. The nurse ultimately completed more of the work that she had previously moved to the physician's work in the past.

In the social realm, providing the teambuilding and connectivity (as noted above in Teambuilding section) is essential. Beyond that, advising and promoting access to resources for on- and off-site interactions and building a culture that supports participation in events and services outside of the daily work environment are important to expand and enhance social relationships. Making a deliberate effort to cultivate social relationship in the workplace can have a positive effect in combating the negative effects of burnout and low job satisfaction [86]. Employees who report having a best friend at work were 43% more likely to report having received praise or recognition for their work in the last seven days; 35% were more likely to report coworker commitment to quality and 21% more likely to report that at work, they have the opportunity to do what they do best every day (www.gallup.com). Underestimating the importance of the social realm, particularly for female physicians [38], may result in worsening levels of fatigue and burnout.

Physical health can decline as female physicians juggle and make time for her many roles while not prioritizing time and attention to individual physical functioning. Adding a treadmill or a piece of exercise equipment to a practice site is a beginning but not an end. What is the plan to open up time to utilize the device? How will physicians be encouraged to use the equipment?

Nutritional counseling and sleep management services are the two remaining core aspects to build into a foundational well-being program. Is there protected time to use the services available or schedule personal medical appointments? What are the messages being given about productivity and time out of the practice? Organizations must be thoughtful about mixed messages and hidden curriculum regarding self-care and the importance of attending to one's personal health needs.

Emotional support and second victim resourcing are often neglected and can serve as ways to enhance the emotional health of physician staff providing direct care to patients. Physicians are taught to work long hours without complaint and to consider loss and trauma as a part of their normal work, often facing heightened levels of stress that would cripple people in the typical work environment. Deliver the needed services based on the knowledge that this exists in health care right now, today. Examples of successful peer support programs and second victim counseling include Brigham and Women's Hospital's "Center for Professionalism and Peer Support," or Johns Hopkins' "Resilience in Stressful Life Events."

The emotional aspects of well-being include a myriad of services and resources. Practical resources for female physicians can also consist of practice support for unexpected absences, breastfeeding options and daycare options, especially for children who are ill, and concierge services to assist with dry cleaning and household requirements. Promoting a culture that truly offers and celebrates disconnected time away for both vacation and CME is needed to reduce potential guilt and embrace actual time away. The stated and unstated messages of the organization make a difference. Avoiding extended work days and the organization produce engaged, healthy female physicians willing to give more than the average employee.

How to Coordinate Efforts and Monitor Outcomes

There is clear evidence that burnout impacts not only well-being of the individual physician but patient care, safety, and finances [64], so how do organizations coordinate and monitor their efforts to mitigate the stress on physicians that occurs as they attempt to successfully translate payer metrics in to the day-to-day work of their front line staff? Given the matrix of our health-care system and the complexity of the burnout problem, many health-care institutions are adding a "Chief Well-being Officer" to the executive suite, along with adequate FTE and administrative support to do the job [66, 67]. The AMA has endorsed this concept with its "Joy in Medicine" recognition program; only those health-care institutions that do so with at least 0.5 FTE can be awarded "Silver" status. Those who also establish a center for physician or workforce well-being can achieve "Gold" status. The thinking is reasonable. We need a team with time and resources dedicated to creating a vision, strategies, and tactics geared to reducing burnout and enhancing professional fulfillment. Consistent with our previous suggestions and specifically inherent in the AMA concept is:

1. Buy-in from organizational leadership on the importance of addressing the systemic drivers of burnout.
2. Conceptualizing a model that can help direct strategy and focus interventions to appropriate targets. The five factor model outlined in this chapter is based on the literature and our experience, but there are also many more established models to choose from such as the Stanford WellMD Model of Professional Fulfillment [9], Shanafelt's drivers of burnout and engagement [65], National Academy of Medicine Model of Factors Affecting Clinician Well-Being and Resilience [10], and several others [74]
3. Utilizing adequate measures to monitor for
    (a) Distress and/or well-being, for example, burnout [42], Well-being Index [19], Professional Fulfillment Index [81], or known proxies of burnout such as decreasing FTE, staff turnover rates [11, 62, 63, 88], "intent to leave" [26], declining quality or safety measures [80], and EHR-related measures [17].
    (b) Effectiveness of any given intervention.
4. Ongoing communication with all leaders and staff to keep them engaged in efforts to improve professionalism, satisfaction, and meaning at work [79].
5. Responding to staff surveys with meaningful actions ([78]).

6. Recognition that one size does not fit all [87].
7. Liaising with governmental bodies, medical boards, insurance carriers, and professional organizations to advocate for actions that, in the quest for maintaining patient care and safety standards, will ease rather than increase burnout and not deter physicians from seeking mental health treatment.

Conclusion

Never before has the proverb "Physician, heal thyself" been so clearly difficult to achieve without the physician having to retire early or cut back on their FTE. The idea that a physician can work independently to prevent or cure their own burnout seems remote today. However, if the physician is aligned with an institution that is driven to improve efficiency, that is set on engaging their workforce, that actively encourages career growth, and that contributes to the space and guidance a team requires to mature and become one unit, and through it all is supportive of a woman's health and well-being, healing will be achieved.

References

1. Al-Ma'mari NO, Naimi AI, Tulandi T. Prevalence and predictors of burnout among obstetrics and gynecology residents in Canada. Gynecol Surg. 2016;13(4):323–7.
2. An PG, Manwell LB, Williams ES, Laiteerapong N, Brown RL, Rabatin JS, Schwartz MD, Lally PJ, Linzer M. Does a higher frequency of difficult patient encounters lead to lower-quality care? J Fam Pract. 2013;62(1):24–9.
3. Andrienie J, Udwin M. Three phases to remedy physician burnout. Med Econ. 2018.
4. Arndt BG, Beasley JW, Watkinson MD, Temte JL, Tuan WJ, Sinsky CA, Gilchrist VJ. Tethered to the EHR: primary care physician workload assessment using EHR event log data and time–motion observations. Ann Fam Med. 2017;15(5):419–26.
5. Ashton M. Getting rid of stupid stuff. N Engl J Med. 2018;379(19):1789–91.
6. Blendon RJ, Benson JM, Hero JO. Public trust in physicians—U.S. medicine in international perspective. N Engl J Med. 2014;371(17):1570–2.

7. Bluni R. Oh no...Not more of that fluffy stuff! The power of engagement. Gulf Breeze: Fire Starter Publishing; 2013.
8. Bodenheimer T, Sinsky C. From triple to quadruple aim: care of the patient requires care for the provider. Ann Fam Med. 2014;12:573–6.
9. Bohman B, Dyrbye L, Sinsky CA, Linzer M, Olson K, Babbott S, Murphy M, DeVries PP, Hamidi MS, Trockel M. Physician well-being: the reciprocity of practice efficiency, culture of wellness, and personal resilience. NEJM Catalyst. 2017.
10. Brigham T, Barden C, Dopp AL, Hengerer A, Kaplan J, Malone B, Martin C, McHugh M, Nora LM. NAM perspectives. Discussion paper, National Academy of Medicine, Washington, DC, 2018.
11. Buchbinder SB, Wilson M, Melick CF, Powe NR. Primary care physician job satisfaction and turnover. Am J Manag Care. 2001;7(7):701–13.
12. Cantlupe J. The rise (and rise) of the healthcare administrator. AthenaInsight. 2017. https://www.athenahealth.com/insight/expert-forum-rise-and-rise-healthcareadministrator. Accessed 20 July 2019.
13. Carter SB. High octane woman: how superachievers can avoid burnout. 2011. p. 18.
14. Cheeseborough JE, Gray SS, Bajaj AK. Striking a better integration of work and life: challenges and solutions. Plastic Reconstr Surg. 2017;139:495.
15. Covey SR. The 7 habits of highly effective people. Restoring the character ethic. 7th ed. New York: Simon and Schuster; 1989.
16. Deci EL, Ryan RM. Intrinsic motivation and self-determination in human behavior. New York: Plenum Press; 1985.
17. DiAngi YT, Lee TC, Sinsky SA, Bohman BD, Sharp CD. Novel metrics for improving professional fulfillment. Ann Intern Med. 2017;167:740–1.
18. Downing NL, Bates DW, Longhurst CA. Physician burnout in the electronic health record era: are we ignoring the real cause? Ann Intern Med. 2018;169(1):50–1.
19. Dyrbye LN, Satele D, Sloan J, Shanafelt TD. Utility of a brief screening tool to identify physicians in distress. J Gen Intern Med. 2013;28(3):421–7.
20. Dyrbye LN, Shanafelt TD, Gill PR, Satele DV, West CP. Effect of a professional coaching intervention on the well-being and distress of physicians: a pilot randomized clinical trial. JAMA Intern Med. 2019;79(10):1406–14.
21. Dyrbye LN, Hanafelt TD, Balch CM, Satele D, Sloan J, Freischlag J. Relationship between work-home conflicts and burnout among American surgeons. A comparison by sex. Arch Surg. 2011;146(2):211–7.
22. Gazelle G, Liebschut JM, Riess H. Physician burnout: coaching a way out. J Gen Intern Med. 2014;30(4):508–13.
23. Gidwani R, Nguyen C, Kofoed A, Carragee C, Rydel T, Nelligan I, Sattler A, Mahoney M, Lin S. Impact of scribes on physician satisfaction, patient

satisfaction and chart efficiency: a randomized controlled trial. Ann Fam Med. 2017;15:427–33.

24. Gleichgerrcht E, Decety J. Empathy in clinical practice: how individual dispositions, gender, and experience moderate empathic concern, burnout and emotional distress in physicians. PLoS One. 2013;8(4):e61526.

25. Gupta K, Murray SG, Sarkar U, Mourad M, Adler-Milstein J. Differences in ambulatory EHR use patterns for male vs. female physicians. NEJM Catalyst. 2019.

26. Hamidi MS, Bohman B, Sandborg C, Smith-Coggins R, de Vries P, Albert MS, Murphy ML, Welle D, Trockel MT. Estimating institutional physician turnover attributable to self-reported burnout and associated financial burden: a case study. BMC Health Serv Res. 2018;18(1):851.

27. Han S, Shanafelt TD, Sinsky CA, Awad KM, Dyrbye LN, Fiscus LC, Trockel M, Goh J. Estimating the attributable cost of physician burnout in the United States. Ann Intern Med. 2019;170(11):784–90.

28. Harrison LH. Elevating women in leadership. A study exploring how organizations can crack the code to make real progress. 2017.

29. Helfrich CD, Simonetti JA, Clinton WL, et al. The association of team specific workload and staffing with odds of burnout among VA primary care team members. J Gen Intern Med. 2017;32(7):760–6.

30. Hotchkiss N, Early S. The differences in keeping both male and female physicians healthy. Health Care Manag. 2009;28(4):299–310.

31. Hubbard SD. Suicide among physicians. Am J Public Health. 1922;12:857.

32. Goleman D. Emotional Intelligence. New York: Bantam Books; 1995.

33. Johnson LW, Garrido T, Christensen K, Handley M. Successful practices in the use of secure e-mail. Perm J. 2014;18(3):50–4.

34. Kaiser RB, ed. Consulting Psychology Journal, Practice and Research. Special issue: fatigue in the workplace. Guest Editors: Kenneth Nowack and Jennifer J. Deal. 2017;69(2).

35. Kassam A, Horton J, Shoimer I, Patten S. Predictors of well-being in resident physicians: a descriptive and psychometric study. J Grad Med Educ. 2015;7:70–4.

36. Leiter MP, Frank E, Matheson TJ. Demands, values and burnout: relevance for physicians. Can Fam Physician. 2009;55:1224–1225.e5.

37. Linzer M, Harwood E. Gendered expectations: do they contribute to high burnout among female physicians? J General Inter Med. 2018;33(6):963–5.

38. Luthar SS, Curlee A, Tye SJ, Engelman JC, Stonnington CM. Fostering resilience among mothers under stress: "authentic connections groups" for medical professionals. Womens Health Issues. 2017;27(3):382–90.

39. Lyon C, English AF, Chabot Smith P. A team-based care model that improves job satisfaction. Am Acad Fam Phys. 2018;25(2):6–11.

40. Magitbay DL, Chesak SS, Coughlin K, Sood A. Decreasing stress and burnout in nurses, efficacy of blended learning with stress management and resilience training program. J Nurs Admin. 2017;47(7/8):391–5.

41. Mark G, Gudith D, Klocke U. The cost of interrupted work: more speed and stress. CHI "08: proceedings of the SIGCHI conference on Human Factors in Computing Systems. 2008;4:107–10.
42. Maslach C, Jackson SE. The measurement of experienced burnout. J Occup Behav. 1981;2:99–113.
43. Maslach C, Jackson SE. Burnout in organization settings. Appl Soc Psychol Annu. 1984;5:133–53.
44. Maume DJ. Gender differences in restricting work efforts because of family responsibilities. J Marriage Fam. 2006;68(4):859–69.
45. Medscape national physician burnout, depression and suicide report 2019.
46. Montori VM. Turning away from industrial health care toward careful and kind care. Acad Med. 2019;94(6):768–70.
47. Morrison JB, Rudolph J. Learning from accident and error: avoiding the hazards of workload, stress, and routine interruptions in the emergency department. Acad Emerg Med. 2011;18:1246–54.
48. Mosley K, Miller O. Our fragile, fragmented physician workforce: how to keep today's physicians engaged and productive. J Med Pract Manage. 2015;31(2):92–5.
49. Nicola R, McNeeley MF, Bhargava P. Burnout in radiology. Curr Probl Diagn Radiol. 2016;44:389–90.
50. Patterson K. Crucial conversations: tools for talking when stakes are high. New York: McGraw-Hill; 2012.
51. Pelley E, Danoff A, Cooper DS, Becker C. Female physicians and the future of endocrinology. J Clin Endocrinol Metab. 2016;101(1):16–22.
52. Porath C. Half of employees don't feel respected by their bosses. Harv Bus Rev. 2014.
53. Purvanova RK, Muros JP. Gender differences in burnout: a meta-analysis. J Vocat Behav. 2010;77:168–85.
54. Rath KS, Huffman LB, Phillips GS, Carpenter KM, Fowler JM. Burnout and associated factors among members of the society of gynecologic oncology. Am J Obstet Gynecol. 2015;213:824e1–9.
55. Richter A, Kostova P, Harth V, Wegner R. Children, care, career – a cross-sectional study on the risk of burnout among German hospital physicians at different career stages. J Occup Med Toxicol. 2014;9:41.
56. Roth M, Morrone K, Moody K, Kim M, Wang D, Moadel A, Levy A. Career burnout among pediatric oncologists. Pediatr Blood Cancer. 2011;57:1168–73.
57. Sandberg S. Lean In. 2013. p. 40.
58. Sambunjak D, Strause SE, Marusic A. Mentoring in academic medicine; a systematic review. JAMA. 2006;296(9):1103–15.
59. Sieja A, Markley K, Pell J, Gonzalez C, Redig B, Kneeland P, Lin C. Optimization sprints: improving clinician satisfaction and teamwork by rapidly reducing electronic health record burden. Mayo Clin Proc. 2019;94(5):793–802.

60. Shanafelt TD, West CP, Sloan JA, et al. Career fit and burnout among academic faculty. Arch Intern Med. 2009;169(10):990–5.
61. Shanafelt TD, Gorringe G, Menaker R, et al. Impact of organizational leadership on physician burnout and satisfaction. Mayo Clin Proc. 2015;90:432–40.
62. Shanafelt TD, Dyrbye LN, Sinsky C, Hasan O, Satele D, Sloan J, West CP. Relationship between clerical burden and characteristics of the electronic environment with physician burnout and professional satisfaction. Mayo Clin Proc. 2016a;91(7):836–48.
63. Shanafelt TD, Mungo M, Schmitgen J, Storz KA, Reeves D, Hayes SN, Sloan JA, Swensen SJ, Buskirk SJ. Longitudinal study evaluating the association between physician burnout and changes in professional work effort. Mayo Clin Proc. 2016b;91(4):422–31.
64. Shanafelt TD, Goh J, Sinsky D. The business case for investing in physician Well-being. JAMA Intern Med. 2017;177:1826–32.
65. Shanafelt TD, Noseworthy JH. Executive leadership and physician Well-being: nine organizational strategies to promote engagement and reduce burnout; Mayo Clinic proceedings, 2019. Mayo Clin Proc. 2017b;92(1):129–46.
66. Shanafelt T, Trockel M, Ripp J, Murphy ML, Sandborg C, Bohman B. Building a program on Well-being: key design considerations to meet the unique needs of each organization. Acad Med. 2019a;94(2):156–61.
67. Shanafelt T, West C, Sinsky C, Trockel M, Tutty M, Satele DV, Carlasare LE, Dyrbye LN. Changes in burnout and satisfaction with work-life integration in physicians and the general US working population between 2011 and 2017. Mayo Clin Proc. 2019b;94:1681–94.
68. Shapiro DE, Duquette C, Abbott L, Babineau T, Pearl A, Haidet P. Beyond burnout: a physician wellness hierarchy designed to prioritize interventions at the systems level. Am J Med. 2019;132:556–63.
69. Shenoi AN, Kalyanaraman M, Pillai A, Raghava P, Day S. Burnout and psychological distress among pediatric critical care physicians in the United States. Crit Care Med. 2018;46:116–22.
70. Sood A, Prasad K, Schroeder D, Varkey P. Stress management and resilience training among Department of Medicine Faculty: a pilot randomized clinical trial. J Gen Intern Med. 2011;26:858–61.
71. Salovey P, Mayer JD. Emotional Intelligence. Imagin Cogn Pers. 1990;9(3):185–211.
72. Speed BC, Goldstein BL, Goldfried MR. Assertiveness training: a forgotten evidence-based treatment. Clin Psychol Sci Pract. 2017. Literature Review. Issue March 13, 2018. Amercian Psychological Association.
73. Spataro BM, Tilstra SA, Rubio DM, McNeil MA. The toxicity of self-blame: sex differences in burnout and coping in internal medicine trainees. J Women's Health. 2016;25(11):1147–52.
74. Stewart MT, Reed S, Reese J, Galligan MM, Mahan JD. Conceptual models for understanding physician burnout, professional fulfillment, and Well-being. Curr Probl Pediatr Adolesc Health Care. 2019 Nov;49(11):100658.

75. Stucke RS, Kelly JL, Mathis KA, Hill MV, Barth RJ Jr. Association of the use of a mandatory prescription drug monitoring program with prescribing practices for patients undergoing elective surgery. JAMA Surg. 2018;153(12):1105–10.
76. Studer Q. Healing physician burnout. Pensacola: Fire Starter Publishing; 2015. p. 56.
77. Thomas RT, Ripp JA, West CP. Charter on physician well being. JAMA. 2018;319(15):1541–2.
78. Swensen S. Physician-organization collaboration reduces physician burnout and promotes engagement: the Mayo Clinic experience. J Healthc Manag. 2016;61(2):105–27.
79. Swensen S, Gorringe G, Caviness J, Peters D. Leadership by design: intentional organization development of physician leaders. J Manag Dev. 2016;35(4):549–70.
80. Tawfik DS, Profit J, Morgenthaler TI, Satele DV, Sinsky CA, Dyrbye LN. Physician burnout, Well-being, and work unit safety grades in relationship to reported medical errors. Mayo Clin Proc. 2018;93(11):1571–80.
81. Trockel M, Bryan B, Lesure E, Hamidi MS, Welle D, Roberts L, Shanafelt T. A brief instrument to assess both burnout and professional Fulfillment in physicians: reliability and validity, including correlation with self-reported medical errors, in a sample of resident and practicing physicians. Acad Psychiatry. 2018;42:11–24.
82. Tsugawa U, Jena AB, Figueroa JF, Orav EJ, Blumenthal DM, Jha AK. Comparison of hospital mortality and readmission rates for Medicare patients treated by male vs female physicians. JAMA Intern Med. 2017;177:206–12.
83. Turner TB, Dilley SE, Smith HJ, Huh WK, et al. The impact of physician burnout on clinical and academic productivity of gynecologic oncologist. Gynecol Oncol. 2017;146:642–6.
84. Van Dyke M. Battling clinician burnout: fighting the epidemic from within. Healthc Exec. 2019;34(1):10–9.
85. Walsh J. Gender, the work-life Interface and wellbeing: a study of hospital doctors. Gend Work Organ. 2013;20(4):439–53.
86. West CP, Dyrbye LN, Rabatin JT, Call TG, Davidson JH, Multari A, Romanski SA, Hellyer JM, Sloan JA, Shanafelt TD. Intervention to promote physician Well-being, job satisfaction, and professionalism. A randomized clinical trial. J Intern Med. 2014;174(4):527–33.
87. West CP, Dyrbye LN, Shanafelt TD. Physician burnout: contributors, consequences and solutions. J Intern Med. 2018;283:516–29.
88. Williams ES, Skinner AC. Outcomes of physician job satisfaction: a narrative review, implications, and directions for future research. Health Care Manag Rev. 2003;28(2):119–39.
89. Williams C. Empathy and burnout in male and female helping professionals. Res Nurs Health. 1989;12:169–78.
90. Wright AA, Katz IT. Beyond burnout – redesigning care to restore meaning and sanity for physicians. N Engl J Med. 2018;378:309–11.

Index

© Springer Nature Switzerland AG 2020
C. M. Stonnington, J. A. Files (eds.), *Burnout in Women Physicians*,
https://doi.org/10.1007/978-3-030-44459-4